Pericardial Diseases

OTHER CARDIOVASCULAR CLINICS BOOKS

Pericardial Diseases

DAVID H. SPODICK, M.D., D.Sc. | Editor

CARDIOVASCULAR CLINICS
ALBERT N. BREST, M.D. | Editor-in-Chief

 F. A. DAVIS COMPANY, PHILADELPHIA

Library of Congress Cataloging in Publication Data
Main entry under title:

Pericardial diseases.

(Cardiovascular clinics ; v. 7, no. 3)
Includes bibliographical references and index.
1. Pericarditis.   2.   Pericardium – Diseases
I.   Spodick, David H.   II.   Series.   [DNLM: 1.   Pericar-
ditis.   2.   Pericardium.   W1 CA77N v. 7 no. 3 / WG275
P441]
RC681.A1C27   vol. 7, no. 3 [RC685.P5]   616.1'008s
ISBN 0-8036-8090-2   [616.1'1]   76-41260

Editor's Commentary

The broad aspects of pericardial diseases tend to be neglected in the medical literature. This neglect stands out in sharp contrast to the overly abundant coverage given to certain other cardiologic topics. Yet the proper understanding and management of pericardial disorders requires a comprehensive knowledge of anatomy, pathology, and pathophysiology of the pericardium in addition to the cataloging of clinical manifestations, diagnostic methods, and natural history. The purpose of this volume is to examine the subject comprehensively. I am extremely grateful to David Spodick for his invaluable guidance in the formulation of this issue, and both of us are deeply indebted to the individual contributors whose painstaking efforts illumine these pages.

ALBERT N. BREST, M.D.

Contributors

George E. Burch, M.D.
Henderson Professor of Medicine, Tulane University School of Medicine, New Orleans, Louisiana

Juan J. Canoso, M.D.
Assistant Professor of Medicine, Boston University School of Medicine, and Chief, Arthritis Section, Boston Veterans Administration Hospital, Boston, Massachusetts

Alan S. Cohen, M.D.
Conrad Wesselhoeft Professor of Medicine, Boston University School of Medicine, and Director, Thorndike Memorial Laboratory, and Chief of Medicine, Boston City Hospital, Boston, Massachusetts

Joseph L. Cohen, M.D.
Associate Professor of Medicine, Tufts University School of Medicine, and Chief of Medicine and Co-Director, Oncology Division, Lemuel Shattuck Hospital, Boston, Massachusetts

Christina M. Comty, M.D.
Associate Professor of Medicine, University of Minnesota, Minneapolis, Minnesota

C. Richard Conti, M.D.
Professor of Medicine and Chief, Division of Cardiology, University of Florida, Gainesville, Florida

Marvin Dunn, M.D.
Professor of Medicine and Director, Division of Cardiovascular Diseases, University of Kansas Medical Center, Kansas City, Kansas

Kathryn H. Ehlers, M.D.
Professor of Pediatric Cardiology, Cornell Medical Center, New York, New York

Mary Allen Engle, M.D.
Professor of Pediatrics and Director of Pediatric Cardiology, Cornell Medical Center, New York, New York

Richard A. Gleckman, M.D.
Assistant Professor of Medicine, Boston University School of Medicine, Boston, Massachusetts

Dwight Emary Harken, M.D.
Clinical Professor of Surgery, Emeritus, Harvard Medical School, Boston, Massachusetts

Seymour Hepner, M.D.
Fellow, Pediatric Cardiology, Cornell Medical Center, New York, New York

Florencio A. Hipona, M.D.
Professor of Radiology, Harvard Medical School, and Associate Director of Radiology, Boston City Hospital, Boston, Massachusetts

Arthur A. Klein, M.D.
Fellow, Pediatric Cardiology, Cornell Medical Center, New York, New York

Leslie A. Kuhn, M.D.
Associate Clinical Professor of Medicine and Director, Ames Coronary Care Unit, Mt. Sinai School of Medicine, New York, New York

Navin C. Nanda, M.D.
Assistant Professor of Medicine and Radiology, University of Rochester School of Medicine and Dentistry, Rochester, New York

William K. Nasser, M.D.
Clinical Associate Professor of Medicine, Indiana University School of Medicine, and Director, Cardiac Catheterization Laboratory, St. Vincent Hospital, Indianapolis, Indiana

Santiago Paredes, M.D.
Associate Professor of Radiology, Boston University School of Medicine, Boston, Massachusetts

Robert L. Rinkenberger, M.D.
Fellow, Cardiovascular Disease, University of Kansas Medical Center, Kansas City, Kansas

William C. Roberts, M.D.
Chief, Section of Pathology, National Heart and Lung Institute, National Institutes of Health, Bethesda, Maryland; and Clinical Professor of Pathology and Medicine (Cardiology), Georgetown University School of Medicine, Washington, D.C.

Ralph Shabetai, M.D.
Professor of Medicine, University of California, San Diego, California, and Chief, Cardiology Service, Veterans Administration Hospital, La Jolla, California

Pravin M. Shah, M.D.
Professor of Medicine and Associate Professor of Pediatrics, University of Rochester School of Medicine and Dentistry, Rochester, New York

Fred L. Shapiro, M.D.
Professor of Medicine, University of Minnesota, Minneapolis, Minnesota

David H. Spodick, M.D., D. Sc.
Professor of Cardiovascular Medicine and Professor of Medicine, University of Massachusetts Medical School, and Director, Cardiology Division, St. Vincent Hospital, Worcester, Massachusetts

Thomas L. Spray, M.D.
Staff Associate, Section of Pathology, National Heart and Lung Institute, National Institutes of Health, Bethesda, Maryland

Ronald L. Wathen, M.D.
Assistant Professor of Medicine, University of Minnesota, Minneapolis, Minnesota

Daniel E. Wise, M.D.
Assistant Professor of Medicine and Director, Noninvasive Laboratory, Division of Cardiology, University of Florida, Gainesville, Florida

Contents

The Pericardium: Structure, Function, and Disease Spectrum

David H. Spodick, M.D., D.Sc.

The pericardium has fascinated physicians since antiquity, largely because pericardial syndromes can produce spectacular clinical and physiologic abnormalities and because pericardial susceptibility to involvement by every kind of disease has two important consequences—mimicry of many nonpericardial syndromes and common difficulty in identifying the pericardium as a site of illness.

ANATOMIC SPECIALIZATION OF THE PERICARDIUM

The pericardium encloses the heart and the proximal few centimeters of the great vessels in a unicellular serous sac (serosa) closely clasped on its outside by a dense fibrous envelope (fibrosa). The serosa contains 15 to 20 ml. of clear fluid; it is applied directly to the heart surface (visceral pericardium or epicardium, Figs. 1 and 2) and is reflected over the inside of the fibrous envelope to form with it the parietal pericardium. Serosal cells are involved in fluid-electrolyte exchange with the vascular system. The fibrosa consists of fibrous tissue bundles and strands with a distinct functional design: they are oriented in relation to cardiac and vascular stresses and thicker over the thinner portions of the heart. Throughout the fibrosa are elastic fibers which vary with age in number, distribution, and waviness.

PHYSIOLOGY OF THE PERICARDIUM

While men and animals appear to get along quite well after removal of the pericardium, it appears to play a physiologic role particularly during cardiovascular stresses. Pericardial physiology is divided into three major categories: mechanical function—promotion of cardiac efficiency, especially during stress; membrane function—shielding the heart against outside influences plus complex effects of a closed chamber with specialized receptors in its wall; ligamentous function—limitation of undue cardiac displacement. A detailed outline follows:*

A. Mechanical function: Promotion of cardiac efficiency, especially during stress
    1. Limitation of excessive acute dilatation
        a. Defense of the integrity of the Starling curve: Starling mechanism operates uniformly at all intraventricular pressures because of pericardium

---

*Modified from Spodick, D.H.: Chronic and Constrictive Pericarditis. Grune & Stratton, New York, 1964.

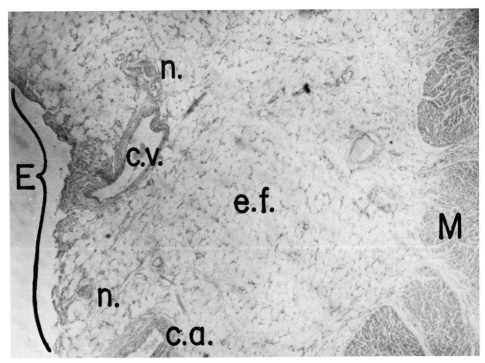

Figure 1. The epicardium: architecture (low power view). E-bracket: serosa. e.f.:subepicardial fat. M: myocardium. n.: nerve. c.v.: coronary venule. c.a.:coronary arteriole. (From Spodick.[8])

    (1) Maintenance of output response to venous inflow loads
    (2) Protection against excessive ventriculoatrial regurgitation. Pericardium:
       (a) Maintains ventricular function curves
       (b) Limits effect of increased left ventricular end-diastolic pressure
       (c) Favors equality of transmural end-diastolic pressure throughout ventricle, therefore uniform stretch of muscle fibers (preload)
    (3) Limits right ventricular stroke work during increased impedance to left ventricular outflow
    (4) Hydrostatic system (with pleural fluid) which constantly compensates for changes in gravitational and inertial forces
   b. Maintenance of output response to rate fluctuations
  2. Maintenance of functionally optimum heart shape
  3. Provision of a closed chamber in which:
   a. The level of transmural cardiac pressures will be low
   b. Pressure changes aid atrial filling via negative pericardial pressure during ventricular systole
  4. ? Mutually restrictive chamber favoring equality of output from right and left ventricles over several beats
  5. Maintenance of normal ventricular compliance (volume-elasticity relationship)
  6. Limits hypertrophy associated with chronic exercise
B. Membrane function: Shielding the heart
  1. Reduction of external friction due to heart movements
  2. Barrier to inflammation from contiguous structures
  3. Buttressing of thinner portions of the myocardium
   a. Atria

2

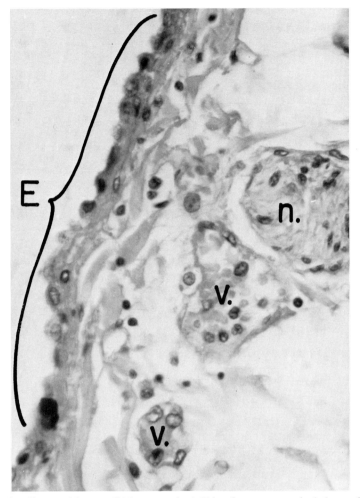

Figure 2. The epicardium: architecture (high power view). E-bracket: serosa, a single layer of cuboidal cells. n.: nerve. v.: blood vessels. (From Spodick.[8])

      b. Right ventricle
    4. "Feedback" circulatory regulation. Stimulation of:
      a. Neuroreceptors (via vagus): lower heart rate and blood pressure
      b. Mechanoreceptors: lower blood pressure and contract spleen
C. Ligamentous function: Limitation of undue cardiac displacement

DISEASES OF THE PERICARDIUM

The diseases of the pericardium are outlined below.
  I. Acute and subacute inflammatory pericardial disease
    A. Acute pericarditis and myopericarditis
      1. Noneffusive
      2. Effusive
        a. Without cardiac compression
        b. With tamponade of the heart

3

    3. Pneumohydropericardium
- B. Recurrent acute pericarditis
- C. "Subacute pericarditis"
- D. Pericardial fat necrosis

II. Noninflammatory excess pericardial contents
- A. Hydropericardium
- B. Hemopericardium
  1. Traumatic
  2. In association with pathologic bleeding
     - a. Hemorrhagic states
     - b. Rupture of contiguous organs
- C. Chylopericardium
- D. Pneumopericardium
- E. Intrapericardial herniation of other organs

III. Chronic and constrictive pericardial disease
- A. Granulomatous
- B. Pericardial scarring
  1. Pericardial fibrosis/adhesions
  2. Pericardial calcification/ossification
  3. Inflammatory cysts and diverticula
- C. Chronic pericardial effusion
- D. Amyloidosis of pericardium

IV. Congenital pericardial abnormalities
- A. Congenital pericardial defects
  1. Partial
     - a. Incidental
     - b. With herniation of portions of the heart
  2. Total
- B. Congenital cysts of the pericardium

The largest group clinically and at necropsy in the preceding outline is category I, acute and subacute inflammatory pericardial disease. The exact incidence of various forms of pericardial disease is difficult to establish because of geographic and demographic factors as well as different kinds of hospital referral patterns, plus the availability of postmortem material in only a relatively small percentage of cases in which death was due to pericardial disease itself. There is, however, strong evidence for a changing picture of acute pericarditis with a decrease in bacterial forms and an increase in the recognition of viral, "immune," neoplastic, and iatrogenic varieties.

Nil nocere!! Iatrogenic pericarditis

Surgical
  Direct
  Postpericardiotomy
  Transplant rejection
Cardiac hypothermia
V-A shunt tubing (Torkildsen)
Pacemaker implant
Transvenous pacemaker
Kirchner wire (sternoclavicular joint)
Esophageal bypass erosion
Cardiac resuscitation

4

Drug reactions
   Radiation
   Hydralazine (LE)
   Procainamide (LE)
   Phenylbutazone
   Psicofuranine
   ?Anticoagulants
Transseptal catheter
Sternal bone marrow tap
Percutaneous LV puncture

Acute and Subacute Inflammatory Pericardial Disease

Acute Pericarditis and Myopericarditis

The largest single group of clinically important pericardial disease is acute pericarditis, which, when it is accompanied by significant involvement of the underlying myocardium may be termed *myopericarditis* (the involvement of one or the other organ often dominating the picture). The following is an outline of the etiology of acute pericarditis, from which it is evident that *the pericardium can be involved in every category of disease, medical and surgical.**

A. Idiopathic pericarditis (syndrome)
B. Pericarditis due to living agents
    1. Bacterial
      a. Suppurative
      b. Tuberculous
    2. Viral
      a. Coxsackie
      b. Influenza
      c. Other
    3. Mycotic (fungous)
    4. Rickettsial
    5. Parasitic
    6. Spirochetal
    7. Spirillum infection
    8. Mycoplasma pneumoniae
    9. Infectious mononucleosis
    10. Leptospira
    11. Listeria
C. Pericarditis in the vasculitis-connective tissue disease group
    1. Rheumatic fever
    2. Systemic lupus erythematosus (LE; See also Iatrogenic pericarditis.)
      a. Naturally occurring
      b. Drug reaction
    3. Rheumatoid arthritis
    4. Ankylosing spondylitis
    5. Systemic scleroderma

*Modified from Spodick, D.H.: Differential diagnosis of acute pericarditis, in Friedberg, C., and Donoso, E. (eds.): Pathophysiology and Differential Diagnosis in Cardiovascular Disease. Grune & Stratton, New York, 1971.

      6. Dermatomyositis
      7. Panmesenchymal reaction of steroid hormone withdrawal
      8. Polyarteritis
      9. Thrombohemolytic thrombocytopenic purpura
D. Pericarditis in "hypersensitivity" states, immune reactions
      1. Drug reactions
      2. Serum sickness
      3. Allergic granulomatosis
      4. Giant urticaria
      5. Other sensitivity reactions
E. Pericarditis in diseases of contiguous structures
      1. Myocardial infarction
         a. Acute myocardial infarction
         b. Postmyocardial infarction syndrome
         c. Ventricular aneurysm
      2. Dissecting aortic aneurysm
      3. Pleural and pulmonary diseases
         a. Pneumonia
         b. Pulmonary embolism
         c. Pleuritis
F. Pericarditis in disorders of metabolism
      1. Renal failure
         a. Acute
         b. Chronic
      2. Myxedema
      3. Cholesterol pericarditis
      4. Gout
G. Neoplastic pericarditis
      1. Secondary (metastatic, hematogenous, or by direct extension): carcinoma, sarcoma, lymphoma, leukemia, other
      2. Primary: (mesothelioma)
H. Traumatic pericarditis
      1. Direct
         a. Pericardial perforation
            1. Penetrating chest injury
            2. Esophageal perforation
            3. Gastric perforation
         b. Cardiac injury
            1. Cardiac surgery
            2. During catheterization
               a. Pacemaker insertion
               b. Diagnostic
         c. "Foreign body" pericarditis
      2. Indirect
         a. Radiation pericarditis
         b. Nonpenetrating chest injury
I. Pericarditis of uncertain origin or in association with various syndromes
      1. Postpericardiotomy syndrome
      2. "Postoperative pericarditis"
      3. Reiter's syndrome
      4. Behçet's syndrome
      5. Inflammatory bowel disease

  a. Colitis (ulcerative; granulomatous)
  b. Segmental enteritis
  c. Whipple's disease
 6. Löffler's syndrome
 7. Sjögren's syndrome
 8. Thalassemia (and other anemias)
 9. "Specific" drug reaction (Psicofuranine, ? others)
10. Pancreatitis
11. Polyserositis
  a. Paroxysmal ("Mediterranean")
  b. Other
12. ? Sarcoidosis
13. ? Silicosis
14. ? Myeloid metaplasia
15. Fat embolism
16. Bile fistula (to pericardium)
17. Wissler's syndrome
18. "P. I. E." syndrome
19. Stevens-Johnson syndrome
20. Gaucher's disease
21. Diaphragmatic hernia
22. Atrial septal defect
23. Giant cell aortitis
24. Takayasu's syndrome

Thus, pericarditis can be an apparently primary illness or may appear in the course of almost any other syndrome. This is evident in pericarditis due to living agents in which any organism that can reach the pericardium can infect or infest it.

Processes and agents acutely inflaming the pericardium reach it by direct extension (e.g., myocardial infarction), through blood or lymph stream dissemination, or by traumatic irritation. The pericardial response to acute inflammation includes exudation of fibrin plus various amounts of serous fluid and infiltration by inflammatory cells of types characteristic for the particular disease process. Large amounts of serous fluid result in detectable pericardial effusion. When the effusion is an inflammatory exudate the greatest quantity exudes through the visceral pericardium owing to inflammation of the subepicardial myocardium (subepicardial myocarditis, myopericarditis). The inflammatory process obstructs pericardial venous and lymphatic drainage with consequent pouring into the pericardial sac of protein rich exudate, analogous to production of ascites from the liver surface. If the disease process permits air to enter the pericardium (by communication with the bronchi, esophagus, or stomach) or if the agent is a gas producing organism, a pneumopericardium or pneumohydropericardium results.

Chronic Pericardial Effusion

Chronic pericardial effusion may follow a known attack of acute pericarditis and may occur with or without compression of the heart. Compression occurs either as a form of chronic tamponade or as a combined form with constriction of the epicardium, the parietal pericardium, or both. Clinically, these patients tend to present as "resistant congestive heart failure." Usually the etiology is unknown although tuberculosis can produce this picture. The syndrome may resemble mild acute tamponade, congestive heart failure, or constrictive pericarditis. Occasional patients with chronic tamponade progress to frank constriction after removal of fluid by pericardiocentesis.

Inflammatory Cysts and Diverticula

Occasionally pericardial scarring and adhesions cause loculation or partial loculation of fluid. Total loculation results in an inflammatory cyst, and partial loculation (with an opening communicating with the general pericardial cavity) causes a diverticulum. These disorders produce abnormalities in the chest x-rays but usually no important clinical findings. In parts of the world with large numbers of sheep, echinococcosis is endemic and echinococcosis may cause hydatid cysts of the pericardium; these cysts may produce severe disease.

Congenital Pericardial Abnormalities

Congenital cysts usually produce abnormal bulges of the cardiac silhouette at the right or left cardiophrenic angle. They are uncommon and accidental discoveries in the course of other conditions for which the patient has chest x-rays. Total and partial absence of the parietal pericardium are relatively rare congenital abnormalities. Most of these have been incidental findings at autopsy, yet characteristic roentgenologic findings may permit clinical recognition. Total absence of the parietal pericardium is compatible with entirely normal catheterization studies. Partial absence may incur the risk of herniation and strangulation of a portion of the heart (usually the left atrium or its appendage) through the pericardial defect, which is usually on the left side. It is more frequently associated with other congenital anomalies than is total or near-total pericardial absence.

Recurrent Acute Pericarditis

Most attacks of acute pericarditis are isolated events. However, certain forms may recur one or more times without being chronic. These disorders are summarized as follows:*
A. Idiopathic pericarditis (syndrome)
B. Pericarditis due to living agents (especially tuberculous, viral)
C. Postmyocardial and pericardial injury syndromes
    1. Following myocardial infarction
    2. Following myocardial trauma
    3. Postpericardiotomy syndrome
    4. Foreign body pericarditis
D. Systemic disorders involving the pericardium
    1. Vasculitis-connective tissue disease group
    2. Hypersensitivity/immune states
    3. Reiter's disease
    4. Periodic ("Mediterranean") polyserositis
    5. Thalassemia major

Chronic and Constrictive Pericarditis

Chronic and constrictive diseases of the pericardium (see Diseases of Pericardium, pp. 3–4) are sequelae of acute or recurrent acute pericarditis and have for etiology most of the conditions enumerated on pp. 5–7 (with the conspicuous exception of rheumatic fever). A number of these represent granulomatous inflammation of the pericardium, particularly tuberculosis, occasionally rheumatoid arthritis with typical rheumatoid

---

*Modified from Spodick, D. H.: Chronic and Constrictive Pericarditis. Grune & Stratton, New York, 1964.

granulomata, and rarely fungi. The usual manifestation of this kind of illness is pericardial scarring which involves fibrosis with or without smaller or larger amounts of pericardial fluid, pus, and cellular detritus, as shown in the following classification:*

(Pericardial scarring varies greatly both in extent and in clinical importance. In general, tight or rigid pericardial scars measurably impair cardiocirculatory function and loose scars, regardless of extent and distribution, do not. Accordingly, separate anatomic and clinical groupings may be made.)

Anatomic classification
1. Pericardial thickening without adhesions
   a. Visceral
   b. Parietal
   c. Visceral and parietal
2. Internal pericardial adhesions
   a. Obliterative
      1. Complete
      2. Incomplete
   b. Focal
      1. "Milk spots"
      2. Individual strands, bridges, and bands
      3. Inflammatory pseudocysts and diverticula
3. External pericardial adhesions
4. Perivascular pericardial adhesions
5. Combined adhesions (two or more of the preceding)
6. Pericardial calcification: alone or with any of the preceding

Clinical consequences
1. Clinically and hemodynamically silent
2. Producing clinical signs without dynamic significance
3. Dynamically significant
   a. Constriction of the heart and/or
   b. Constriction of one or more great vessels
4. With other findings (usually etiologically related)
   a. Endocardial (especially valvular) lesions
   b. Mediastinal lesions
   c. Lesions of other serosae
   d. Pericardial calcification
5. Combinations of the preceding

Pericardial calcification and ossification may occur following the more severe inflammations. Frequently, however, pericardial calcification exists without clinical effects. (Inflammatory cysts and diverticula of the pericardium can coexist with other scarring but are quite uncommon and are the residua of scarring which closes off either completely or incompletely a portion of the pericardial cavity). The effects of scarring are innocent in the largest number of patients. For example, over 40 percent of patients with rheumatoid arthritis have pericardial adhesions but these usually are incidental postmortem findings.

Constrictive Pericarditis

Constrictive pericarditis may be acute, subacute, or chronic. Formerly chronic constriction was the usual form. However, with earlier and better diagnosis the subacute variety seems most common. Constriction has been observed to develop within a few

---

*Modified from Spodick, D. H.: Chronic and Constrictive Pericarditis. Grune & Stratton, New York, 1964.

weeks after an attack of acute pericarditis (*acute constriction*), sometimes so quickly that the patient never leaves the hospital. In other cases, a number of weeks or months go by before signs of chronic cardiac compression appear; these represent *subacute constrictive pericarditis*. Some patients are found in an advanced state of circulatory congestion with either a remote acute phase or no recollection of an acute pericarditis or, occasionally, after recurrent acute pericarditis; these cases represent *chronic constrictive pericarditis*.

REFERENCES

1. HOLT, J.P.: *The normal pericardium*. Am. J. Cardiol. 26:455, 1970.
2. SHABETAI, R., FOWLER, N. O., AND GUNTHEROTH, W. G.: *The hemodynamics of cardiac tamponade and constrictive pericarditis.* Am. J. Cardiol. 26:480, 1970.
3. SPODICK, D.H.: *Acoustic phenomena in pericardial disease*. Am. Heart J. 81:114, 1971.
4. SPODICK, D.H.: *Differential diagnosis of acute pericarditis*. Prog. Cardiovasc. Dis. 14:192, 1971.
5. SPODICK, D.H.: *Pericardial friction: characteristics of pericardial rubs in 50 consecutive, prospectively studied patients*. New Engl. J. Med. 278:1203, 1968.
6. SPODICK, D.H.: *Acute cardiac tamponade: pathophysiology, diagnosis and management*. Prog. Cardiovasc. Dis. 10:64, 1967.
7. SPODICK, D. H.: *Chronic and Constrictive Pericarditis*. Grune & Stratton, New York, 1964.
8. SPODICK, D.H.: *Acute Pericarditis*. Grune & Stratton, New York, 1959.

Pericardial Heart Disease:
A Study of Its Causes, Consequences,
and Morphologic Features

William C. Roberts, M.D., and Thomas L. Spray, M.D.

"Probably no serious disease is so frequently overlooked by the practitioner. Post-mortem experience shows how often pericarditis is not recognized, or goes on to resolution and adhesion without attracting notice."

William Osler (1892)[1]

Pericardial heart disease* from the clinical standpoint is one of the more infrequent cardiac diseases, but from the morphologic standpoint, it is common. Nevertheless, many publications have appeared on clinical aspects of pericardial disease, and surprisingly few have dealt with its morphologic aspects. The present report focuses on the morphologic features of pericardial heart disease.

CLINICAL AND MORPHOLOGIC SPECTRUM
OF PERICARDIAL HEART DISEASE

Although its exact frequency from either clinical or necropsy standpoints is uncertain, pericardial heart disease, as Osler emphasized above, is observed more often at necropsy than during life. Pericardial heart disease has been found clinically in less than 1 percent of patients admitted to one large general hospital[2] and in about 5 percent of consecutive necropsies at another large general hospital.[3] These figures were produced, however, in the era before cardiac catheterization or operation, renal dialysis, or widespread use of antibiotics. The present clinical and necropsy frequencies of pericardial heart disease are entirely unknown. Better diagnostic tools and prolonged longevity in systemic illness, however, have almost certainly increased the clinical recognition of pericardial heart disease in recent years. Nevertheless, as shown in Figure 1, pericardial heart disease is more often subclinical than clinical, and, even when clinical manifestations are present, evidence of myocardial compression, the worst form of pericardial disease, is uncommon. Myocardial compression from pericardial disease may result from pericardial effusion without pericardial thickening or from pericardial thickening

---

*Although the term "pericarditis" is applied to many, indeed, most pericardial disorders, relatively few of the disorders are actually associated with inflammatory cell reaction and therefore probably most do not warrant the designation "pericarditis." Fibrinous deposits without inflammatory cells, as occur in most patients with uremia, for example, do not justify a diagnosis of "pericarditis." The presence of inflammatory cells in the pericardia rather than an acute clinical course or a pericardial friction rub should determine whether the term "pericarditis" is appropriate. "Pericardial heart disease" is a better general term.

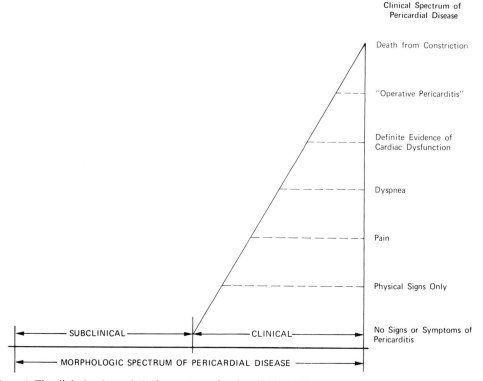

Clinical Spectrum of
Pericardial Disease

Death from Constriction

"Operative Pericarditis"

Definite Evidence of
Cardiac Dysfunction

Dyspnea

Pain

Physical Signs Only

No Signs or Symptoms of
Pericarditis

Figure 1. The clinical and morphologic spectrum of pericardial heart disease.

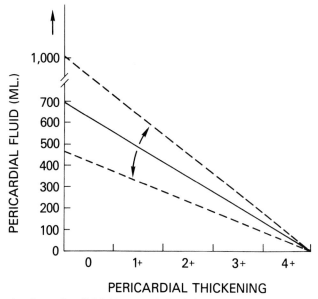

Figure 2. Graph showing that pericardial fluid accumulation is in general not proportional to pericardial thickening: the more the pericardial fluid, the less the pericardial thickening and vice versa. The dashed lines on either side of the uninterrupted line indicate that the latter may be shifted by an acute or chronic course. Less fluid is needed to produce tamponade if the fluid accumulation is rapid than if it is slow. Likewise, less pericardial thickening is needed to produce constriction if the thickening occurs rapidly as opposed to slowly.

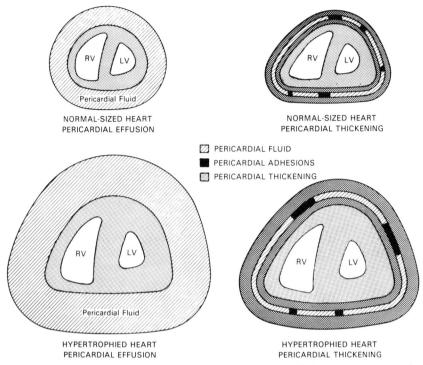

Figure 3. Diagrams showing that more pericardial fluid or thicker pericardia is necessary to constrict a hypertrophied heart than a normal sized one. RV = right ventricle; LV = left ventricle.

without pericardial fluid or from both. As shown in Figures 2 and 3, among patients with "pericardial" compression (in actuality it is the myocardium which is compressed, not the pericardium), the larger the amount of pericardial fluid the thinner the pericardia, and conversely, the thicker the pericardia the less the amount of pericardial fluid.

The type of clinical presentation of pericardial heart disease, that is, whether acute or chronic, does not necessarily correlate with the type of morphologic derangement present. The person with thick constricting pericardium (obvious evidence of chronic disease) may present clinically with an acute picture (Fig. 4). Probably more often than not, however, the clinical course follows the morphologic picture or vice versa.

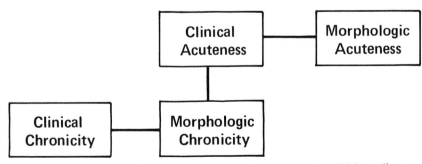

Figure 4. Relationship between the clinical and morphologic features in pericardial heart disease. Although clinical and morphologic acuteness and clinical and morphologic chronicity often go together, an obvious chronic morphologic process often presents acutely clinically.

NORMAL PERICARDIUM

The normal *parietal pericardium* (fibrous sac or fibrous pericardium), the bag which encloses the heart, consists of a 1 mm. thick layer of dense collagen (fibrous layer), devoid of elastic fibrils, and covered by a layer of mesothelial cells (serous layer) (Fig. 5). The *visceral pericardium* (epicardium or serous pericardium) is the surface of the

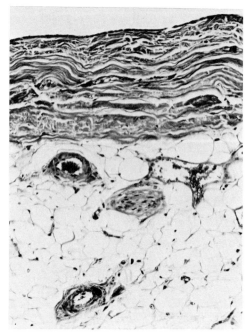

Figure 5. Normal parietal pericardium. A single layer of mesothelial cells covers the layer of dense fibrous tissue on the cardiac side. On the mediastinal side of the fibrous layer is adipose tissue and in it are located vascular channels and nerves. Masson stain; reduced 25% from ×185.

heart itself and consists of a thin (< 1 mm.) layer of loose fibrous tissue covered by mesothelial cells (serous layer). The serous layer of parietal pericardium is continuous with the serous layer of visceral pericardium at or near sites of attachment of the great vessels to the heart. The portion of epicardium which covers the vessels is arranged in the form of two tubes: the ascending aorta and pulmonary trunk are enclosed in one *(arterial mesocardium)* and the superior and inferior vena cavae and the four pulmonary veins are enclosed in the second *(venous mesocardium)*. The attachment of the latter to the parietal pericardium is in the shape of an inverted U and the cul-de-sac enclosed between the limbs of the U lies behind the left atrium and is known as the *oblique sinus*. The passage between the venous and arterial mesocardia, that is, that between the aorta and pulmonary trunk anteriorly and the atria posteriorly, is the *transverse sinus*.

The flask shaped bag of parietal pericardium is closed at its neck by fusion with the adventitia of the great vessels; its base is attached to the tendinous and muscular portions of the left-sided diaphragm. It is also attached to the posterior surface of the sternum by the *superior* (to manibrium) and *inferior* (to xiphoid process) *pericardiosternal ligaments*. Between the left main pulmonary artery and subjacent pulmonary vein is a triangular fold of visceral pericardium known as the *ligament of the left vena cava,* a remnant of the lower part of the left superior vena cava. The sinus node is located near the attachment of the parietal pericardium to the superior vena cava and consequently it may be "irritated" by a pericardial process producing an arrhythmia or a conduction disturbance.

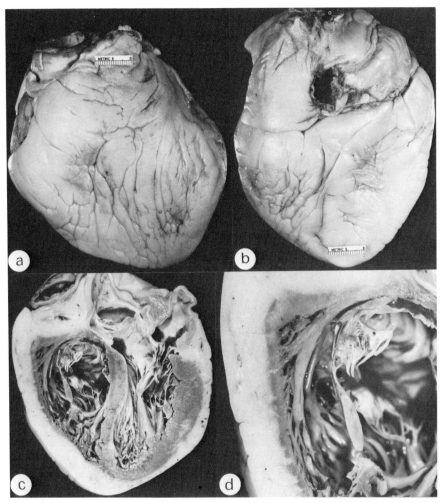

Figure 6. Massive increase in subepicardial adipose tissue in an 82-year-old man (A70-12) with idiopathic hemochromatosis. The myocardium is completely covered exteriorly by fat. The heart weighed 500 grams. a, Anterior view. b, Posterior view. c, Longitudinal section showing the thickness of fat compared to the thickness of the myocardial wall. d, Close-up view of right ventricular wall. The cause of the massive subepicardial adiposity in this patient is uncertain.

Beneath the visceral pericardium is either myocardium or adipose tissue. The amount of subepicardial adipose tissue increases, up to a point, with age. Large quantities are rare in persons under age 10 years and in persons over 90 years of age. The deposits are largest in the atrioventricular sulci and next, about the anterior and posterior descending coronary arteries. At times, the entire surface of the heart is covered by fat (Fig. 6). In general, the amount of subepicardial adipose tissue is proportional to the amount of fat present in other body tissues. At times, however, considerable quantities of subepicardial adipose tissue are present in persons of normal body weight, and the amount may not be excessively increased in persons of huge body weight

15

($>$ 135 kg. [300 lb.]).[4] Corticosteroid therapy causes the subepicardial adipose tissue to increase in amount.[5] In persons with debilitating diseases, for example malignant neoplasms or chronic starvation, the subepicardial fat may atrophy, giving it a watery, gelatinous appearance.

When subepicardial adipose tissue is excessive, strands of fat cells also extend into adjacent myocardium. This occurrence is most frequent in the right ventricle and right atrium. The fat may extend through the myocardial wall and infiltrate endocardium. Although there is no hemodynamic documentation, most older writers believed that excessive subepicardial adipose tissue could cause cardiac dysfunction. Flint,[6] writing in 1870, stated that when ". . . the accumulation (of subepicardial fat) is excessive . . . its weight . . . leads to enfeebled muscular action and consequent weakness of the circulation." He also believed that the excess fat led to myocardial atrophy and cavity dilatation. Osler,[1] writing in 1892, stated that excessive subepicardial fat *(cor adiposum)* ". . . occasionally leads to dangerous or even fatal impairment of the contractile power of the heart."

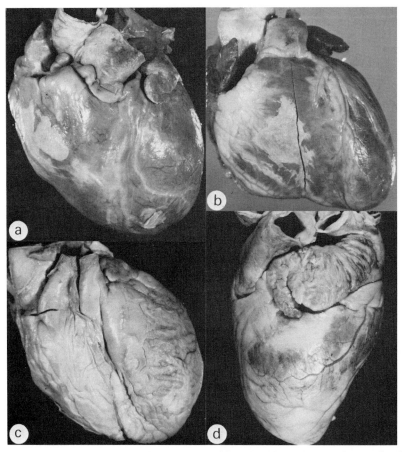

Figure 7. Epicardial collagen plaques (soldier's plaques, milk spots). Shown here are hearts of 4 different patients. a, Collagen plaques are present over the right ventricle and over the left ventricular apex. b, A discrete collagen plaque is visible over the right ventricle. c, Virtually the entire right ventricle and pulmonary trunk are covered by a collagen plaque in this patient. d, Lateral view showing collagen plaques just beneath the left atrial appendage and over the left ventricular apex. Note that the subepicardial adipose tissue is relatively sparse in the 4 patients. The more subepicardial fat present the less the likelihood of epicardial collagen plaques being present.

16

Although normally the serous layer of parietal pericardium contacts the serous layer of visceral pericardium, up to 50 ml. of fluid, which has a chemical composition similar to that of serum, normally is present in the pericardial sac. The pericardial fluid in essence serves as a lubricating oil to diminish the amount of friction between the moving heart and the adjacent tissues.

In the adipose tissue beneath the visceral pericardium and on the mediastinal aspect of the parietal pericardium are located vascular channels, including arteries, veins, and lymphatics, and also nerves. None of these structures, however, is located within the fibrosa component of the parietal pericardium.[7] The arteries of the pericardium arise from the internal mammary artery, and its musculophrenic branch, and from the descending thoracic aorta. Branches of the vagus and phrenic nerves, and branches from the sympathetic trunk supply the pericardium.

Normally, the visceral pericardium is translucent and the underlying subepicardial tissue or myocardium is readily visible. In many individuals the epicardium is focally white (Fig. 7) and then the underlying structures are obscured. These foci (variously called milk spots, soldiers' spots, tendinous patches, and maculae tendinae) most commonly are present over the anterior surface of the right ventricle, are often multiple, and increase in incidence and size with age and with cardiac enlargement. Histologically, these foci consist of dense collagen, occasionally with underlying small collections of mononuclear cells (lymphocytes). Consequently, we prefer calling them "collagen plaques." They are usually absent in the first decade, and nearly always present by the sixth decade. When the right ventricle is enlarged, the collagen plaques over its anterior surface may be quite prominent and presumably result from contact of the beating heart with the undersurface of the sternum. In conditions producing considerable enlargement of the right atrium, for example atrial septal defect, chronic lung disease, or cardiomyopathy, the collagen plaques may occur over the right atrium[8] (Fig. 8). In kyphoscoliosis, the plaques often are found on the posterior surface of the heart, presumably due to contact with the vertebral bodies during cardiac motion. In conditions which cause left ventricular enlargement, particularly systemic hypertension and left ventricular outflow tract obstruction, collagen plaques are often present over the apex of the left ventricle. Plaques in this location may be anatomic expressions of the "point of maximal impulse," and result from contact of the left ventricular apex with the undersurface of the anterior ribs during ventricular systole. In patients with large amounts of subepicardial adipose tissue, collagen plaques may be less numerous, presumably since the epicardial fat acts as a cushion for the underlying myocardium.

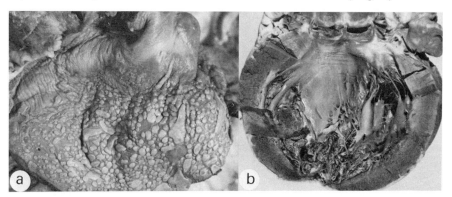

Figure 8. Collagen plaques — multiple discrete — over right atrium in a patient (72A-50) with idiopathic cardiomyopathy of the ventricular dilated type. a, Right atrium exteriorly. b, Dilated and hypertrophied left ventricle containing a thrombus. This type of collagen plaque over the right atrium occurs in patients with dilated right atria from any cause, particularly atrial septal defect.

MORPHOLOGIC RESPONSES OF THE PERICARDIA TO INJURY

Although there are many causes of pericardial disease, the morphologic reaction of the pericardia to injury is rather limited. The pericardium reacts to acute injury by exuding fluid, fibrin, or cells or combinations of these three. The type of fluid and/or cells exuded is determined by the cause of the pericardial disease. There is no pericardial reaction to either serous fluid or to blood in the pericardial sac. If, however, the lipid component of pooled lysed erythrocytes is injected into the pericardial sac, a fibrinous reaction may result and fibrous pericarditis or even cholesterol pericarditis may develop.[9] Blood in the pericardial space of injured pericardia, however, may lead to fibrous pericardial adhesions. Isolated injury to the serosal pericardia of rabbits without associated bleeding causes only a fibrinous reaction; if blood is injected after the serosal injury, pericardial adhesions may result.[10] Deposits of fibrin alone on the pericardial surfaces apparently cause no permanent reaction. If microorganisms enter the pericardial space or tissues, the reaction appears to depend on the type of infecting organism. Viruses, the presumed cause of acute benign pericarditis, generally produce only a transient pericardial reaction which usually resolves.[11, 12] Acid-fast organisms produce a mononuclear cell reaction and generally go on to cause severe fibrous thickening of the pericardia. Pyogenic organisms cause a violent polymorphonuclear cell reaction which also may progress to fibrous thickening with or without constriction.

Eight general morphologic responses to injury are listed in Tables 1 and 2. Although their occurrence in pure form is unusual, the recognition of the dominant morphologic component is useful in determining the cause of "pericarditis" in any particular patient. The causes of each of the primary morphologic components will be discussed more thoroughly in the remainder of this report.

TABLE 1

PERICARDIAL HEART DISEASE: Morphologic Classification

Primary Morphologic Component	Potential for Constriction	Clinical Presentation
1. Fibrin	0	"Acute"
2. Fluid	+	
A. Serous		"Acute"
B. Blood		or
C. Lymph		"Chronic"
3. Purulent	+	
4. Fibrous Tissue	+	"Acute"
5. Neoplasm	+	or
6. Granuloma	+	"Chronic"
7. Calcium	+	
8. Cholesterol	+	

TABLE 2

PERICARDIAL HEART DISEASE: Etiologic and Morphologic Classifications

Etiologic	Morphologic							
	Fibrinous	Effusion	Infective	Fibrous	Neoplastic	Granulomatous	Calcific	Cholesterol
1. Idiopathic	++	+	0	++	0	0	++	++
2. Infective								
A. Pyogenic (Purulent)	+	+	++	+	0	0	0	0
B. Tuberculous	+	+	+	++	0	++	+	+
C. Viral or "Acute Benign Nonspecific"	++	0	+	+	0	0	0	0
D. Parasitic	+	+	++	+	0	+	+	0
E. Fungal	+	+	++	+	0	+	+	0
3. Associated with Systemic Disease								
A. Collagen disease								
1. Rheumatic fever	++	0	0	0	0	0	0	0
2. Rheumatoid arthritis	+	0	0	++	0	+	0	+
3. Systemic lupus erythematosis	+	+	0	++	0	0	0	0
4. Scleroderma	+	0	0	++	0	0	0	0
B. Renal disease	++	+	0	+	0	0	0	0
C. Thyroid disease	0	+	0	0	0	+	+	++
D. Sarcoidosis	0	0	0	0	0	++	0	0
4. Associated with Other Disease of Heart or Aorta								
A. Acute myocardial infarction	++	0	0	+	0	0	0	0
B. Ascending aortic aneurysm	+	++	0	0	0	0	0	0
5. Trauma and Iatrogenic								
A. Penetrating and non-penetrating injury	+	++	0	++	0	0	0	+
B. Cardiac catheterization	++	+	0	0	0	0	0	0
C. Cardiac operation and post pericardiotomy syndrome	+	+	+	++	0	0	0	0
D. Resuscitation	+	+	0	++	0	0	0	0
E. Radiation	+	+	0	++	0	0	0	0
F. Drugs and hypersensitivity states	++	+	0	0	0	0	0	0
G. Talc	+	0	0	+	0	++	0	0
6. Neoplastic	+	+	0	0	++	0	0	. 0
7. Congenital								
A. True and false (diverticulae) cysts	–	–	–	–	–	–	–	–
B. Complete and partial absence	–	–	–	–	–	–	–	–

FIBRINOUS "PERICARDITIS" (TABLE 3)

Fibrin deposits on the pericardial surfaces are commonly observed at necropsy. The deposits may be focal or diffuse, and they may or may not be associated with an increased quantity of pericardial fluid. Every type of pericardial disease probably is associated with fibrinous deposits at one time and probably most resolve without residua. Fibrinous deposits are not capable by themselves of causing myocardial constriction. The causes of fibrinous "pericarditis" include the following:

19

TABLE 3

PERICARDIAL HEART DISEASE:

Etiology of <u>Fibrinous</u> "Pericarditis"

1. Acute Myocardial Infarction
2. Iatrogenic and Traumatic
     A. Cardiovascular Operation
     B. Complications of Catherization
     C. Irradiation
     D. Chemical Agents
     E. Penetrating and Non-penetrating Injury
3. Infectious Agents
4. Idiopathic ("Acute Benign Nonspecific")
5. Neoplasm
6. Associated with Systemic Disease
     A. Renal Disease ("Uremia")
     B. Collagen Disease
          1. Acute Rheumatic Fever
          2. Rheumatoid Arthritis
          3. Systemic Lupus Erythematosis
     C. Hypersensitivity States and Drug-induced

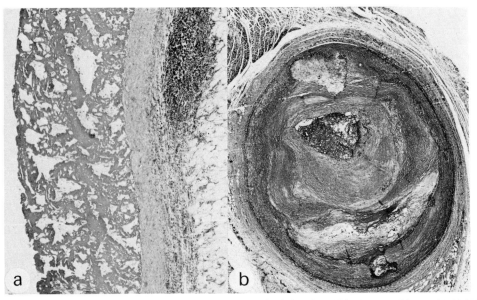

Figure 9. Diffuse fibrinous pericarditis from acute myocardial infarction. This 56-year-old man (A66-171) developed a precordial friction rub on day 6 following infarction and died on day 16. a, A deposit of fibrin covers the midly thickened epicardium. Hematoxylin and eosin stain. b, Left circumflex coronary artery completely occluded by both atherosclerotic plaque and thrombus. Movat stain. Reduced 15% from ×28 (a) and ×14(b).

ACUTE MYOCARDIAL INFARCTION (AMI). Fibrinous pericarditis occurs in virtually all patients with transmural AMI (Fig. 9). The deposits may be limited to the visceral and parietal pericardium immediately overlying the area of transmural necrosis or they may spread to involve the pericardial surfaces diffusely. The mechanism of development of diffuse fibrinous pericarditis in these patients is unclear but it may be related to the presence of an associated serosanguinous effusion. The parietal pericardium may adhere to the underlying visceral pericardium at the site of the transmural AMI. If the pericardial adherence occurs before left ventricular free wall rupture occurs (as a consequence of the AMI), then extravasation of blood into the pericardial space may be prevented and a false left ventricular aneurysm may result (Figs. 10–12).[13, 14]

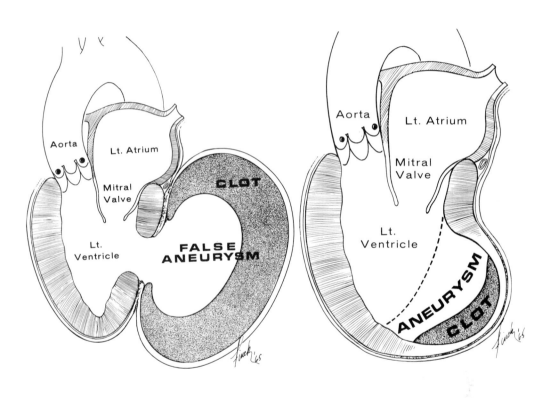

Figure 10. Left ventricular aneurysms with adherent parietal pericardia. This diagram shows differences between false and true left ventricular aneurysm. The wall of the false one is parietal pericardium which had become adherent to epicardium before left ventricular rupture occurred. In the true aneurysm (right) the parietal pericardium adheres to the scarred left ventricular myocardium but the actual wall of the aneurysm had been, at one time, myocardium.

21

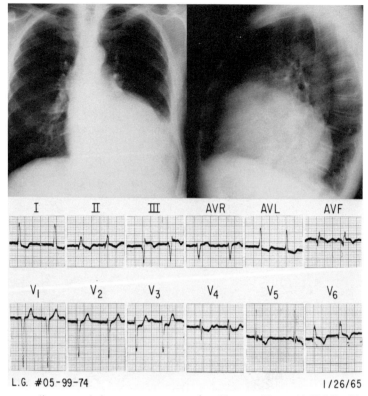

I II III AVR AVL AVF

V1 V2 V3 V4 V5 V6

L.G. #05-99-74   1/26/65

Figure 11. Electrocardiogram and chest roentgenograms in a 53-year-old man (A65-24) with a huge false left ventricular aneurysm.[13] The acute myocardial infarction had occurred 4 years earlier. The electrocardiogram does not allow distinction between a true and false aneurysm. The heart weighed 800 gm. and the false left ventricular aneurysm with its intra-aneurysmal thrombus weighed 850 gm.

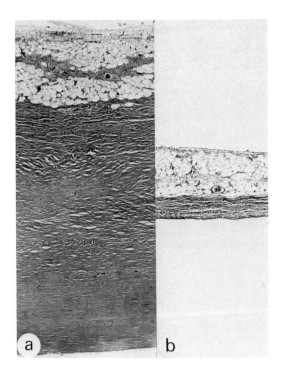

a   b

Figure 12. Parietal pericardium (a) in a 53-year-old man (A65-24, Fig. 11) with a false left ventricular aneurysm. The parietal pericardium, which is the wall of the aneurysm, is much thicker than is the normal parietal pericardium (b) (from another patient). Hematoxylin and eosin stains; each reduced 20% from ×40.

22

IATROGENIC. *Cardiac surgery* is certainly one of the most common causes of "pericarditis" today. Whenever the mesothelial cells of the pericardia are "rubbed off," a fibrinous reaction ensues. As healing of the injured pericardia occurs, the fibrin disappears and the two serous layers of pericardium remain adherent by fibrous adhesions. Despite this adherence, however, the parietal pericardium rarely is thickened by operative intervention. Obviously, blood and its products enter the pericardial space during any cardiac operation and organization of the blood products may be more responsible for the eventual fibrous pericardial obliteration than the fibrinous deposits.[10] Perforation of a cardiac wall by a catheter may lead to a pericardial reaction similar to that produced by cardiac surgery.[15] Blunt or penetrating trauma also may cause a fibrinous pericardial reaction, which on rare occasion may progress to constriction.[16]

Irradiation to the mediastinum and *chemical agents* initially cause a fibrinous pericardial reaction which also may heal by fibrous obliteration.

INFECTIOUS AGENTS. These will be discussed under infective pericarditis.

IDIOPATHIC. Although abundant clinical information is available on acute benign pericarditis, morphologic information on this entity is lacking because of its self-limited character and rare association with pericardial constriction.[11, 12, 17, 18] A viral etiology of this entity has been implicated on the basis of viral shedding, a rise in viral titers, and the presence of lymphocytes and virus in aspirated pericardial fluid.[19, 20] A virus, however, has never to our knowledge been observed ultrastructurally in pericardium, although viral antigen has been located in pericardium by immunofluorescence.[21]

NEOPLASM. A fibrinous pericardial reaction is common whenever the pericardium is infiltrated by a neoplasm, but the fibrin deposits, obviously, are of minor consequence in this circumstance.

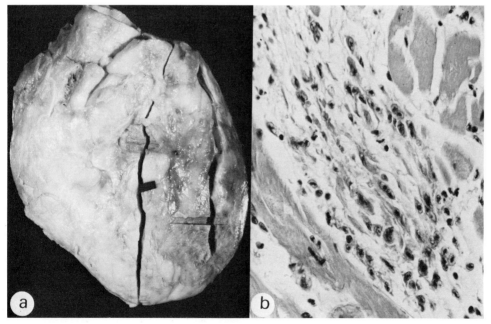

Figure 13. Diffuse fibrinofibrous pericarditis in acute rheumatic fever. This 41-year-old woman (A68-20) developed acute pharyngitis about 7 weeks before death, followed by polyarthritis and finally congestive cardiac failure. At no time was a precordial murmur or a friction rub heard. The antistreptolysin 0 titer was elevated (833 Todd units; normal less than 150 units). At necropsy, the pericardial space was obliterated by fibrinofibrous adhesions (a) and Aschoff bodies were present in the sections of myocardium (b). Hematoxylin-eosin stain; reduced 20% from ×400 (b).

ASSOCIATED SYSTEMIC DISEASE. *Uremic pericarditis* at least initially is always fibrinous in type and is found at necropsy in over 50 percent of patients with fatal acute or chronic renal disease.[22, 23] Its cause remains unclear. The term "uremic pericarditis" is a misnomer because, to our knowledge, injection of neither urea nitrogen nor creatinine into the pericardial space will result in a fibrinous pericardial reaction. Furthermore, uremic pericarditis may occur in patients with chronic renal disease whose levels of urea nitrogen and creatinine have been made normal for long periods by frequent dialysis.[24, 25] Usually the amount of pericardial fluid is increased in patients with renal failure in addition to the fibrinous pericardial deposition. On occasion, the pericardia may become quite thick by fibrous proliferation and lead to constriction with or without associated serous or hemorrhagic effusion.[26, 27]

Acute rheumatic fever is usually associated with a fibrino-mononuclear cell reaction which usually is subclinical (Fig. 13).[28, 29] This pericardial reaction apparently usually resolves because evidence of previous pericardial disease is rarely observed at necropsy in patients with rheumatic heart disease (Fig. 14). Calcific pericardial deposits also may occur in patients with rheumatic heart disease, but they too are extremely rare[30] and when present, focal, and never associated with myocardial constriction.

Fibrinous pericarditis was common (about 60 percent) in patients with *systemic lupus erythematosus* seen in the precorticosteroid era.[31] Today, however, a fibrous obliterative pericardial reaction is more commonly observed.[5] A fibrinous pericardial reaction also is observed at necropsy in about 40 percent of patients with *rheumatoid arthritis*.[32, 33]

The morphologic features of pericardial disease resulting from *hypersensitivity states* and *drug reactions* is uncertain, but it is presumed that the reaction is of a fibrinous type.

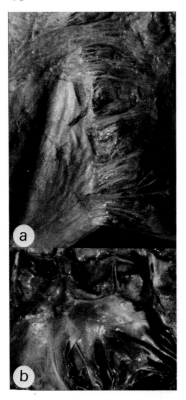

Figure 14. Diffuse fibrous obliterative pericarditis in rheumatic heart disease. This 44-year-old woman (72A-153), who had mitral stenosis and aortic regurgitation, never had clinical evidence of pericardial disease. a, Close-up view of exterior of heart showing total adherence of the parietal to the visceral pericardia by the fibrous adhesions. b, Opened left ventricular outflow tract showing diffuse fibrous thickening of the mitral and aortic valves.

TABLE 4

PERICARDIAL HEART DISEASE:

Etiology of <u>Effusion</u> (>50 ml.) into Pericardial Space

SEROUS
1. Congestive Cardiac Failure
2. Hypoalbuminemia
3. Irradiation

BLOOD (Hematocrit >10%)
1. Iatrogenic
   - A. Cardiac Operation
   - B. Cardiac Catheterization
   - C. Trauma (penetrating and non-penetrating)
   - D. Anticoagulant Agents
   - E. Chemotherapeutic Agents
2. Neoplasm
3. Trauma
4. Acute Myocardial Infarction
5. Cardiac Rupture
6. Rupture of Ascending Aorta or Major Pulmonary Artery
7. Coagulopathy
   - A. Thrombocytopenia
   - B. Hypoprothrombinemia
   - C. Other (Hemophilia, Gaucher's, etc.)
8. Renal Disease

LYMPH OR CHYLE
1. Neoplasm
2. Iatrogenic
   - A. Cardiothoracic Surgery
3. Congenital
4. Idiopathic ("Primary Chylopericardium")
5. Non-neoplastic Obstruction of Pulmonary "Hilum" or Superior Vena Cava

EFFUSION INTO PERICARDIAL SAC (TABLE 4)

Excessive (> 50 ml.) effusion into the pericardial sac is extremely common, probably far more common than generally appreciated because the amounts are rarely accurately measured at necropsy. Serous effusions up to 200 ml., as commonly occur in patients with congestive cardiac failure or hypoalbuminemia, may be overlooked entirely at necropsy.

The amount of pericardial fluid necessary to cause ventricular constriction is highly variable and dependent on several factors: (1) the time period required to accumulate the fluid; (2) the amount of thickening of the underlying or overlying pericardia; (3) the amount of muscle mass (weight) of the cardiac ventricles; and (4) the blood volume. The more rapidly fluid accumulates, the greater the chance that myocardial dysfunction (constriction) will result. Fluid volumes of many times the normal amount (< 50 ml.) may be present without myocardial constriction if the accumulation is slow (see Fig. 2).

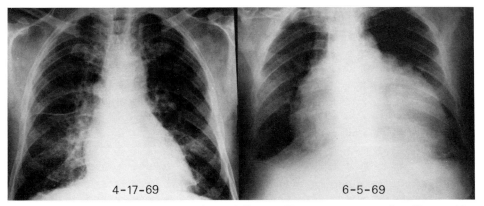

Figure 15. Hemorrhagic pericarditis in chronic renal disease. Chest roentgenograms in a 60-year-old man (A69-201) who died with cardiac tamponade on June 24, 1969.[40] He developed hypotension and severe right-sided cardiac failure associated with rapid enlargement of the cardiac silhouette beginning 28 days before death.

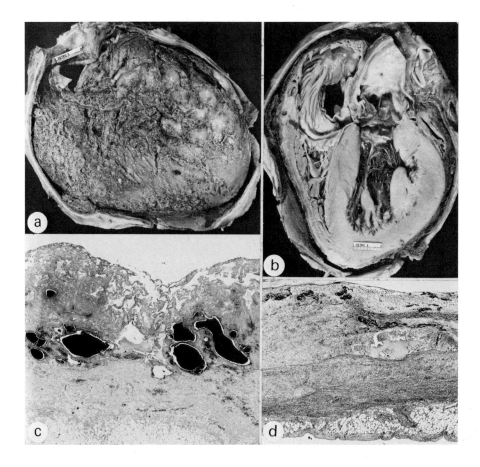

Figure 16. Hemorrhagic pericarditis in chronic renal disease in the patient described in Figure 15. A 50 ml. hemorrhagic effusion was present and the pericardial surfaces contain diffuse fibrin deposits and blood clots. In addition, the pericardia were thickened by fibrous tissue. a, Anterior surface of the heart. b, Longitudinal cut showing the thickened pericardia in relation to the thickness of the walls of the cardiac chambers. c, Visceral pericardium containing many dilated vessels; rupture of one or more of them is the presumed cause of the hemorrhagic effusion. d, Parietal pericardium. Hematoxylin and eosin stain; reduced 30% from ×16 (d).

26

The greater the thickness of the parietal or visceral pericardia or both the less fluid is necessary to produce signs or symptoms of constriction (see Fig. 3). The thicker the ventricular walls, the more fluid required for constriction. More fluid is required, for example, to constrict the hypertensive ventricle than the normotensive ventricle (see Fig. 3).

SEROUS EFFUSION. These are most common in patients with congestive cardiac failure and hypoalbuminemia. Irradiation (usually > 4000 rads) to the mediastinum may produce a large effusion with tamponade.[34]

BLOODY EFFUSION. These most commonly result from acute myocardial infarction; rupture of the heart or aorta;[13, 14, 35] neoplasms;[36] cardiac operations or other procedures;[15] drugs which alter clotting mechanisms;[37] and chronic renal disease.[38, 39] That renal disease may be associated with large bloody effusions is largely unappreciated;[40] this circumstance may occur in the natural history of renal disease (Figs. 15 – 17) as

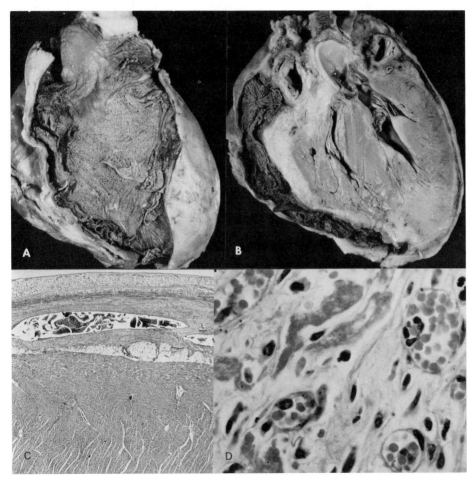

Figure 17. Hemorrhagic pericarditis in chronic renal disease. This 26-year-old woman (A67-256) had renal failure and pericardial effusion on admission 3 weeks before death.[40] Pericardiocentesis was performed twice but cardiac tamponade progressed. At necropsy, 800 ml. of hemorrhagic fluid was present and the pericardia are diffusely thickened and covered by fibrin deposits and blood clots. a, Exterior view of heart anteriorly. b, Longitudinal section of heart. The pericardial space over the left ventricle is obliterated. c, Photomicrograph showing adherence of parietal pericardium to underlying visceral pericardium over left ventricle. d, Close-up of portion of epicardium showing many vascular channels, the presumed source of the hemorrhagic pericardial effusion. c, Phosphotungstic acid hematoxylin stain. d, Hematoxylin and eosin stain. [Reduced 20% from ×7.5 (c) and ×628 (d).]

27

well as that prolonged by chronic dialysis. Gaucher's disease also may be associated with large pericardial effusions[41, 42] (Fig. 18). Hemopericardium is always an ominous sign because malignancy is one of its more common causes. Hemorrhages into epicardium are common in patients with thrombocytopenia (Fig. 19).

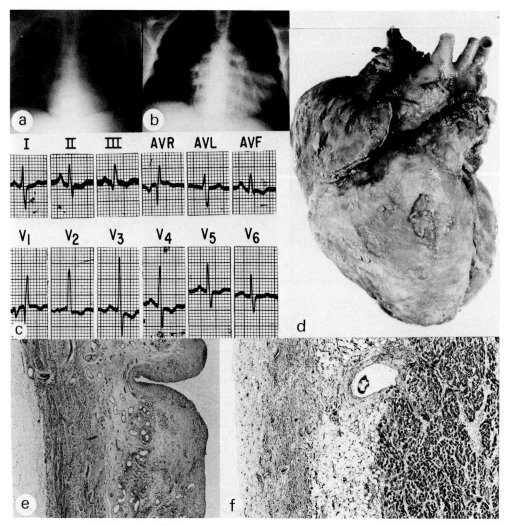

Figure 18. Hemorrhagic pericarditis in a 30-year-old man (A62-4) with Gaucher's disease and pulmonary hypertension (from Gaucher cells plugging pulmonary capillaries).[41] a and b, Chest radiographs. a, Two months before death. b, Day of death demonstrating marked enlargement of the cardiac silhouette. About 750 ml. of blood were present in the pericardial sac. c, Electrocardiogram recorded 1 hour before death. d, Exterior of heart showing diffuse fibrinous pericarditis and marked enlargement of the right atrium and ventricle. e, Thickened parietal pericardium containing large vascular channels. f, Thickened visceral pericardium. The cause of the hemorrhagic pericardial effusion was not determined. Periodic acid-Schiff stains; reduced 25% from ×22 (e) and ×33 (f).

LYMPHATIC AND CHYLOUS EFFUSION. Most reports concerning lymph or chyle within the pericardial space concern only isolated patients because this condition is rare.[43-47] *Chylopericardium*, that is, milky effusion, most commonly results from obstruction of, or injury to, the thoracic duct.[47] At other times its cause is not discernible,

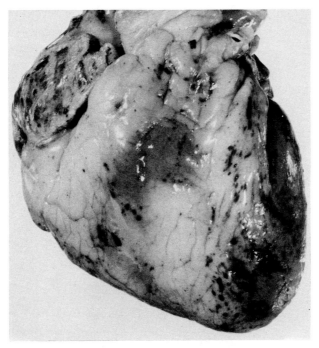

Figure 19. Focal epicardial hemorrhages in hypothrombocytopenia. Anterior surface of heart showing focal hemorrhages in a 56-year-old man (A65-71) with acute myelogenous leukemia. The epicardial hemorrhages seen here are typical of those observed in many patients with severe hypothrombocytopenia from any cause. This man's platelet count 2 days before death was 500 per cu. mm.

but, nevertheless, hemipericardiectomy and ligation of pericardial lymphatics may result in disappearance of the chylous effusion.[43] Lymphangiomatous hamartoma (cystic hygroma) of the mediastinum associated with a communication between the thoracic duct and pericardial space[44, 45] also has caused chylopericardium. Chylous fluid may accumulate rapidly, estimated in one patient to be 5 ml. per minute.[43] Lymphopericardium, that is, clear fluid, which is even less common than chylopericardium, usually results from pericardial lymphangiomas which may be part of a generalized lymphangiectasia.[46]

TABLE 5

PERICARDIAL HEART DISEASE:

Etiology of <u>Infective</u> (Purulent) Pericarditis

1. Infectious Agent
    A. Bacterium
    B. Fungus
    C. Parasite
    D. Virus

INFECTIVE (PURULENT) PERICARDITIS (TABLE 5)

Infective pericarditis is the presence of pus or microorganisms or both in the pericardial sac or tissues. Nontuberculous infective pericarditis is infrequent. In the preantibiotic and prethoracic surgical eras it usually was the result of direct spread of an acute infection from the lung, pleura, mediastinum, or abdomen or a complication of a generalized septicemia.[48] Today, however, the most common predisposing factors are cardiothoracic operations, immunosuppressive therapy, trauma, rupture of the esophagus into the pericardial sac secondary to neoplasm (Fig. 20), and infective endocarditis with rupture of a ring abscess, septic coronary embolus, or rupture of a myocardial abscess (Figs. 21 and 22).[49] The expected increase in frequency of purulent pericarditis with the advent of cardiothoracic operations has been offset by the widespread use of antibiotics and the decrease in bacterial infections in general.[36, 50] Indeed, purulent pericarditis is less frequent today than in the preantibiotic and prethoracic surgical eras.[51] The occurrence of infective pericarditis as a consequence of infective endocarditis is not widely appreciated.[52] Among 1284 patients with fatal infective endocarditis reviewed by Buchbinder and Roberts,[52] 172 (13 percent) had pericarditis at necropsy. The pericarditis in this circumstance, however, need not be purulent. Several mechanisms of formation of pericarditis in patients with infective endocarditis are shown in Figure 21.

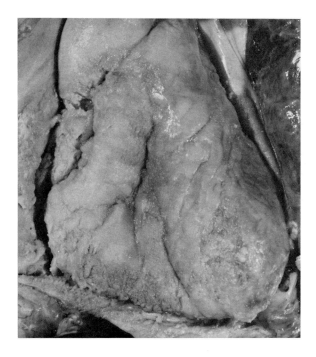

Figure 20. Purulent pericarditis. Exterior of heart in a 56-year-old man (A60-30) with squamous cell carcinoma arising in the floor of the mouth. He developed a neoplastic abscess cavity in the left posterior mediastinum and it opened into esophagus, bronchus, left pleural cavity and pericardial sac. *Candida albicans* was cultured from the purulent material in the pericardial sac.

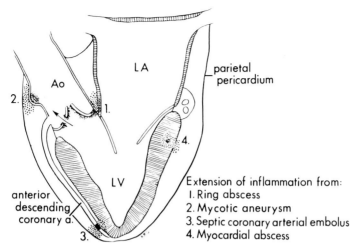

Figure 21. Schematic portrayal of the pathogenesis of pericarditis in infective endocarditis. Ao = aorta; LV = left ventricle; LA = left atrium.

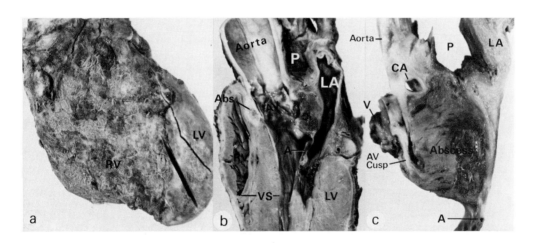

Figure 22. Fatal hemorrhagic pericarditis with tamponade secondary to *Escherichia coli* endocarditis in a 51-year-old woman (72A-22) with previous systemic hypertension and portal cirrhosis. The infective endocarditis was not suspected clinically. a, Exterior of heart showing diffuse fibrino-hemorrhagic exudate. b, Longitudinal section showing a ring abscess (abs) in the angle between the aortic valve (AV) and anterior mitral leaflet (A). The abscess represents extension of the vegetations (V) which have destroyed one of the aortic valve cusps. c, Close-up view of ring abscess and site of rupture into the pericardial space (P). RV = right ventricle; LV = left ventricle; LA = left atrium; CA = coronary artery; and VS = ventricular septum.

The organisms responsible for nontuberculous infective pericarditis have changed considerably since the introduction of antibiotics, cardiothoracic surgery, and immunosuppression. In the preantibiotic era a Gram-positive bacterium was responsible in 80 percent and a Gram-negative bacterium in 4 percent (Table 6). These figures were from the study by Cabot of 186 necropsy patients with purulent pericarditis.[29] In a recent study from the same hospital (Massachusetts General) of 26 patients with purulent pericarditis, Gram-positive bacteria were responsible in 42 percent, Gram-negative bacteria in 39 percent, and fungi in 19 percent (Table 6).[49] In none of Cabot's patients were fungi the causative agent. Furthermore, the types of Gram-positive bacteria causing

31

TABLE 6

ORGANISMS RESPONSIBLE FOR NON-TUBERCULOUS INFECTIVE PERICARDITIS

		Pre-antibiotic Era (1896-1919)[*]	Early Antibiotic Era (1949-59)[**]	Antibiotic Era (1960-74)[***]
I.	Gram-positive			
	Staphylococcus aureus	14	7	8
	Staphylococcus epidermidis	3	0	0
	Staph. (species unspecified)	4	0	0
	Streptococcus	39	1	1
	Pneumococcus	33	0	2
II.	Gram-negative			
	Escherichia coli	3	1	0
	Klebsiella pneumoniae	1	0	0
	Hemophilus influenzae	0	0	2
	Neisseria meningitidis	0	0	1
III.	Multiple bacteria	7	0	0
IV.	Fungi	0	0	5
V.	Unspecified or unproved	9	2	7[****]
VI.	Negative cultures	73	0	0
	Totals	186	11	26

[*]From Cabot, Massachusetts General Hospital, 1896-1919 (29).
[**]From Boyle, et al., Wadsworth General Hospital. 1949-1959 (51).
[***]From Rubin and Moellering, Massachusetts General Hospital. 1960-1974 (49).
[****]All of these may be Gram-negative organisms.

infective pericarditis have changed considerably: streptococcus and pneumococcus were most common in the preantibiotic era, and staphylococcus in the recent antibiotic era (Table 6).

Purulent pericarditis with or without antibiotic treatment has a poor prognosis. It nearly always also indicates a widespread infection of mediastinum and lung. Although tamponade and constriction may occur, drainage of the pericardial pus usually is not lifesaving because the infective process is so extensive.

Although parasites can infect pericardium, all are rare. About 80 patients with amebic pericarditis have been reported, and in each spread was from a hepatic abscess.[53-56] Before actual perforation into the pericardial space, an amebic abscess can cause a local pericardial reaction with fluid accumulation; later, the effusion becomes purulent. The pericardial fluid in amebic pericarditis is described classically as "anchovy-sauce" pus, but *Entamoeba histolytica* organisms are infrequently found in it.[57] A rapid course to contriction may occur.[54] Pericardial involvement by toxoplasmosis and echinococcosis is extremely rare,[58] and cases of pericardial involvement by dracunculosis have been reported.[59]

Fungal pericarditis has increased in frequency with the use of immunosuppressive agents. Although usually granulomatous, fungal pericarditis may be purulent. *Coccidiodes immitis* has been found in pericardium, and clinical evidence of pericarditis occurs in about 15 percent of patients with pulmonary coccidiodomycosis.[60, 61] Pericarditis occurred in 2 percent of 470 necropsied patients with actinomycosis[62, 63] but sulfur granules were rare.[62] Pericardial calcific deposits may occur in patients exhibiting positive reactions to histoplasmin and no response to other fungal antigens;[64] but acute pericarditis has not been reported in patients with histoplasmosis. Pericardial candidiasis has been observed in patients with leukemia receiving immunosuppressive drugs (Fig. 23).[65]

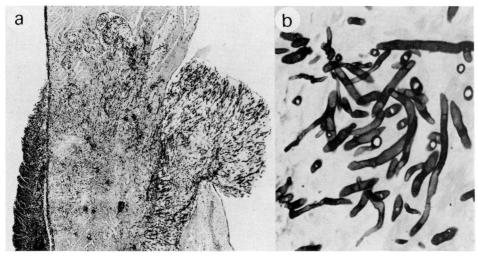

Figure 23. *Candida tropicalis* pancarditis in a 7-year-old girl (A63-246) with acute lymphocytic leukemia and a 21 month illness. The child never had signs or symptoms of cardiac disease, but died of disseminated candidiasis. a, Section of right atrial wall with fungi extending from epicardium through myocardium into endocardium. b, Close-up of candida organisms. Methenamine silver stains; reduced 15% from ×12 (a) and ×520 (b).

Pericarditis has been seen in association with several viral diseases including infectious mononucleosis, atypical pneumonia, mumps, measles, smallpox, and influenza.[19, 20] Although viral titers may rise, morphologic confirmation of a viral etiology is lacking.

Percarditis is probably most frequent from Coxsackie viruses;[10, 19, 66] biopsy of parietal pericardium, however, has not revealed intracellular virions, although viral antigens may be present.[21] Indeed, almost no morphologic information is present on viral pericarditis in humans. "Acute benign idiopathic pericarditis" may in actuality be "Coxsackie pericarditis."

FIBROUS "PERICARDITIS" (TABLE 7)

Fibrous "pericarditis" is thickening of the pericardia or the presence of adhesions between the visceral and parietal pericardia or both. Either the thickening or the adhesions may be focal or diffuse. The thickening may involve both visceral and parietal pericardia or only one of them. The collagen plaque, for example, is a form of fibrous pericarditis with focal thickening often limited to epicardium. Pericardial thickening may occur in the absence of pericardial adhesions or adhesions may occur in the absence of pericardial thickening or the two may occur together. When pericardial adhesions are diffuse the pericardial space is obliterated and this circumstance has been called *obliterative pericarditis*. Obliterative pericarditis may occur in the absence of thickening of the parietal pericardium. Obviously, since its space is no longer present, pericardial effusion, by definition, cannot be present in the patient with obliterative pericarditis. A pericardial effusion may be present, however, in patients with focal pericardial adhesions or in patients with diffuse pericardial thickening with either no adhesions or only focal adhesions.

There are many causes of pericardial thickening and pericardial adhesions. The most common are listed in Table 7.

TABLE 7

PERICARDIAL HEART DISEASE:

Etiology of <u>Fibrous</u> (Adhesive) "Pericarditis"

1. Healing of Hemopericardium (of any cause) in the presence of serosal injury

    A. Cardiac Operation

    B. Trauma — blunt and penetrating

2. Irradiation

3. Associated with Another Disease

    A. Renal Disease

    B. Rheumatoid Arthritis

    C. Systemic Lupus Erythematosis

    D. Scleroderma

4. Infectious Agent

5. Idiopathic

HEALING OF HEMOPERICARDIUM (OF ANY CAUSE). As mentioned earlier, the presence of blood within the pericardial sac by itself leaves no residua. The presence of blood, however, superimposed on injured pericardial surfaces (mesothelial layer "rubbed off," for example) generally leads to adhesions between the pericardia with or without thickening of the pericardia themselves.[10] After cardiac operations the pericardia become adherent to one another by fibrous adhesions. In this circumstance, it is presumed that manipulation of the pericardia at operation damaged the pericardial surfaces. The adherence of the two layers, therefore, represents an "overreaction" of a healing process. Interestingly, in this situation (postcardiotomy), the parietal pericardium is not thickened. Blunt external trauma from, for example, resuscitation may produce a similar reaction. Nonpenetrating blunt trauma may also simply "bruise" the pericardial surfaces, producing a focal fibrinous reaction which may resolve or go on to fibrous adhesions if blood exudes into the pericardial space at the site of the contusion.[16]

IRRADIATION. "Radiation always produces injury, and repair of that injury may cause [fibrous] proliferation."[67] Although the endocardium, myocardium, and pericardium may be injured by high-dose irradiation, the portion of the heart most frequently damaged by this means is the pericardium. Experimentally, mediastinal irradiation to rabbits (in a dosage equivalent to 4000 rads to mediastinum of humans) initially produces a polymorphonuclear reaction in the pericardia followed in one or two days by a mononuclear reaction.[68-71] Damage to the endothelial cells of both lymphatic and blood capillaries leads to luminal obstruction of these channels, which, in turn, leads to peri-

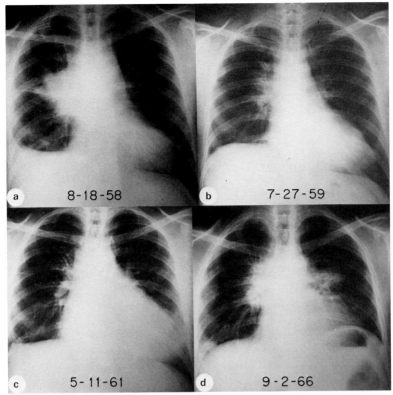

a 8-18-58	b 7-27-59
c 5-11-61	d 9-2-66

Figure 24. Pericardial Hodgkin's disease causing right ventricular outflow obstruction. This 36-year-old man, who died on Sept. 24, 1966, was found to have a mediastinal mass on routine chest roentgenogram (a) in August 1958, and biopsy of the mass disclosed Hodgkin's disease. A pericardial effusion was present at the time of thoracotomy, but no tumor nodules were observed within the pericardium. A pericardiopleural window was created. Postoperatively, he received 3,000 rads to the mediastinum, and during the ensuing 3 months the mass disappeared. Four months after operation a supraclavicular mass appeared, and it was treated with 3,000 rads. He then was asymptomatic until March 1959 when cough, malaise, and episodes of pressing substernal pain and dyspnea after exertion appeared. Large pulsations (a wave) developed in the jugular veins, and when examined in July 1959 the heart was enlarged (b), a grade 3/6 ejection-type systolic murmur was audible along the upper left sternal border and the liver was enlarged and pulsatile.

Cardiac catheterization in May 1961 disclosed significant systolic pressure gradients between the right ventricular body, infundibulum, and pulmonary trunk (Fig. 25). There was also partial A-V block. Injection of contrast material into the right ventricle disclosed a large mass which compressed the pulmonary trunk and right ventricular outflow tract. No fluid was obtained at pericardiocentesis. Chest roentgenogram at this time revealed increased cardiac enlargement (c). During the 10 days after catheterization he received 1,480 rads to the mediastinum. Within a month the 2:1 A-V block had disappeared, the P-R interval had returned to normal, the a wave in the jugular venous pulse had diminished, the intensity of the precordial murmur had decreased, and he was asymptomatic with good tolerance to exercise. Repeat catheterization showed a normal right ventricular systolic pressure (Fig. 25).

The patient was well thereafter until December 1962 when exertional dyspnea and periodic precordial chest pain recurred, and he was digitalized. The precordial systolic ejection murmur was grade 3/6 intensity again, a ventricular gallop was present, but there was no right ventricular hypertrophy by electrocardiogram, which showed sinus rhythm, low voltage, abnormal P waves consistent with both right and left atrial enlargement, and periodic T wave inversion in the lateral precordial leads. In October 1965 he received 2,000 rads to the left hilar region of the lung because of radiodensities in this region. Also, at this time the dyspnea worsened but was lessened by treatment with vincristine and nitrogen mustard. In December 1965 the dyspnea worsened abruptly and he retained fluid. He was now cachectic and dyspneic while sitting. The chest roentgenogram was interpreted as showing radiation pneumonitis and fibrosis. With diuretic therapy the dyspnea lessened, the excess fluid disappeared, and thereafter he was able to walk up two flights of stairs with only mild dyspnea until May 1966 when acute pneumonitis, which responded to antibiotics, caused the return of severe dyspnea. From July until his death in September 1966 he was always mildly dyspneic and had mild subcutaneous edema. The neck veins terminally were only mildly distended. Hepatic failure from serum hepatitis was the immediate cause of death. The roentgenogram in d was taken 22 days before death.

cardial effusion.[72] The pericardia also are thickened by fibrous tissue but its mechanism of development is uncertain.

Mediastinal irradiation in high doses in humans with resulting pericardial injury occurs primarily in patients with Hodgkin's disease,[68, 69, 73] because it is the most common mediastinal tumor irradiated in sufficient doses to cause cardiac disease (Figs. 24–29).

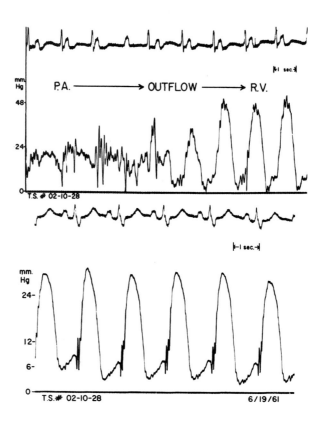

Figure 25. Same case as Figure 24. Right-sided cardiac pressure tracings. The upper panel (May 1961) shows the pressure during withdrawal of the catheter from the pulmonary artery (P.A.) (24/10 mm Hg) through the right ventricular outflow tract (34/6 mm Hg) into the right ventricular body (R.V.) (52/6 mm Hg). The lower panel shows the right ventricular pressure (30/8 mm Hg) at catheterization one month after upper tracing and after therapy. The electrocardiogram during the first catheterization (upper) showed second degree heart block, which had disappeared by the second study (lower).

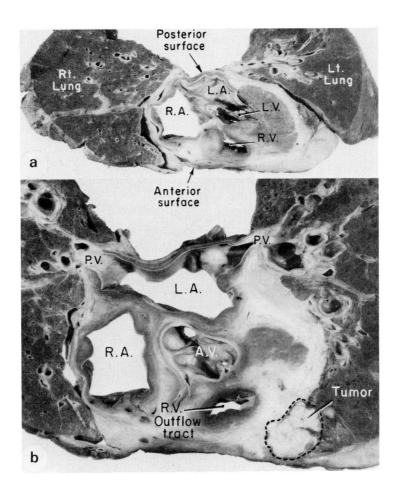

Figure 26. Same case as Figure 24. Radiation fibrosis of the heart. a, Transverse section of the heart and lung demonstrating severe fibrous thickening of the epicardium and fibrosis of the outer walls of the right (R.V.) and left (L.V.) ventricles. The body of the right ventricle is very small. b, Close-up of transverse section of the heart at the level of the right ventricular outflow tract (infundibulum), which is severely narrowed. The only residual of Hodgkin's disease is at the junction of the right ventricle and left lung (enclosed by the dashed lines). R.A. = right atrium; L.A. = left atrium; A.V. = aortic valve; and P.V. = pulmonary vein.

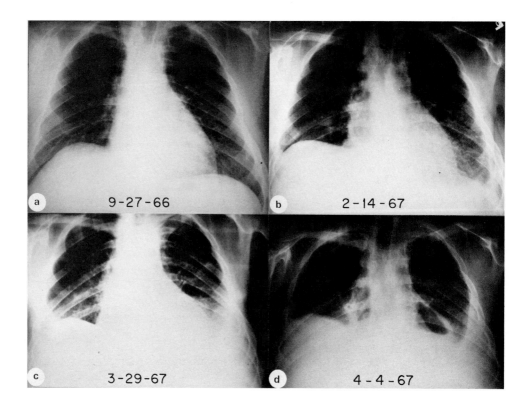

Figure 27. Chest roentgenograms in a 26-year-old man who died on April 5, 1967, of cardiac tamponade and Hodgkin's disease. In September 1964 biopsy of a painless unilateral swelling in the neck disclosed Hodgkin's disease. The heart and lungs appeared normal on chest roentgenogram in December 1964. In January 1965 he received 6,000 rads to the upper chest and neck, 6,000 to the lower mediastinum, 6,000 to the abdominal periaortic regions, 2,000 to the splenic area, and 1,800 to the pelvis. Except for acute esophagitis in February 1965, presumably secondary to the irradiation, he was asymptomatic until January 24, 1967, when exertional and nocturnal dyspnea, precordial pain, and swelling of the legs and abdomen suddenly appeared. Examination on February 1, 1967 disclosed dyspnea on sitting up in bed, a 25 mm Hg decrease in the brachial arterial systolic pressure during inspiration, rapid respirations (40/min.), distended neck veins, a pericardial friction rub, sinus tachycardia (150/min.) with atrial premature contractions, ascites, pitting lower leg edema, and large pleural effusions. No murmurs or gallops were audible and a precordial impulse was not palpable. Left thoracentesis yielded 1,200 ml. serous fluid and pericardiocentesis yielded 200 ml. of bloody fluid. The patient then felt better and the heart sounds were louder on precordial auscultation.

His last two months were characterized by repeated reaccumulations of pleural fluid (a total of 9,200 ml. was removed from the pleural spaces during 9 thoracenteses) and continued evidence of right-sided and left-sided cardiac failure. A second pericardiocentesis yielding 210 ml. of fluid was performed on February 7, 1967, and he then was digitalized. Approximately eight days before death the dyspnea worsened, hypotension, oliguria, and hyperkalemia appeared and he gained weight. Pericardiocentesis was repeated on April 4 and 330 ml. of fluid was obtained. Several hours later he died.

At necropsy, 350 ml. of fluid was present in the pericardial sac, 2,500 ml. in each pleural space, and 1,200 in the peritoneal cavity.

The date of each roentgenogram shown is indicated. Eighty ml. of air was injected into the pericardial sac (d) after the third and final pericardiocentesis, and this study demonstrates the thickened parietal pericardium.

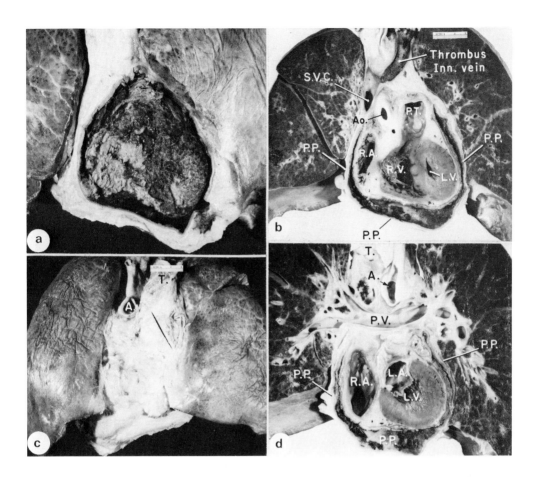

Figure 28. Same case as Figure 27. Exterior and interior of the heart. a, the anterior portion of the parietal pericardium has been excised, exposing the ragged hemorrhagic epicardial surface of the heart. The parietal pericardium is tightly adherent to the left lung. c, posterior surface of the heart and lungs showing severe fibrosis of the mediastinal structures. Both lungs are adherent posteriorly to the parietal pericardium. A. = aorta at level of isthmus; T. = trachea. b, frontal section of heart and lungs. The parietal pericardium (P.P.) and epicardium are thick. An antemortum thrombus occludes the innominate (Inn.) vein. Ao. = ascending aorta; S.V.C. = superior vena cava; R.A. = right atrium; R.V. = right ventricle; L.V. = left ventricle; and P.T. = pulmonic trunk. d, another section of heart and lungs, but it is more posterior than view b. There is marked fibrosis of the tissues adjacent to the pulmonary veins. The lymph nodes adjacent to the trachea (T.) are large. L.A. = left atrium.

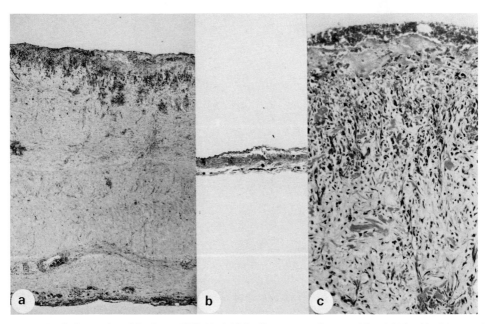

Figure 29. Radiation pericarditis. Stage IIIB Hodgkin's disease was diagnosed in 1965 in this 54-year-old man (S67-3079) and he then received radiation therapy to mediastinum. In June 1967 (18 months later) he developed recurrent pericardial effusion and signs of pericardial constriction including elevated venous pressure and congestive cardiac failure. He underwent pericardiectomy in August 1967 and at operation the pericardial sac contained about 150 ml. of fluid. The parietal and visceral pericardia were focally adherent by fibrinous adhesions. After excision of the anterior portion of parietal pericardium, which was up to 1.0 cm. in thickness, the central venous pressure dropped from 15 to 8 cm. of water. The patient had an uneventful recovery and no further symptoms of myocardial constriction. a, Section of parietal pericardium, showing diffuse fibrous thickening with fibroblast proliferation. Plasma cells and lymphocytes are present. b, Section of normal pericardium for comparison. c, Higher power view of parietal pericardium in this patient showing fibroblasts, lymphocytes, and plasma cells. These changes are characteristic of radiation pericarditis. Hematoxylin and eosin stains; reduced 20% from ×27 (a and b) and ×160 (c).

Pericardial injury probably occurs in most patients receiving 4000 or more rads to mediastinum.[72] Fibrous thickening of the pericardia combined with pericardial effusion (usually serous) has been the most frequent consequence of this irradiation. Clinical evidence of cardiac dysfunction resulting from pericardial disease occurs in about 5 percent of patients with Hodgkin's disease treated with high-dose mediastinal irradiation.[73] Cardiac tamponade, usually resulting from combined pericardial effusion and fibrous thickening of the parietal pericardium, may occur.[72, 74] The coronary arteries lying in the subepicardial adipose tissue also may be damaged by irradiation with resulting coronary arterial luminal narrowing and symptomatic or fatal ischemic heart disease.[75]

ASSOCIATED WITH ANOTHER DISEASE. Although fibrinous "pericarditis" is the most common type of pericardial involvement in the patients with *chronic renal disease,* fibrous thickening of the pericardia with or without associated fibrous adhesions or pericardial effusion also may occur in patients not treated with dialysis (see Figs. 15–17). Fibrous pericarditis, however, appears to be more frequent in the patients on chronic dialysis than in patients with chronic renal disease not treated in this fashion.

Nearly 50 percent of patients with *rheumatoid arthritis* at necropsy have fibrous obliterative pericarditis, and, rarely, calcific or cholesterol pericardial disease.[76] Usually, no functional consequence results from the obliterative pericarditis.

Among 36 patients with *systemic lupus erythematosus* (SLE) studied at necropsy in our laboratory,[5] 19 had pericardial heart disease: fibrinous in 4, purulent in 2, and fibrous in 13. Before corticosteroids were introduced, however, fibrinous pericarditis was the most common type of pericardial disease seen in patients with SLE. Among patients with SLE treated with corticosteroids, fibrous pericarditis is the most common. Among our 19 SLE patients with pericardial heart disease at necropsy, none had evidence of myocardial dysfunction as a consequence of the pericardial involvement. Eleven of the 19 had pericardial friction rubs. Pericarditis, however, in patients with SLE serves as an excellent marker indicating the presence of associated endocarditis. Endocarditis was present at necropsy in 18 of our 19 SLE patients with and in none of the 17 SLE patients without pericardial disease.

Although uncommon clinically, pericardial heart disease is commonly found at necropsy in patients with *scleroderma*. Of 31 necropsy patients collected by Oram and Stokes,[77] 22 (71 percent) had morphologic evidence of pericardial disease. Fibrous obliterative pericarditis is the most frequent type of pericardial involvement in scleroderma. Fibrinous pericarditis, less commonly seen, may result from associated renal failure (uremia) rather than scleroderma per se.[77-79] Among 14 necropsy patients with scleroderma studied in our laboratory, five had pericardial involvement, fibrous type in each.

INFECTIOUS AGENT. See section on infective (purulent) pericarditis.

IDIOPATHIC. Fibrous pericardial disease of unknown etiology is the most common cause today of chronic constrictive pericarditis (see Table 7).[80-85] Among 137 reported patients undergoing pericardiectomy because of constrictive pericarditis, no cause was found on histologic study of the excised pericardia in 106 (82 percent) (Table 8).[85]

TABLE 8

ETIOLOGY OF CONSTRICTIVE PERICARDITIS IN USA TREATED BY PERICARDIECTOMY

Type "Pericarditis"	Detering + Humphreys 1930-1954 (81)	Chambliss 1939-1951 (80)	Gimlette -1959 (82)	Conti + Friesinger 1961-1966(83)	Lange -1967 (84)	Wychulis, Connolly + McGoon 1936-1969 (85)	Totals
Idiopathic	12	35	39	11	10	106	213 (68%)
Tuberculous	8	20[†]	17	0	6	12	63 (20%)
Traumatic	4	0	0	0	0	2	6 (2%)
Rheumatic	1	1**	0	0	0	0	2 (1%)
Neoplasm	0	0	3	0	0	0	3 (1%)
Pyogenic	0	2	1	0	0	1	4 (1%)
Irradiation	0	0	2	0	0	2	4 (1%)
Post-cardiotomy	0	0	0	0	2	0	2 (1%)
Rheumatoid arthritis	0	0	0	0	0	2	2 (1%)
Viral	0	0	0	0	0	1	1 (0%)
Acute non-specific	0	3	0	0	0	11	14 (4%)
Total	25	61	62	11	18	137*	314 (100%)

*Eleven patients with intracardiac disease in addition to pericardial disease were excluded: 5 had atrial septal defect and 6 had valvular heart disease (probably rheumatic in origin in 5).

**Considered as etiology but not proven; had recurrent rheumatic fever preceding and following development of constriction.

†Includes 4 patients with "suggestive evidence" for tuberculosis on pathologic specimen.

TABLE 9

PERICARDIAL HEART DISEASE:

Etiology of <u>Neoplastic</u> "Pericarditis"

1. Metastatic
    - A. Lung
    - B. Breast
    - C. Lymphoma
    - D. Leukemia
    - E. Miscellaneous

2. Primary
    - A. Benign
        1. Teratoma
        2. Fibroma
        3. Lipoma
        4. Angioma
    - B. Malignant
        1. Mesothelioma
        2. Sarcoma
            - a. Differentiated
            - b. Undifferentiated

NEOPLASTIC "PERICARDITIS" (TABLE 9)

As seen from Figure 30, the heart is involved in approximately 10 percent of patients with malignant neoplasms and of the patients with cardiac involvement 85 percent have tumor in pericardium. Furthermore, only about 10 percent of patients with cardiac involvement by neoplasm have clinical evidence of cardiac disease and in 90 percent of those with clinical dysfunction it is the result of pericardial involvement, usually constriction by either pericardial effusion or neoplastic thickening of pericardia or both. The most common neoplasms in absolute numbers with cardiac metastases are lung (in males), breast (in females), followed by leukemia and lymphoma. Nearly any tumor, however, may metastasize to the heart. Among patients with carcinoma of the breast or lung about 10 percent have neoplastic involvement of the heart.[86, 87] Because spread of these two tumors to the heart appears to be by direct extension, the pericardia are virtually always involved (Fig. 31).

Among specific malignant neoplasms, the ones with the highest percentage of metastases to the heart are melanoma (70 percent) (Fig. 32),[88] leukemia (37 percent) (Fig. 33),[65] and lymphoma (24 percent).[89] As with the tumors which spread by direct extension, melanoma, leukemia, and lymphoma invade the pericardia in 85 percent of the patients with cardiac metastases and spread of these tumors appears to be by the hematogenous route.

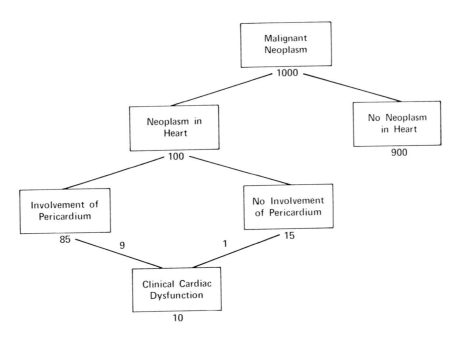

Figure 30. Diagram depicting the frequency of pericardial involvement in malignant neoplasms.

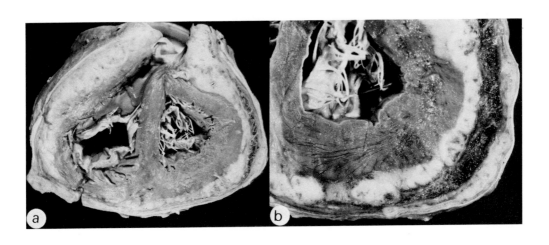

Figure 31. Heart of a 61-year-old man (67A-531) who died of carcinoma of the lung. A pericardial friction rub was heard when the scalene node biopsy showed squamous carcinoma. The pericardial rub gradually diminished in intensity and pulsus paradoxicus (10 mm. Hg) appeared. Cardiac tamponade with hypotension and oliguria followed. At necropsy, the entire heart and great vessels were encased in tumor. a, Transverse section of cardiac ventricles just caudal to the atrioventricular valves showing tumorous encasement of the heart. b, Close-up of left ventricle and adhering pericardium. The white tumor in the epicardium and visceral pericardium is separated by blood clots.

43

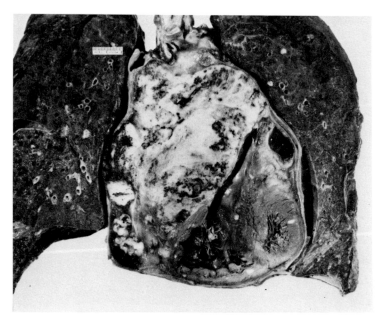

Figure 32. Neoplastic pericarditis. Longitudinal section of heart and lungs in a 53-year-old man (A75-41) with metastatic melanoma. During life a pericardial friction rub was audible and the neck veins were quite distended. There was no evidence, however, of myocardial constriction. The parietal pericardium is adherent everywhere to the epicardium; the superior vena cava, right atrium, right ventricle and pulmonary trunk are compressed by the overlying mass of tumor.

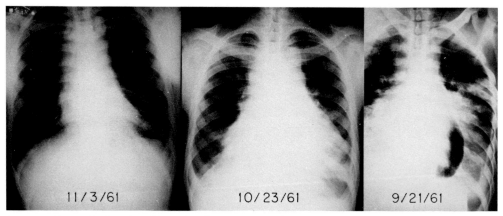

Figure 33. Hemorrhagic pericarditis and cardiac tamponade. Chest roentgenograms in a 22-year-old man with acute lymphocytic leukemia (A61-258). During the last week of life (he died on November 4, 1961) severe dyspnea developed with signs of increased central venous pressure, hepatic tenderness, and marked paradoxic pulsation. The electrocardiogram showed low voltage and sinus tachycardia. Pericardiocentesis, performed two days before death, yielded 100 ml. of serous fluid, which contained 102,000 lymphocytes per cu. mm. and virtually no erythrocytes; the total protein was 6.6 gm. with albumin 3.6 gm per 100 ml. After removal of this fluid, 100 ml. of air was injected into the pericardial space (right). At necropsy, the heart weighed 350 gm., and 200 ml. of bloody fluid was present in the pericardial space. The parietal pericardium measured 4 cm. in thickness and was massively infiltrated by leukemic cells. No leukemic cells were seen in the epicardium, which was covered by fibrin.

44

Although pericardial effusions, often bloody, are frequent in patients with cardiac metastases, pericardial effusions also are common in patients with malignant neoplasms without cardiac metastases.[89] Pericardial effusions (> 50 ml.) were recorded in 17 percent of 48 patients with cardiac lymphoma studied in this laboratory, [89] and in 14 percent of 148 patients with lymphoma but without cardiac metastases. In both groups, the effusions were serous and probably the result of hypoalbuminemia (< 3.5 gm percent) which was present in 95 percent of the 196 necropsy patients with lymphoma.[89]

Pericarditis may occur in patients with malignant neoplasms who do not have involvement of the heart (including pericardia) by tumor. Pericarditis of varying types was present in 21 percent of 48 patients with cardiac lymphoma and in 7 percent of 148 patients with lymphoma but without metastases to the heart.[89]

Symptoms and signs in patients with cardiac metastases are often attributed to cardiac involvement by the tumor but this often may not be justified. Dyspnea, for example, was present in 27 percent of our 48 patients with cardiac lymphoma but it also occurred in 24 percent of the 148 patients with lymphoma and no cardiac metastases.[89] Pleural effusion appeared to be the most common explanation and among the 196 patients with lymphoma they were present in 52 percent of 48 patients with and in 52 percent of 148 patients without cardiac lymphoma.[89] Likewise, precordial or substernal chest pain was present in the same frequency (6 percent) and precordial murmurs in the same frequency (35 percent) among patients with lymphoma irrespective of the presence or absence of cardiac metastases. Furthermore, ventricular gallops were present also in equal frequencies (5 percent) in the two groups. Surprisingly, electrocardiographic abnormalities were present in identical frequencies among patients with lymphoma with and without cardiac tumor deposits: 62 percent in each of the two groups.

Primary pericardial neoplasms are extremely rare and about one half of them are benign.[90] The most common is teratoma[91-93] and although usually histologically benign it can produce fatal compression of a cardiac chamber (Fig. 34). Hemangioma (Fig. 35), leiomyofibroma, lipoma, and fibroma are other "benign" pericardial neoplasms. The hemangioma may rupture to cause hemorrhagic pericardial effusion with or without tamponade.[94]

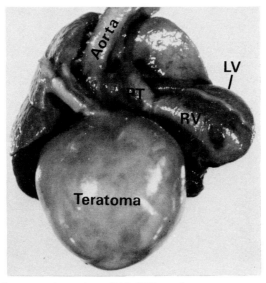

Figure 34. Intrapericardial teratoma in newborn (74A-126) causing severe compression of the right atrium, right ventricle (RV) and ascending aorta. Although histologically benign, the tumor was larger than the heart and it caused fatal cardiac compression. PT = pulmonary trunk; LV = left ventricle.

45

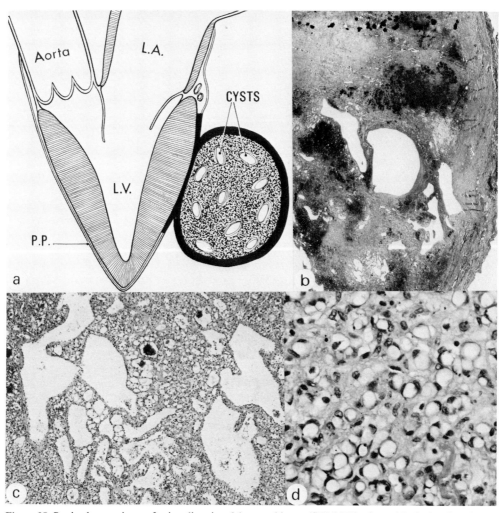

Figure 35. Benign hemangioma of epicardium in a 36-year-old man (S68-2017) who suddenly developed transient but severe anterior chest pain a few hours after playing basketball. When examined after the pain had disappeared, there was a 3 × 3 cm. area of precordial pulsation and a grade 2/6 short systolic murmur, which could not be recorded by phonocardiogram. Fluoroscopy disclosed a mass along the left cardiac border and it enlarged during ventricular systole. Left ventricular angiography, however, showed a smooth endocardial surface and no aneurysm. Coronary angiography showed the left circumflex artery to be dilated and tortuous and the left anterior descending and right to be normal. The pressures in mm Hg were: pulmonary artery, 28/14; right ventricle 28/9; right atrial mean, 9; pulmonary artery wedge mean, 13; left ventricle 118/19; and aorta 118/80. The elctrocardiogram showed left axis deviation (+120°). At thoracotomy, a nonexpansile, solid, 7 × 3 × 2 cm. mass was found on the posterolateral surface of the left ventricle (a). The tumor was covered by a capsule attached to the epicardium of the left ventricle, which was uninvolved by the tumor. On sectioning, the tumor was cystic, hemorrhagic, and firm. Histologically (b, c, and d), the tumor consisted of numerous small and large vascular channels lined by either mesothelial or endothelial cells. Between the vascular channels was fibrous tissue containing hemosiderin deposits. The tumor was judged to be benign. Hematoxylin and eosin stains; reduced 30% from ×15 (b), ×63 (c), and ×400 (d).

Among the primary malignant pericardial neoplasms, mesothelioma is by far the most frequent. It may totally encase the heart resulting in fatal myocardial constriction.[95]

46

TABLE 10

PERICARDIAL HEART DISEASE:

Etiology of <u>Granulomatous</u> Pericarditis

1. Infectious Agent
    A. Tuberculosis
    B. Fungus
    C. Parasite
2. Cholesterol
    A. Idiopathic
    B. Associated with another condition
        1. Hypothyroidism
        2. Rheumatoid Arthritis
        3. Tuberculosis
        4. Hypercholesterolemia
3. Iatrogenic
    A. Talc
    B. Other Foreign Body
4. Sarcoidosis

GRANULOMATOUS "PERICARDITIS" (TABLE 10)

INFECTIOUS AGENT. Among the causes of granulomatous pericarditis, *tuberculosis* is by far the most important. Pericardial involvement by tuberculosis was initially described by Rokitansky in 1852, and it was he who noted the "association with, and dependence upon, an earlier tuberculous lesion."[96] Since that time there has been much debate over whether primary tuberculous pericarditis is a separate clinicopathologic entity, or whether it is the recognizable result of an earlier, resolved or inactive, primary lesion.

The frequency of tuberculous pericarditis has diminished in recent years, presumably paralleling the reduction in incidence of pulmonary tuberculosis. Osler observed tuberculosis in 215 (21 percent) of 1000 necropsies, and 7 (3 percent) of the 215 had pericardial involvement.[97] More recent studies[98, 99] have shown pericarditis to be present at necropsy in 8 percent of patients with pulmonary tuberculosis.

The pathogenesis of pericardial involvement by tuberculosis is not clear. Pericardial disease probably results from early dissemination following a primary infection. The infection appears to reach the pericardium either from the blood (miliary) or, more commonly, by retrograde lymphatic spread from infected mediastinal glands. The pericardial infection rarely arises from direct spread from the lung or pleura.

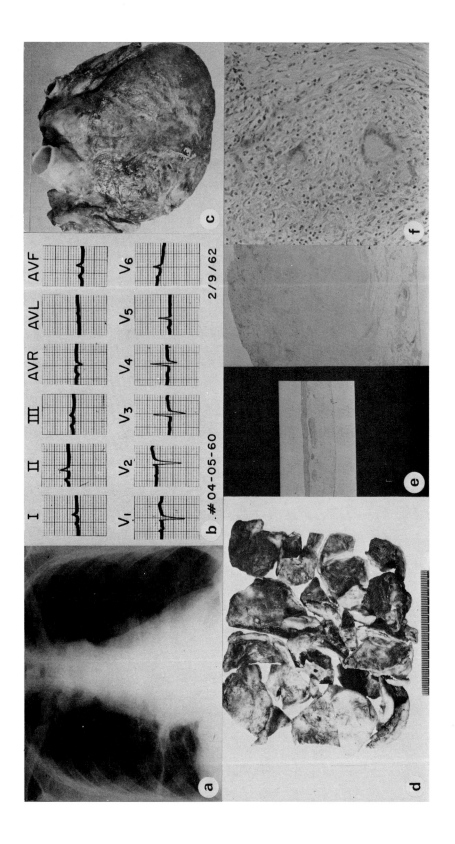

AVF AVL AVR Ⅲ Ⅱ I

V6 V5 V4 V3 V2 V1

2/9/62

b . # 04-05-60

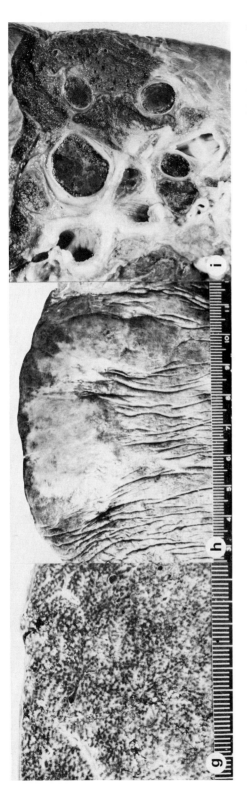

Figure 36. Tuberculous constrictive pericarditis in a 54-year-old man (A62–41) who was asymptomatic until the onset of cough, fever, weight loss, chest pain, exertional dyspnea, and subcutaneous edema in November 1961. He was admitted to the National Heart and Lung Institute in February 1962. Chest radiograph (a) showed bilateral pleural effusions and only mild enlargement of the cardiac silhouette. Electrocardiogram (b) showed decreased voltage and T-wave abnormalities. Pericardiocentesis yielded a small amount of fluid that grew out *M. tuberculosis* (human). Cardiac catheterization disclosed the following pressures in mm Hg: pulmonary trunk, 20/8; right ventricle 25/13; right atrial mean, 12; systemic artery, 114/72 (inspiration) and 84/12 (expiration) yielding a 30 mm Hg paradox. Pericardiectomy was performed. During the procedure episodes of hypotension requiring vasopressors occurred. Shortly after operation he suddenly stopped breathing; electrocardiogram showed ventricular fibrillation which was not converted.

At necropsy the exterior of the heart was covered by fibrinofibrous material (c). The parietal pericardium had been excised except over the left atrium. The parietal pericardium (d) removed at operation was up to 0.5 cm. thick and leathery. In e, the parietal pericardium from this patient (right) is compared to normal parietal pericardium (from another patient) at the same magnification. Granulomas containing giant cells and epitheloid elements were found in sections of pericardium (f). Ventricular myocardial sections showed hypertrophy. The liver showed severe congestion (g). A large antemortem thrombus was found in the superior vena cava proximal to the innominate vein, and postmortem examination of the lungs showed a large pulmonary infarct (h) and pulmonary arteries filled with clot (i). Hematoxylin and eosin stains; reduced 30% from ×8 (e) and ×170 (f).

49

TABLE 11

TUBERCULOUS PERICARDITIS: 4 Stages

		Tb Organisms
1.	Fibrinous	–
2.	Effusive (non-constrictive)	20%
3.	Fibrous (non-constrictive)	0
4.	Fibrous (constrictive)	0

Four stages of tuberculous pericarditis have been described[100] (Table 11). The *fibrinous* stage is characterized by diffuse deposits of fibrin associated with a granulomatous reaction. This stage actually is rarely observed and there is some debate as to whether it can resolve or whether it always goes on to the second stage which is characterized by *effusion* into the pericardial sac. The effusions, which may be massive (> 2000 ml.), are usually serous or serosanguinous but they may be bloody or turbid. Many lymphocytes may be present in the effusion but tuberculous organisms are uncommonly observed morphologically in the fluid or cultured from it.

By stage 3 the parietal pericardium is considerably thickened by both *fibrous* tissue and granulomas and most of the fluid has resolved. If the parietal pericardium becomes markedly thickened, myocardial *constriction* may occur and this is considered stage 4. By this time the pericardial space may be completely obliterated by diffuse fibrous adhesions (Fig. 36). Eventually the granulomas apparently can be replaced entirely by fibrous tissue and if observed morphologically at this point the pericardial disease would have to be called "idiopathic" rather than granulomatous (tuberculosis). Calcific deposits with or without bone formation may occur in the markedly thickened pericardia. Progression from stage 3 to stage 4 may occur despite antituberculous therapy.

Tuberculous pericarditis, however, by no means always progresses to the constrictive fibrous stage (Fig. 37). Heimann and Binder[101] described 31 patients with granulomatous pericarditis; in none of them was it constrictive and all had tuberculous hilar lymph nodes.

Among patients with "chronic" constrictive pericarditis, however, tuberculosis remains an important cause accounting for nearly 20 percent of the cases in the United States (see Table 8).[80-85] In some areas of the world a tuberculous cause of constrictive pericarditis is more common than a nontuberculous cause. Among 61 patients with constrictive pericarditis undergoing pericardectomy in India, the etiology was tuberculous in 37 (61 percent) and nontuberculous in 24 (39 percent).[102]

Fungi and parasites are rare causes of granulomatous pericarditis.

CHOLESTEROL. So-called "cholesterol pericarditis" always produces a granulomatous reaction, and it will be discussed separately below.

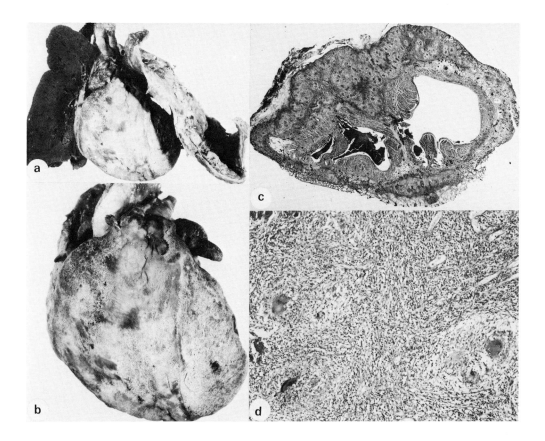

Figure 37. Tuberculous pericarditis. Heart of a 45-year-old dyspneic man (A68-162) whose chest roentgenogram showed complete loss of volume of the left lung and massive left pleural effusion. Congestive cardiac failure and respiratory insufficiency led to death. At necropsy, the entire left lung was collapsed and the left hemithorax was filled with pus. The left pleura was markedly thickened and focally calcified. No granulomas or foci of caseation necrosis were observed in either lung or in the hilar lymph nodes. a, Heart and lungs showing loss of left lung, cardiomegaly (600 gm.) and diffuse pericarditis. b, Closer view of exterior of heart showing fibrinous exudate covering the entire myocardial surface. c, Section of left atrial appendage showing complete involvement of the epicardium by caseating granulomas and giant cells. Fibrinous pericardial exudate also covers most of its surface. d, High-power view of granulomas covering left atrial appendage. No acid fast organisms were found. c, Hematoxylin and eosin stain. d, Periodic acid-Schiff stain. [Reduced 30% from ×5 (c) and ×80 (d).]

IATROGENIC. The sprinkling of *talc* in the pericardial space, a procedure introduced by Beck and by Thompson and Raisbeck in the early 1940s[103, 104] as a form of treatment for ischemic heart disease, produces an extensive granulomatous reaction resulting in obliteration of the pericardial space[105] (Fig. 38). A similar type of granulomatous reaction occurs in the lungs of persons who inject intravenously drugs intended for oral use because virtually every tablet contains talc.[106] A foreign-body type granulomatous reaction results from deposition of starch granules within the pericardial space, a minor complication of cardiac operations.[107, 108]

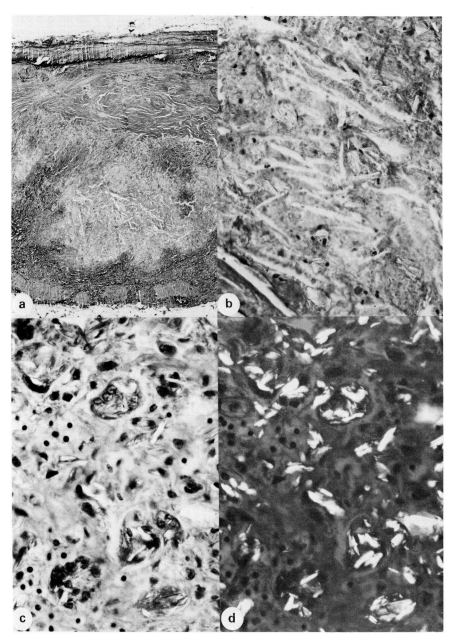

Figure 38. Talc-induced granulomatous pericarditis in a 92-year-old woman (71A-405) who was stated to have had angina pectoris beginning at age 63. At age 67 (1946), she underwent talcum-powder sprinkling on her pericardium (Beck or Thompson procedure). Immediately preoperatively, she was in congestive heart failure with atrial fibrillation and a slow ventricular response. At necropsy, an old healed anterolateral apical infarct was present but no myocardial necrosis was observed. The striking finding, however, was a diffuse fibrous and granulomatous pericarditis secondary to talc with complete obliteration of the pericardial space. a, Section of parietal pericardium showing large foci of acellular debris containing multiple cholesterol clefts. b, Higher power view showing cholesterol clefts and talc. c, Multinucleated foreign-body giant cells with intracellular talc granules. A few monomuclear cells are present. d, Same field as in c with polarization showing highly refractile talc particles both intracellularly and extracellularly. Hematoxylin and eosin stains; reduced 25% from ×23 (a), ×250 (b), and ×380 (c and d).

SARCOIDOSIS. Not generally recognized as a cause of pericarditis because clinical evidence of pericardial involvement is rare, focal, noncaseating pericardial granulomas are observed at necropsy in patients with sarcoidosis.[109] Among 34 patients with cardiac sarcoidosis studied at necropsy by Roberts and associates,[110] 12 (36 percent) had granulomas involving epicardium (Fig. 39). None, however, had clinical signs. In addition, another patient had obliterative fibrous pericarditis causing no clinical signs. Only three patients had excessive pericardial fluid measured at necropsy but it was < 300 ml. in each.

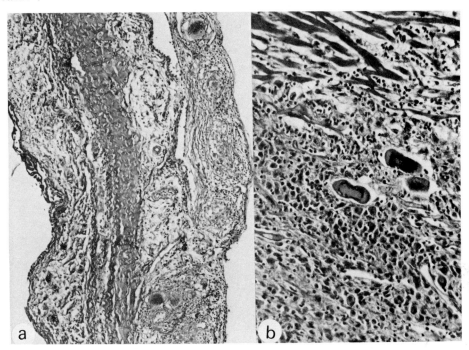

Figure 39. Sarcoidosis of pericardium in a 47-year-old woman (74A-223) who was well until 16 months before death when exertional dyspnea appeared. Thereafter, there was evidence clinically of recurring pleural and pericardial effusions. She died of progressive respiratory insufficiency. At necropsy, both lungs were extensively infiltrated by noncaseating granulomas devoid of microorganisms. Grossly, the pericardium and myocardium contained no focal lesions except in the left ventricular papillary muscles. On histologic examination, however, noncaseating granulomas were found in the parietal pericardium (a) and visceral pericardium (b). In addition to the noncaseating granulomas in the papillary muscles, similar microscopic-sized granulomas were observed in the walls of all 4 cardiac chambers. Hematoxylin and eosin stains; reduced 20% from ×80 (a) and ×220 (b).

CALCIFIC "PERICARDITIS" (TABLE 12)

The occurrence of calcific deposits in pericardia constitutes calcific pericarditis. The calcific deposits may vary in size from microscopic, that is, visible only by histologic examination, to massive, in other words, encircling all or most of the heart and readily visible by roentgenographic examination. Calcific deposits appear to represent the end-stage of organization of a pericardial process and in themselves are not indicative of any specific etiology. Because they represent an end-stage process, histologic examination of calcified pericardia rarely provides specific diagnoses. Conditions predisposing to calcific pericarditis are listed in Table 12. The etiology is based on historical data or an

TABLE 12

PERICARDIAL HEART DISEASE:

Etiology of <u>Calcific</u> "Pericarditis"

1. Idiopathic
2. Tuberculous
3. Purulent
4. Rheumatic Fever
5. Trauma

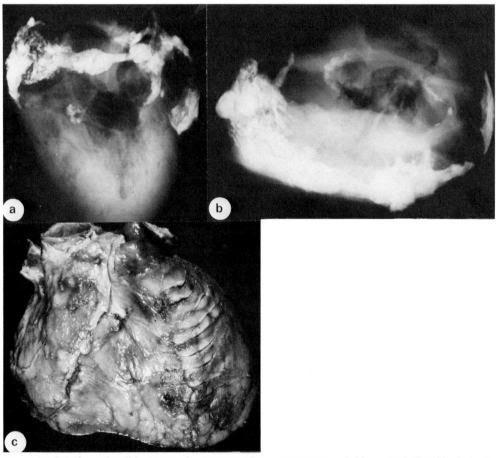

Figure 40. Calcific pericarditis. Heart of a 78-year-old man (A69-130), a habitual alcoholic with cirrhosis, esophageal varices, and chronic pancreatitis, who died from a gastrointestinal hemorrhage. No evidence of cardiac dysfunction was ever present clinically. At necropsy, the pericardial space was obliterated by fibrous adhesions. The adherence of the parietal to the visceral pericardia could not be separated over the right atrio-ventricular (A-V) sulcus. The cardiac chambers, valves, and coronary arteries were normal. The right A-V sulcus was extensively infiltrated by calcific deposits. a and b, Radiographs of heart specimen at necropsy: a, anteroposterior view; b, cephalad-caudal view. Calcific deposits also are present in the mitral anulus. c, Exterior of heart. The parietal pericardium has been stripped off except for the area over the right A-V sulcus.

associated abnormality rather than on specific pericardial alteration. There is strong suggestive evidence that large calcific pericardial deposits most frequently represent "burnt out" pericardial tuberculosis.

At times (Fig. 40), huge calcific deposits may be present in the pericardia without evidence of myocardial constriction or other myocardial dysfunction.[111, 112] For myocardial constriction to occur, the calcific deposits must encircle both ventricles (Figs. 41 and 42). Localized bands of calcium, however, may cause cardiac dysfunction. The occurrence of a large band of calcium traversing the right ventricular conus has led to right ventricular outflow obstruction.[30] An anular band of calcium in the right or left atrioventricular sulcus may delay or inhibit ventricular filling and consequently simulate tricuspid or mitral stenosis.[30]

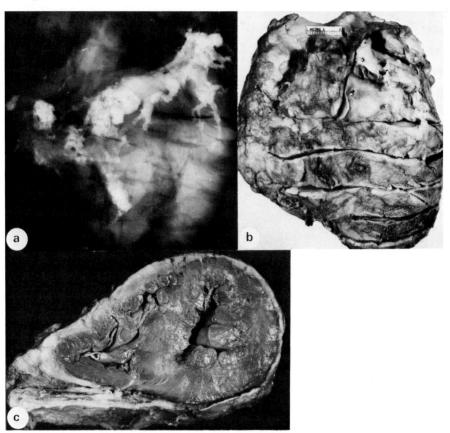

Figure 41. Calcific constrictive pericarditis in a 54-year-old man (70A-27) who at age 36, was stated to have had an acute myocardial infarct, but recovered without difficulty and remained asymptomatic until age 50 when he noted pedal edema. Diuretics initially cleared the edema, but at age 53 it recurred along with ascites and exertional dyspnea. Chest roentgenogram showed extensive pericardial calcification and examination disclosed a 10 mm Hg paradox. A pericardial friction rub and a diastolic pericardial knock were audible. Electrocardiogram showed a plus 90 degree axis and inverted T waves in leads II, III, and AVF. Catheterization revealed the following pressures in mm Hg; right atrial mean, 10; right ventricular end-diastolic, 14; and mean pulmonary-artery wedge, 12. The anterior parietal pericardium was then excised. Thereafter, he was well until a year later when he had an acute anterior wall myocardial infarct shortly after a hemorrhoidectomy. a, Postmortem roentgenogram of the heart showing heavy calcific deposits in the right atrioventricular sulcus. b, Exterior of heart showing diffuse fibrous obliterative pericardial disease. c, Transverse section of ventricles showing thickening of the parietal pericardium posteriorly over the right ventricle and obliteration of the pericardial sac by fibrous tissue. The cause of the pericardial disease was never determined.

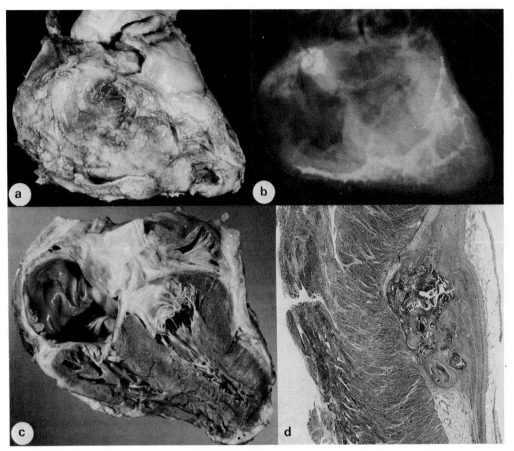

Figure 42. Calcific constrictive pericarditis in a 68-year-old man (A67-287) who had had pericardiectomies for relief of constriction 15 and 7 years respectively before death. Terminally, evidence of myocardial constriction reappeared again. Chylous ascites secondary to obstruction of the thoracic duct by carcinoid tumor also was present. At necropsy, the heart weighed 530 gm. Diffuse obliterative constrictive pericarditis was present and the remaining parietal pericardium was bound down to the epicardium by fibrous tissue. The inferior and superior vena cavae were enlarged and the right atrium was dilated. The pulmonary trunk was dilated. Yellow intimal streaks were seen in the pulmonary arteries, suggesting pulmonary arterial hypertension. Histologic sections showed fibrous thickening with calcific deposits of the pericardia with occasional collections of lymphocytes, plasma cells and histiocytes, but no granulomas. The intrapulmonary arteries had thickened walls. No granuloma were found in the lungs. The cause of the pericardial constriction was never determined. a, Exterior of the heart. b, Roentgenogram of the heart showing residual calcific deposits over the ventricles. c, Longitudinal section of the heart showing right atrial dilatation and right ventricular hypertrophy. d, Section of left ventricle compressed by overlying calcific deposit. Hematoxylin and eosin stain; reduced 25% from ×3.

CHOLESTEROL "PERICARDITIS" (TABLE 13)

Clinically, cholesterol pericarditis is most often characterized by slowly developing, nonconstricting large effusions.[113] Although the pericardial fluid may be turbid or clear, cholesterol crystals give the effusion a "gold paint" appearance. The parietal and visceral pericardia may become markedly thickened; histologic examination shows giant cells containing cholesterol clefts, mononuclear cells including foam cells, and fibrous tissue (Fig. 43).

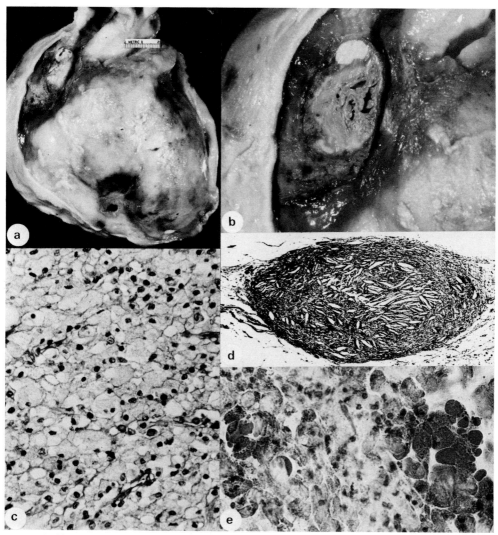

Figure 43. Cholesterol pericarditis in a 34-year-old woman (A69-202) who had hypothyroidism, probably from birth. She was short and stocky, had enlarged ear lobes, bilateral hypoplastic fourth toes, receding hairline with brittle coarse hair, small tongue, underdeveloped breasts, no menstruation, and juvenile external genitalia. She had orthopnea, pedal edema, and hypoactive deep tendon reflexes. Laboratory studies showed hypothyroidism. Chest roentgenogram showed a globular-shaped cardiac silhouette and clear lung fields. A CO_2 angiogram showed an 18 mm. thick pericardial effusion. Electrocardiogram showed low voltage but a normal QRS axis. Diabetes mellitus also was found. Despite diuresis, the pedal edema persisted and the blood urea nitrogen and creatinine levels rose. Pleuritic-type anterior chest pain appeared associated with increased orthopnea and a 15 mm. paradoxical pulse pressure was measured. Pericardiocentesis produced 500 ml. of cloudy golden-colored fluid. The polyethylene catheter was left in place and over the next 5 days 2 liters of fluid were removed. Cholesterol content of the fluid was 165 mg. per 100 ml. (The serum cholesterol was 355 mg. per 100 ml.) The other chemistries were similar to the respective serum levels. She improved following pericardiocentesis, but became anuric following aortography to evaluate her renal disease, and died. a, Exterior surface of heart and pericardium showing thickening of the parietal pericardium and focal deposits of cholesterol (yellow in color) over the right ventricle. b, View of thickened parietal pericardium over right atrial appendage and also an epicardial cholesterol deposit. c, Foam cells in the cholesterol deposit shown in b. d, Cholesterol granuloma in pericardium showing cholesterol clefts and foreign body reaction. e, Frozen section of epicardial deposits stained for lipid. The foam cells stain strongly for lipid. c and d, hematoxylin and eosin stains. e, Oil-red 0 stain. [Reduced 30% from ×400 (c), ×50 (d), and ×400 (e).]

57

TABLE 13

PERICARDIAL HEART DISEASE:

Etiology of <u>Cholesterol</u> "Pericarditis"

1. Idiopathic
2. Associated with Another Condition
    A. Hypothyroidism
    B. Rheumatoid Arthritis
    C. Tuberculosis
    D. Hypercholesterolemia (from any cause)

Cholesterol pericarditis may be seen in many different conditions (Table 13), but most commonly in patients with *hypothyroidism, rheumatoid arthritis,* and *tuberculosis.*[114]

The cause of the increased cholesterol content of the pericardial fluid in these patients is unclear but several theories have been presented:[114] (1) that necrosis of superficial cells of the pericardia liberates intracellular cholesterol; (2) that lysis of erythrocytes following hemopericardium yields the cholesterol; and (3) that pericardial inflammation decreases lymphatic drainage of pericardia causing decreased reabsorption of cholesterol with ultimate precipitation and crystallization. The cholesterol crystals then incite a vigorous cellular reaction enhancing fluid production and pericardial thickening. Chronic exudation and diminished reabsorption of cholesterol might increase its concentration and allow crystallization. The total lipid content of the pericardial fluid, however, is approximately the same as that of serum.[115]

In hypothyroid patients the primary effusion may contain sufficient cholesterol to incite a local pericarditis which then further increases the cholesterol concentration as less is reabsorbed. Large effusions with resulting high levels of cholesterol are produced. In hypothyroid patients the pericarditis appears to be a secondary phenomenon, while cholesterol pericarditis in euthyroid patients must be associated with an actual pericardial inflammation for the cholesterol to accumulate. Experimental studies have shown that small amounts of blood in the presence of pericardial damage from any cause will produce dense adhesions, and it is probably this phenomenon which accounts for cases of constriction in cholesterol pericardial disease.[10]

CONGENITAL ANOMALIES OF PERICARDIUM

These include *cysts* and *absence of all or portions (defects) of parietal pericardia.* All are rare. Cysts are of two types: true and false (diverticulae). The true ones are located within the pericardial sac but have no communication with it; the false ones or diverticulae are protrusions of parietal pericardium and consequently have direct communication with it.[116] Of 72 cysts reported by Wychulis and associates, 88 percent were true and 12 percent were false.[92] The cysts are thin-walled, translucent, lined by mesothelial cells, contain watery-yellow fluid, usually are attached by a thick fibrous pedicle, and most commonly are located in the right cardiophrenic angle (Figs. 44 and 45).[92] The cysts ranged in size from 2 to 16 cm. in largest diameter in one series.[92] Although most

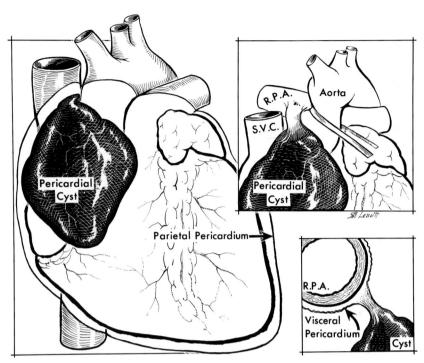

Figure 44. Pericardial cyst, an incidental necropsy finding in a 75-year-old woman (A240-68). The cyst, which contained serous fluid, overlies the right atrium and arises from a pedicle attached to the right main pulmonary artery (R.P.A.). S.V.C. = superior vena cava.

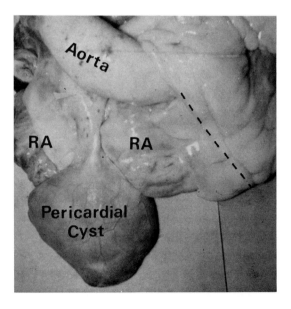

Figure 45. Photograph of the pericardial cyst shown diagramatically in Figure 44. RA = right atrium.

are multilobulated, 99 percent are unilocular. The fluid within the cysts is similar to normal pericardial fluid. The cysts produce signs or symptoms of cardiac dysfunction in 25 percent of the patients, and no evidence of dysfunction in the other 75 percent.[92] The larger the size the more likely will symptoms result. The mechanism of formation of pericardial cysts is unclear. Failure of the pericardial mesenchymal lacunae to unite with the pericardial coelom has been suggested.[117]

Absence of, or defects in, parietal pericardium may be classified into three major types:[118] (1) heart and left lung in a common cavity (60 percent); (2) defect or foramen in parietal pericardium providing communication between pericardial sac and pleural sac (20 percent) (nearly always the left one); and (3) totally absent or rudimentary parietal pericardium (20 percent). These defects may be associated with anomalies of the heart (30 percent), lungs, pleura, peritoneum, or kidney and are more common in males. Cardiac enlargement occurs in about one half of the patients, and commonly the heart is displaced to the left and abnormally mobile. Total absence of parietal pericardium usually produces no functional disturbance. Partial absence, however, may result in herniation of the entire heart or a part of the left atrium through the defect or allow direct extension of a lung infection to the pericardium via the defect.

DIFFERENTIAL DIAGNOSIS (TABLE 14)

Constrictive pericardial heart disease, either from pericardial effusion or from thickened pericardia or both, may be confused with a number of conditions which are listed in Table 14.[119] An occasional patient with idiopathic cardiomyopathy or extensive cardiac amyloidosis particularly has been subjected in the past to thoracotomy because of

TABLE 14

PERICARDIAL HEART DISEASE:
Differential Diagnosis of Constrictive "Pericarditis"

1. Congestive Cardiac Failure from Other Causes
   A. Idiopathic Cardiomyopathy
      1. Ventricular Dilated Type
      2. Hypertrophic Type
   B. Mitral Stenosis or Left Atrial Tumor
   C. Pulmonary Heart Disease
   D. Restrictive Heart Disease
      1. Amyloid
      2. Endomyocardial Fibrosis
   E. Tricuspid Stenosis or Right Atrial Tumor
2. Hepatic Cirrhosis
3. Mediastinal Neoplasm
4. Obstruction (usually by thrombus) of Portal Vein, Hepatic Vein, or Vena Cava

suspected pericardial constriction. The use of echocardiography will make differentiation of pericardial heart disease from these other conditions easier.

SUMMARY

This report reviews morphologic aspects of pericardial heart disease. A morphologic classification for this condition is presented. An ideal classification of pericardial heart disease obviously would take into account clinical, etiologic and morphologic features of this condition but a single classification combining these three components is lacking. Pericardial heart disease is relatively uncommon clinically, and when present at necropsy it usually had not been recognized during life. The term "pericarditis" is inaccurate because most pericardial diseases are noninflammatory in nature. Morphologically chronic pericardial heart disease may present clinically as an acute illness. Even when clinical symptoms are present, however, few patients develop evidence of cardiac dysfunction (constriction). When pericardial constriction occurs, it is the result of increased pericardial fluid or increased pericardial tissue or both. Increased fluid is treated by drainage; increased tissue is treated by excision. In most patients with chronic constrictive pericarditis the etiology is not apparent even after histologic examination of pericardia.

REFERENCES

1. OSLER, W.: *The Principles and Practice of Medicine*. D. Appleton, Co., New York, 1892, 1079 pp.
2. REEVES, R. L.: *Cause of acute pericarditis*. Am. J. Med. Sci. 225:34, 1953.
3. GRIFFITH, G. C., AND WALLACE, L.: *The etiology of pericarditis*. Am. Heart J. 37:636, 1949.
4. AMAD, K. H., BRENNAN, J. C., AND ALEXANDER, J. K.: *The cardiac pathology of chronic exogenous obesity*. Circulation 32:740, 1965.
5. BULKLEY, B. H., AND ROBERTS, W. C.: *The heart in systemic lupus erythematosus and the changes induced in it by corticosteroid therapy. A study of 36 necropsy patients*. Am. J. Med. 58:243, 1975.
6. FLINT, A.: *A Practical Treatise on the Diagnosis, Pathology, and Treatment of Diseases of the Heart*, ed. 2. Henry C. Lea, Philadelphia, 1870, p. 94.
7. MILLER, A. J., JAIN, S., AND LEVIN, B.: *Radiographic visualization of lymphatic drainage of heart muscle and pericardial sac in the dog*. Chest 59:271, 1971.
8. JUST, H., AND MATTINGLY, T. W.: *Interatrial septal defect and pericardial disease; Coincidence or causal relationship?* Am. Heart J. 76:157, 1968.
9. EHRENHAFT, J. L., AND TABER, R. E.: *Hemopericardium and constrictive pericarditis*. J. Thorac. Surg. 24:355, 1952.
10. CLIFF, W. J., GROBÉTY, J., AND RYAN, G. B.: *Postoperative pericardial adhesions. The role of mild serosal injury and spilled blood*. J. Thorac. Cardiovasc. Surg. 65:744, 1973.
11. SWAN, W. G. A.: *Acute non-specific pericarditis*. Br. Heart J. 22:651, 1960.
12. KROOK, H.: *Acute non-specific pericarditis. Study in 24 cases including descriptions of 2 with later development into constrictive pericarditis*. Acta Med. Scand. 148:201, 1954.
13. ROBERTS, W. C., AND MORROW, A. G.: *Pseudoaneurysm of the left ventricle. An unusual sequel of myocardial infarction and rupture of the heart*. Am. J. Med. 43:639, 1967.
14. GOBEL, F. L., VISUDH-AROM, K., AND EDWARDS, J. E.: *Pseudoaneurysm of the left ventricle leading to recurrent pericardial hemorrhage*. Chest 59:23, 1971.
15. PETER, R., WHALEN, R., ORGAIN, E., ET AL.: *Postpericardiotomy syndrome as a complication of percutaneous left ventricular puncture*. Am. J. Cardiol. 17:86, 1966.
16. GOLDSTEIN, S., AND YU, P. N.: *Constrictive pericarditis after blunt chest trauma*. Am. Heart J. 69:544, 1965.
17. CARMICHAEL, D., SPRAGUE, H. B., WYMAN, S. M., ET AL.: *Acute non-specific pericarditis. Clinical laboratory and follow-up considerations*. Circulation 3:321, 1951.
18. RABINER, S. F., SPECTOR, L. S., GRIPSTEIN, C. B., ET AL.: *Chronic constrictive pericarditis as a sequel to acute benign pericarditis – Report of a case*. N. Engl. J. Med. 251:425, 1954.
19. BURCH, G. E., AND GILES, T. D.: *The role of viruses in the production of heart disease*. Am. J. Cardiol. 29:231, 1972.

20. HIRSCHMAN, S. Z., AND HAMMER, G. S.: *Coxsackie virus myopericarditis, a microbiological and clinical review.* Am. J. Cardiol. 34:224, 1974.

21. BURCH, G. E., AND COLCOLOUGH, H. L.: *Progressive Coxsackie viral pancarditis and nephritis.* Ann. Intern. Med. 71:963, 1969.

22. WACKER, W., AND MERRILL, J. P.: *Uremic pericarditis in acute and chronic renal failure.* J.A.M.A. 156:764, 1954.

23. RICHTER, A. B., AND O'HARE, J. P.: *Heart in chronic glomerular nephritis.* N. Engl. J. Med. 214:824, 1936.

24. SCHUPAK, E., AND MERRILL, J. P.: *Experience with long-term intermittent hemodialysis.* Ann. Intern. Med. 62:509, 1965.

25. ABELLA, R., BLONDEEL, J., ROGUSKA, J., ET AL.: *Periodic dialysis in terminal uremia.* J.A.M.A. 199: 362, 1967.

26. REYMAN, T. A.: *Subacute constrictive uremic pericarditis.* Am. J. Med. 46:972, 1969.

27. LINDSAY, J., JR., CRAWLEY, S., AND CALLAWAY, G. M., JR.: *Chronic constrictive pericarditis following uremic hemopericardium.* Am. Heart J. 79:390, 1970.

28. MOSCHCOWITZ, E.: *Pathogenesis of constrictive pericardium.* J.A.M.A. 153:194, 1953.

29. CABOT, R. C.: *Facts on the Heart.* W. B. Saunders Co., Philadelphia, 1926, 731 pp.

30. SHAPIRO, J. H., JACOBSON, H. G., RUBINSTEIN, B. M., ET AL.: *Calcifications of the Heart.* Charles C Thomas, Springfield, Ill., 1963, 198 pp.

31. SHEARN, M. A.: *The heart in systemic lupus erythematosus.* Am. Heart J. 58:452, 1959.

32. CATHCART, E. S., AND SPODICK, D. H.: *Rheumatoid heart disease. A study of the incidence and nature of cardiac lesions in rheumatoid arthritis.* N. Engl. J. Med. 266:960, 1962.

33. BAUER, W., AND CLARK, W. S.: *The systemic manifestations of rheumatoid arthritis.* Trans. Assoc. Am. Physicians 61:339, 1948.

34. MARTIN, R. G., RUCKDESCHEL, J. C., CHANG, P., ET AL.: *Radiation-related pericarditis.* Am. J. Cardiol. 35:216, 1975.

35. HIRST, A. E., AND BARBOUR, B. H.: *Dissecting aneurysm with hemopericardium.* N. Engl. J. Med. 258: 116, 1958.

36. CORTES, F. M.: *The Pericardium and its Disorders.* Charles C Thomas, Springfield, Ill., 1971, 298 pp.

37. FELL, S. C., RUBIN, I. L., ENSELBERG, C. D., ET AL.: *Anticoagulant-induced hemopericardium with tamponade.* N. Engl. J. Med. 272:670, 1965.

38. BEAUDRY, C. B., NAKAMOTO, S., AND KOLFF, W. J.: *Uremic pericarditis and cardiac tamponade in chronic renal failure.* Ann. Intern. Med. 64:990, 1966.

39. HAGER, E. B.: *Clinical observations on five patients with uremic pericardial tamponade.* N. Engl. J. Med. 273:304, 1965.

40. BUJA, L. M., FRIEDMAN, C. A., AND ROBERTS, W. C.: *Hemorrhagic pericarditis in uremia. Clinicopathologic studies in six patients.* Arch. Pathol. 90:325, 1970.

41. ROBERTS, W. C., AND FREDRICKSON, D. S.: *Gaucher's disease of the lung causing severe pulmonary hypertension with associated acute recurrent pericarditis.* Circulation 35:783, 1967.

42. HARVEY, P. K. P., JONES, M. C., AND ANDERSON, E. G.: *Pericardial abnormalities in Gaucher's disease.* Br. Heart J. 31:603, 1969.

43. NAEF, A.P.: *Primary chylopericardium: its surgical treatment.* Dis. Chest 30:160, 1956.

44. MILLER, S. W., PRUETT, H. J., AND LONG, A.: *Fatal chylopericardium caused by hamartomatous lymphangiomatosis.* Am. J. Med. 24:951, 1959.

45. HUDSON, R. E. B.: *Cardiovascular Pathology.* Williams and Wilkins Co., Baltimore, 1965, 2123 pp.

46. OFFERIJNS, F. G. J., VAN DER VEEN, K. J., DURRER, D., ET AL.: *Lymphopericardium with hypoproteinemia, intestinal loss of protein, and congenital defects of lymphatic system.* Circulation 39:116, 1969.

47. HAWKER, R. E., CARTMILL, T. B., CELEREMAJER, J. M., ET AL: *Chylous pericardial effusion complicating aorta-right pulmonary artery anastomosis.* J. Thorac. Cardiovasc. Surg. 63:491, 1972.

48. ADAMS, R., AND POLDERMAN, H.: *Suppurative pericarditis.* N. Engl. J. Med. 225:897, 1941.

49. RUBIN, R. H., AND MOELLERING, JR., R. C.: *Clinical microbiological and therapeutic aspects of purulent pericarditis.* Am. J. Med. 59:68, 1975.

50. KAUFFMAN, C. A., WATANAKUNAKORM, C., AND PHAIR, J. P.: *Purulent pneumococcal pericarditis: A continuing problem in the antibiotic era.* Am. J. Med. 54:743, 1973.

51. BOYLE, J. D., PEARCE, M. L., AND GUZE, L. B.: *Purulent pericarditis: Review of literature and report of 11 cases.* Medicine 40:119, 1961.

52. BUCHBINDER, N. A., AND ROBERTS, W. C.: *Left-sided valvular active infective endocarditis. A study of forty-five necropsy patients.* Am. J. Med. 53:20, 1972.

53. CARTER, M. G., AND KORONES, S. B.: *Amebic pericarditis. Review of the literature and report of a case.* N. Engl. J. Med. 242:390, 1950.

54. LAMONT, N. MC. E., AND POOLER, N. R.: *Hepatic amoebiasis; A study of 250 cases.* Quart. J. Med. 27: 389, 1958.

55. IBARRA-PÉREZ, C., GREEN, L. S., CALVILLO-JUÁREZ, M., ET AL.: *Diagnosis and treatment of rupture of amebic abscess of the liver into the pericardium.* J. Thorac. Cardiovasc. Surg. 64:11, 1972.

56. COSTA-GUIMARÁES, AZEVEDO-VINHAES, L., SANTOS-FILHO, A., ET AL.: *Acute suppurative amebic pericarditis.* Am. J. Cardiol. 34:103, 1974.

57. MAC LEOD, I. N., WILMOT, A. J., AND POWELL, S. J.: *Amoebic pericarditis.* Quart. J. Med. 35:293, 1966.

58. KEAN, B. H., AND BRESLAU, R. C.: *Parasites of the Human Heart.* Grune & Stratton, New York, 1964, 186 pp.

59. KINARE, S. G., PARULKAR, G. B., AND SEN, P. K.: *Constrictive pericarditis resulting from dracunculosis.* Br. Med. J. 1:845, 1962.

60. LARSON, R., AND SCHERB, R. E.: *Coccidioidal pericarditis.* Circulation 7:211, 1953.

61. CHAPMAN, M. G., AND KAPLAN, L.: *Cardiac involvement in coccidioidomycosis.* Am. J. Med. 23:87, 1957.

62. KASPER, J. A., AND PINNER, M.: *Actinomycosis of the heart: Report of a case with actinomycotic emboli.* Arch. Pathol. 10:687, 1930.

63. LOURIA, D. B., AND GORDON, R. E.: *Pericarditis and pleuritis caused by recently discovered microorganism, Waksmania rosea.* Am. Rev. Resp. Dis. 81:83, 1960.

64. OWEN, G. E., SCHERR, S. N., AND SEGRE, E. J.: *Histoplasmosis involving the heart and great vessels.* Am. J. Med. 32:552, 1962.

65. ROBERTS, W. C., BODEY, G. P., AND WERTLAKE, P. T.: *The heart in acute leukemia: A study of 420 autopsy cases.* Am. J. Cardiol. 21:388, 1968.

66. GIBBONS, J. E., GOLDBLOOM, R. B., AND DOBELL, A. R. C.: *Rapidly developing pericardial constriction in childhood following acute nonspecific pericarditis.* Am. J. Cardiol. 15:863, 1965.

67. WARREN, S.: *The Pathology of Ionizing Radiation.* Charles C Thomas, Springfield, Ill., 1961, 42 pp.

68. COHN, K. E., STEWART, J. R., FAJARDO, L. F., ET AL.: *Heart disease following radiation.* Medicine 46:281, 1967.

69. FAJARDO, L. F., STEWART, J. R., AND COHN, K. E.: *Morphology of radiation-induced heart disease.* Arch. Pathol. 86:512, 1968.

70. FAJARDO, L. F., AND STEWART, J. R.: *Experimental radiation-induced heart disease. I. Light microscopic studies.* Am. J. Pathol. 59:299, 1970.

71. STEWART, J. R., AND FAJARDO, L. F.: *Radiation-induced heart disease: Clinical and experimental aspects.* Radiol. Clin. North Am. 9:511, 1971.

72. RUCKDESCHEL, J. C., CHANG, P., MARTIN, R. G., ET AL.: *Radiation-related pericardial effusions in patients with Hodgkin's disease.* Medicine 54:245, 1975.

73. MARTIN, R. G., RUCKDESCHEL, J. C., CHANG, P., ET AL.: *Radiation related pericarditis.* Am. J. Cardiol. 35:216, 1975.

74. MORTON, D. L., KAGAN, A. R., ROBERTS, W. C., ET AL.: *Pericardiectomy for radiation-induced pericarditis with effusion.* Ann. Thorac. Surg. 8:195, 1969.

75. MC REYNOLDS, R. A., GOLD, G. L., AND ROBERTS, W. C.: *Coronary heart disease after mediastinal irradiation for Hodgkin's disease.* Am. J. Med. (in press).

76. ARTHUR, A., OSKVIG, R., AND BASTA, L. L.: *Calcific rheumatoid constrictive pericarditis with cardiac failure treated by pericardiectomy.* Chest 64:769, 1973.

77. ORAM, S., AND STOKES, W.: *The heart in scleroderma.* Br. Heart J. 23:243, 1961.

78. NASSER, W. K., MISHKIN, M. D., ROSENBAUM, D., ET AL.: *Pericardial and myocardial disease in progressive systemic sclerosis.* Am. J. Cardiol. 22:538, 1968.

79. MC WHORTER, J. E., AND LE ROY, E. C.: *Pericardial disease in scleroderma (systemic sclerosis).* Am. J. Med. 57:566, 1974.

80. CHAMBLISS, J. R., JARUSZEWSKI, E. J., BROFMAN, B. L., ET AL.: *Chronic cardiac compression (chronic constrictive pericarditis): Critical study of 61 operated cases with follow-up.* Circulation 4:816, 1951.

81. DETERLING, R. A. JR., AND HUMPHREYS, G. H.: *Factors in the etiology of constrictive pericarditis.* Circulation 12:30, 1955.

82. GIMLETTE, T. D. M.: *Constrictive pericarditis*. Br. Heart J. 21:9, 1959.

83. CONTI, C. R., AND FRIESINGER, G. C.: *Chronic constrictive pericarditis: Clinical and laboratory findings in 11 cases*. Johns Hopkins Med. J. 120:262, 1967.

84. LANGE, R. L.: *Chronic constrictive pericarditis*. Mod. Treat. 4:1967.

85. WYCHULIS, A. R., CONNOLLY, D. C., AND MC GOON, D. C.: *Surgical treatment of pericarditis*. J. Thorac. Cardiovasc. Surg. 62:608, 1971.

86. YOUNG, J. M., AND GOLDMAN, I. R.: *Tumor metastasis to the heart*. Circulation 9:220, 1954.

87. ONUIGBO, W. I. B.: *The spread of lung cancer to the heart, pericardium, and great vessels*. Jap. Heart. J. 15:234, 1974.

88. GLANCY, D. L., AND ROBERTS, W. C.: *The heart in malignant melanoma: A study of 70 autopsy cases*. Am. J. Cardiol. 21:555, 1968.

89. ROBERTS, W. C., GLANCY, D. L., AND DE VITA, V. T.: *Heart in malignant lymphoma (Hodgkin's disease, lymphosarcoma, reticulum cell sarcoma and mycosis fungoides): A study of 196 autopsy cases*. Am. J. Cardiol. 22:85, 1968.

90. PADER, E., AND KIRSCHNER, P. A.: *Primary sarcoma of the pericardium*. Am. J. Cardiol. 14:399, 1964.

91. WILSON, J. R., WHEAT, M. W., JR., AND AREAN, V. M.: *Pericardial teratoma. Report of a case with successful surgical removal and review of the literature*. J. Thorac. Cardiovasc. Surg. 45:670, 1963.

92. WYCHULIS, A. R., CONNOLLY, D. C., AND MC GOON, D. C.: *Pericardial cysts, tumors, and fat necrosis*. J. Thorac. Cardiovasc. Surg. 62:294, 1971.

93. DEENADAYALU, R. P., TUURI, D., DEWALL, R. A., ET AL.: *Intrapericardial teratoma and bronchogenic cyst*. J. Thorac. Cardiovasc. Surg. 67:945, 1974.

94. WENDER, C., AND ACKER, J. E.: *Constrictive pericarditis associated with hemangioma of the pericardium*. Am. Heart J. 72:255, 1966.

95. RECANT, L., AND LACY, P.: *Pericardial disease with effusion, systemic involvement and pulmonary edema (CPC)*. Am. J. Med. 33:442, 1962.

96. ROKITANSKY, C. K.: *A Manual of Pathological Anatomy*, ed. 4. The Sydeham Society, London, 1852, p. 137.

97. OSLER, W.: *Tuberculous pericarditis*. Am. J. Med. Sci. 105:20, 1893.

98. BELLET, S., MC MILLAN, T. M., AND GOULEY, B. A.: *Tuberculous pericarditis: Clinical and pathologic study based upon a series of 17 cases*. Med. Clin. N. Am. 18:201, 1934.

99. WOODS, J. A.: *Tuberculosis pericarditis: A study based upon a series of 17 cases*. Med. Clin. N. Am. 18:201, 1934.

99. WOODS, J. A.: *Tuberculosis pericarditis: A study of forty-one cases with special reference to prognosis*. Am. Heart J. 42:737, 1951.

100. PEEL, A. A. F.: *Tuberculous pericarditis*. Br. Heart J. 10:195, 1948.

101. HEIMANN, H. L., AND BINDER, S.: *Tuberculous pericarditis*. Br. Heart J. 2:165, 1940.

102. DAS, P. B., GUPTA, R. P., SUKUMAR, I. P., ET AL.: *Pericardiectomy: indications and results*. J. Thorac. Cardiovasc. Surg. 66:58, 1973.

103. SCHILDT, P., STANTON, E., AND BECK, C. S.: *Communications between the coronary arteries produced by the application of inflammatory agents to the surface of the heart*. Ann. Surg. 118:34, 1943.

104. THOMPSON, S. A., AND RAISBECK, M. J.: *Cardio-pericardiopexy. The surgical treatment of coronary arterial disease by the establishment of adhesive pericarditis*. Ann. Intern. Med. 16:495, 1942.

105. EISEMAN, B., SEELING, M. G., AND WOMACK, N. A.: *Talcum powder granuloma: a frequent and serious postoperative complication*. Ann. Surg. 126:820, 1947.

106. ARNETT, E. N., BATTLE, W. E., RUSSO, J. V., ET AL.: *Intravenous injection of talc-containing drugs intended for oral use: A cause of pulmonary granulomatosis and pulmonary hypertension*. Am. J. Med. 60:711, 1976.

107. OSBORNE, M. P., PANETH, M., AND HINSON, K. F. W.: *Starch granules in the pericardium as a cause of the post-pericardiotomy syndrome*. Thorax 29:199, 1974.

108. BATES, B.: *Granulomatous peritonitis secondary to corn starch*. Ann. Intern. Med. 62:335, 1965.

109. KIRCHHEINER, B.: *Sarcoidosis cordis*. Acta Med. Scand. 168:223, 1960.

110. ROBERTS, W. C., MC ALLISTER, H. A., AND FERRANS, V. J.: *Sarcoidosis of the heart; a study of 37 necropsy patients with cardiac sarcoidosis*. (in preparation.)

111. HARVEY, R. M., FERRER, M. I., CATHCART, R. T., ET AL.: *Mechanical and myocardial factors in chronic constrictive pericarditis*. Circulation 8:695, 1953.

112. MATHEWSON, F. A. L.: *Calcification of the pericardium in apparently healthy people. Electrocar-*

diographic abnormalities found in tracings from apparently healthy persons with calcification of the pericardium. Circulation 12:44, 1955.

113. CREECH, O., JR., HICKS, W., JR., SYNDER, H. B., ET AL.: Cholesterol pericarditis. Successful treatment by pericardiectomy. Circulation 12:193, 1955.

114. BRAWLEY, R. K., VASKO, J. S., AND MORROW, A. G.: Cholesterol pericarditis. Considerations of its pathogenesis and treatment. Am. J. Med. 41:235, 1966.

115. BROWN, A. K.: Chronic idiopathic pericardial effusion. Br. Heart J. 28:609, 1966.

116. LOEHR, W. M.: Pericardial cysts. Am. J. Roentgenol. 68:584, 1952.

117. LILLIE, W. I., MC DONALD, J. R., AND CLAGETT, O. T.: Pericardial coelomic cysts and pericardial diverticula. A concept of etiology and report of cases. J. Thorac. Surg. 20:494, 1950.

118. MOORE, R. L.: Congenital deficiencies of the pericardium. Arch. Surg. 11:765, 1925.

119. SOMERS, K., BRENTON, D. P., D'ARBELA, P. G., ET AL.: Haemodynamic features of severe endomyocardial fibrosis of right ventricle, including comparison with constrictive pericarditis. Br. Heart J. 30: 322, 1968.

The Pathophysiology of Cardiac Tamponade and Constriction

Ralph Shabetai, M.D.

Knowledge of the hemodynamics of cardiac tamponade and constrictive pericarditis stems from cardiac catheterization of large numbers of patients with these disorders[1] and from experiments in the animal laboratory[2] In normal physiology, there is very little difference in the intrapericardial pressure and intrapleural pressure, both in regard to wave form and absolute values.[3] Thus during quiet respiration the pericardial pressure is slightly subatmospheric. During the quiescent phase of the respiratory cycle an intrapericardial pressure of minus 2 mm. Hg may be found. During inspiration the intrapericardial pressure drops abruptly to a greater subatmospheric value, e.g., minus 5 mm. Hg (Fig. 1). Experimental work has shown that these respiratory swings in intrathoracic and intrapericardial pressure are faithfully transmitted to the cardiac chambers and to the vessels. In the intact animal and in normal man, or man with pericardial disease, respiratory variation in arterial pressure is a compound phenomenon depending among other things upon the changes in intrathoracic pressure, the ratio of respiratory to cardiac rate, the stroke volume, transit time in the pulmonary circulation, and the intrapericardial pressure.[4] In the catheterization laboratory, pressures are usually measured with reference to atmospheric pressure. Under these circumstances, inspiration is accompanied by a small decline in venous pressure, right ventricular pressure, pulmonary arterial pressure, and pulmonary wedge pressure. Left ventricular systolic pressure, aortic pressure, and peripheral arterial pressures also decline slightly during inspiration. However, respiratory variation in the pulmonary circulation is not exactly in phase with that of the systemic circulation, rather, inspiratory decline of pressures in the pulmonary circulation leads that in the arterial circulation by one or two heart beats.[2, 4]

With transducers leveled to the mid-chest, the right atrial and right ventricular diastolic pressures seldom exceed 4 to 6 mm. Hg. Left ventricular diastolic pressure is usually 1 to 5 mm. Hg higher than right ventricular diastolic pressure. Although the upper limit of normal for left ventricular end diastolic pressure is commonly given as 13 mm. Hg, in most normal subjects this pressure does not exceed 5 to 8 mm. Hg.

The normal left ventricular end diastolic volume averages 70 ± 20 ml./M²[.5] During a normal beat some two thirds of the left ventricular content are ejected, giving an ejection fraction which averages 0.67 ± 0.07. The mean circumferential fiber shortening rate takes into account not only the extent of shortening of the left ventricular circumference but the time taken for the shortening to occur. The normal left ventricle has a mean circumferential fiber shortening rate which exceeds one circumference per second.[6]

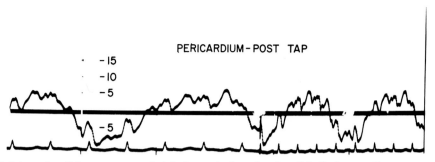

Figure 1. Intrapericardial pressure recorded during aspiration of pericardial effusion to relieve acute cardiac tamponade. Clinically significant compression has been alleviated. During inspiration the pressure is 10 mm. Hg below atmospheric but during expiration is still 7 mm. Hg above atmospheric. This wide pressure swing reflects hyperventilation. The mean intrapericardial pressure is approximately zero.

Indices of cardiac performance which deal with the manner, rate and amount of systolic ejection are referred to as the ejection phase indices of cardiac contractility. They are said to be useful in comparing one patient or group of patients with another.[7] The isovolumic indices of left ventricular contractility deal with the 40 msec. or so period which begins immediatedly after the mitral valve closes and ends immediately before the aortic valve opens. In general, ventricles with good contractility rapidly develop tension and therefore pressure during this period. This is the rationale for using peak dp/dt as a measure of left ventricular contractility. Unfortunately, peak dp/dt is also highly dependent upon both preload and afterload and therefore much effort has been expended in trying to define improved indices of contractility which would be independent of these two variables. Several such indices have been proposed, for instance V_{max}, V_{pm}, and dp/dt at a common isovolumic developed pressure. The relative merits

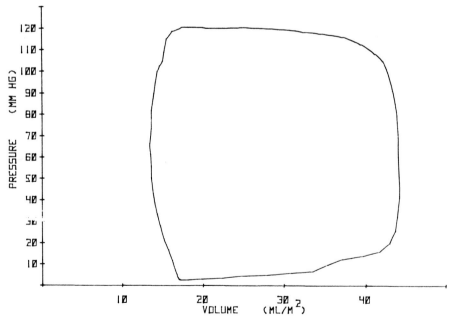

Figure 2. Pressure volume loop of a normal left ventricle. Data points are obtained simultaneously every 13 msec. from a cine left ventriculogram and a high fidelity record of left ventricular pressure.

of these indices lie beyond the scope of this chapter. Here it should be noted that they all depend upon the instantaneous relationship between left ventricular pressure or developed pressure and dp/dt, all are less sensitive than peak dp/dt to preload and afterload but they are less sensitive than peak dp/dt to contractility changes. In general, there is a consensus that these parameters are useful for intrapatient comparisons but not for interpatient comparisons.[7]

Aortic flow begins immediately after opening of the aortic valve, peaks rapidly in early systole but because of inertia ends after ventricular pressure begins to fall. Aortic stroke flow can be measured in intact man by means of catheter tip velocity transducers. During inspiration there normally occurs a 5 to 10 percent decrease in aortic stroke volume.[4]

The concept of ventricular diastolic compliance is a complex one due to the complexity of ventricular diastolic filling, the complex elastic and viscous properties of the myocardium, and the role of the pericardium and endocardium. High quality cine left ventriculograms recorded simultaneously with high fidelity left ventricular pressure tracings permit construction of pressure volume curves for the left ventricle (Fig. 2). When protodiastolic active rapid filling is omitted, this relationship is generally exponential and expresses the continuous change in ventricular diastolic compliance that occurs throughout the slow filling period of diastole (Fig. 3).[8] *Operational compliance* can be determined at any point on the pressure volume curve by taking the tangent to the curve at that point. Most clinical studies of compliance deal with end diastolic com-

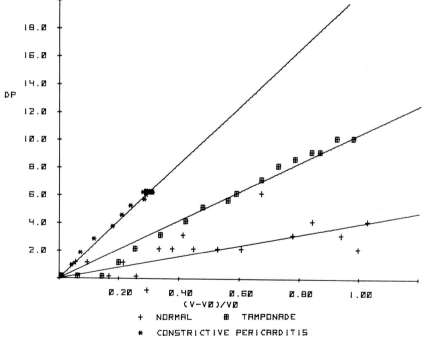

Figure 3. On the ordinate the change of pressure DP, on the abscissa the volume strain, i.e., instantaneous volume minus initial volume divided by initial volume (V-Vo/Vo). The nearest straight line fit passing through zero is plotted by a computer. The normal (+) is the lowest curve representing the most compliant ventricle. The steepest curve* is from a patient with constrictive pericarditis. Note that at the end of this curve the points are superimposed upon each other representing the plateaus of diastolic volume and pressure that characterize this disorder. A case of cardiac tamponade (⊞) demonstrates a compliance between normal and that of constrictive pericarditis.

pliance. Calculations derived only from left ventricular pressure and volume yield information about the pressure volume characteristics of the chamber as a whole but are of no value in considering the compliance of the myocardium. For this, account must be taken of the thickness of the left ventricular wall since left ventricular stress, while increasing with increasing pressure and dimension, decreases with increasing wall thickness. If one is to deal with diastolic myocardial fiber compliance it is necessary to employ normalizing techniques, that is, to substitute left ventricular wall stress for left ventricular pressure and left ventricular strain, or volume strain for left ventricular volume (Fig. 4).[4] Another normalizing technique is to include a term which expresses the ventricular volume/mass ratio in the formulae used to calculate compliance. These complex physiologic and mechanical considerations are the basis of much current work in the study of left ventricular performance. The measurements are difficult and tedious to obtain, the models of left ventricular geometry are poorly understood and many untrue assumptions have to be accepted before it is possible to approximate the elasticity or compliance of the left ventricle.

When one considers pericardial disease the problems of deriving myocardial compliance are compounded, for overlying the left ventricle is a thick or thin peel of virtually inelastic pericardium, or else an incompressible pericardial effusion which may be under various degrees of pressure. This additional consideration complicates even further the difficult and as yet not totally answered question of how to describe and measure left ventricular diastolic compliance. The reader should keep in mind these limitations of the methods, models and concepts when he considers the remainder of this chapter.

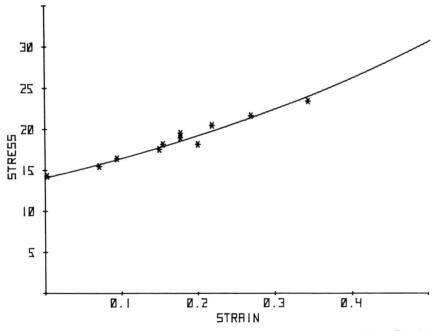

Figure 4. The stress strain relation for a normal ventricle. Stress (σ) is taken as: $\sigma = \frac{P}{h}\left(1 - \frac{B}{2h} - \frac{A^2}{h^2}\right)$ where P is the pressure and A and B are the major and minor semi-axes, and h the wall thickness. Strain (ϵ) is taken as $\epsilon = \frac{B-Bo}{Bo}$ where Bo is the end systolic semi-minor axis. Note that constrictive pericarditis poses a special problem in the calculation of σ because it is not possible to separate the components of h that are myocardial from those which are pericardial.

The normal pericardium is a thin fibrous membrane which is rather inelastic. For this reason it has a steep pressure volume curve (Fig. 5). Most of the pressure volume curves that have been published for normal pericardium have been obtained in the animal laboratory.[10] In these experiments, the pressure in the pericardial sac is monitored while fluid is instilled incrementally and then is removed in aliquots. Some of these experiments have been performed on the dog either with its chest open or closed, and others have been performed in the isolated animal heart. These studies have shown that when the intrapericardial fluid volume is increased from zero to 50 or 60 ml., intrapericardial pressure increases from its normal subatmospheric value up to 3 to 5 mm. Hg. Thereafter the intrapericardial pressure rises extremely steeply and values of 20 or more mm. Hg above atmospheric are achieved following the addition of approximately 200 ml. of fluid into the pericardium of dogs weighing approximately 25 kg. Intrapericardial volume in these studies includes the heart and its contents. The pressure increase produced by the instillation of fluid reflects not only the compliance of the pericardium, but also the effect of diminishing the blood volume of the cardiac chambers. Others experiments have been performed by injecting saline into the pericardial space of the dog immediately following death. In these experiments which reflect the total pericardial volume, 175 ml. of fluid could be injected before the pericardial pressure rose above its control value of zero. Thereafter, intrapericardial pressure rose precipitously to 100 mm. Hg following the addition of another 10 to 20 ml. of fluid. It has been shown that the pericardial pressure volume loop has hysteresis (Fig. 6), that is to say that it does not follow the same slope when fluid is withdrawn from the pericardium as it did when fluid was added to the pericardium. This observation while of interest to the physiologist has little clinical significance.

We have obtained pressure volume curves from the pericardium of patients at the time of pericardiocentesis. Patients with cardiac tamponade have by definition, strik-

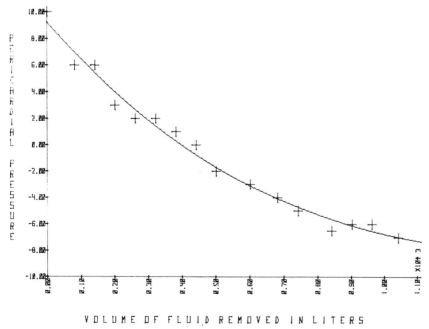

VOLUME OF FLUID REMOVED IN LITERS

Figure 5. The pressure volume relation of the pericardium in a patient with acute cardiac tamponade. Fluid was aspirated via an intrapericardial catheter attached to a Statham P23Db pressure transducer. Pressure was measured after the aspiration of every 50 ml. aliquot.

71

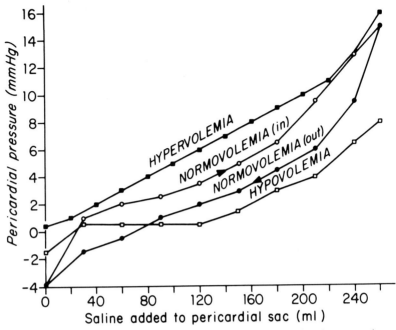

Figure 6. The pressure volume relation of the pericardium in the dog. Note that the curves demonstrate hysteresis, i.e., they do not retrace their paths when fluid is removed (see normovolemia in and out). Of major clinical importance is the observation well illustrated here that for a given volume of pericardial fluid, the pressure is considerably lower in the presence of hypovolemia. Thus, signs of cardiac tamponade may be masked by hypovolemia, e.g., in traumatic cases. (Reproduced from Shabetai et al.[1] with permission.)

ingly elevated intrapericardial pressure when the pericardial space is first entered. When pressure is monitored as each 50 ml. of fluid are aspirated, intrapericardial pressure tumbles rapidly from a typical value of between 15 and 25 mm. Hg to a value of a few mm. Hg above atmospheric. Thereafter as more and more fluid is aspirated, intrapericardial pressure declines slowly and finally achieves its normal subatmospheric value, at first during inspiration and eventually throughout the respiratory cycle (see Figs. 1 and 5). The steepest pressure volume relationships are found in the more acute cases of cardiac tamponade. The clinical and therapeutic implications of the steep nature of the pericardial pressure volume relationship in cardiac tamponade are that removal of only a small portion of a pericardial effusion or hemorrhage results in a drastic fall in intrapericardial pressure and a commensurate improvement in the hemodynamic situation. This important principle will be further elaborated in the sections dealing with cardiac tamponade and pericardiocentesis.

A pericardial effusion which has collected slowly over a matter of weeks or months may gradually stretch the pericardium and thereby alter its compliance. Thus, one may encounter pericardial effusions of two or more liters which are either under normal pressure or in which the intrapericardial pressure is raised to only 2 or 3 mg. Hg above atmospheric.

The changing volume of the heart during the cardiac cycle results in a small decrease in intrapericardial pressure during ventricular ejection and a small increase during ventricular filling. These cardiac variations of the intrapericardial pressure are scarcely noticable when the intrapericardial pressure is normal but are magnified when the intrapericardial pressure is increased.

Venous Pressure

The central venous pressure in man is usually recorded by means of a catheter placed in the superior vena cava or in the right atrium. Clinical measurements of the central venous pressure are not measured transmurally but are referred to atmospheric pressure with the pressure gauge leveled at the mid-chest. Under these circumstances the central venous pressure averages 5 mm. Hg and during quiet respiration exhibits a respiratory variation of 1 to 5 mm. Hg. When the heart rate is 70 or less and the P–R interval is normal, several distinct pulsations can be recognized on a recording of central venous or right atrial pressure. These are the A wave generated by atrial systole, the C wave which is associated with an increase in atrial pressure during isovolumic ventricular contraction, the X descent which occurs at the onset of ventricular ejection, the V wave which represents a gradual increase in venous pressure which occurs during passive filling of the atrium, and the Y descent which is associated with opening of the atrioventricular valve. In the normal subject these waves are smooth, imparting a somewhat rounded contour to the venous pressure tracing. The amplitude of the V wave in the right atrium exceeds that of the A wave whereas in the left atrium, A wave amplitude is greater than V.

The normal venous return is biphasic, a considerable proportion occurring during ventricular systole and a second portion occurring during ventricular diastole.[1, 11] In

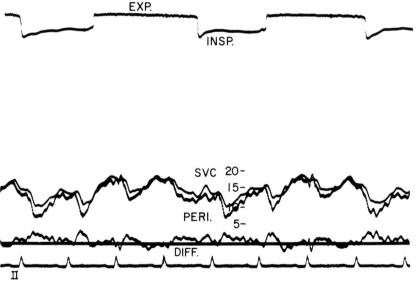

Figure 7. Simultaneous recording of superior vena caval pressure and intrapericardial pressure obtained during pericardiocentesis for the relief of cardiac tamponade complicating idiopathic pericarditis. From top to bottom: respiration, superior vena caval pressure, intrapericardial pressure, SVC minus pericardial pressure, ECG. Note that the central venous pressure declines normally during inspiration. The pressure in the superior vena cava demonstrates a deep x descent, but the y descent is absent. These two findings are characteristic of cardiac tamponade and should be compared with the prominent x and y descent and absent respiratory variations that characterize constrictive pericarditis. Note the close agreement between intrapericardial and venous pressure. At the time of the x descent, when ventricular ejection begins, transmural venous pressure (superior vena cava minus pericardium) achieves a positive value of 2 to 3 mm. Hg. This positive transmural pressure is not affected by respiration. (Reproduced with permission from Shabetai, R.: *Hemodynamics of pericardial disease*, in Grossman, W. (ed.): *Cardiac Catheterization and Angiography*, Lea and Febiger, Philadelphia, 1974.)

general, a reciprocal relationship exists between venous pressure and venous return. Blood flow through the vena cava to the right atrium increases during inspiration[1, 11] when central venous pressure drops, and increases during the X and Y descents of the venous pressure.

Cardiac tamponade imparts several abnormalities to the venous pressure and venous return. Circulation is maintained in the presence of an elevated intrapericardial pressure because the elevation of intrapericardial pressure is transmitted to the great veins and to the cardiac chambers. Thus, in patients with otherwise normal hearts, the intrapericardial pressure and the central venous pressure are equal.[1] In a typical case of severe cardiac tamponade, both may exceed 20 mm. Hg (Fig. 7). Cardiac tamponade in addition to causing an elevation of the central venous pressure, produces characteristic alterations in the wave form and in the pattern of venous return. Thus the Y descent is gradually obliterated with increasing severity of cardiac tamponade and is finally abolished altogether, to be replaced by a positive wave in the venous pressure tracing.[12] As the Y descent disappears, the component of venous return which normally accompanies ventricular diastole is abolished. The normal biphasic pattern of venous return is replaced by a monophasic pattern in which venous return is limited to ventricular systole.[1] Even in the presence of severe cardiac tamponade, inspiration continues to be associated with an increase in venous return[13] and a decrease in central venous pressure (Fig. 8). Thus, Kussmaul's sign is not found in cardiac tamponade. Total venous return is progressively reduced with increasing severity of cardiac tamponade, and this is responsible for a progressively declining cardiac output.

A somewhat different situation is found in constrictive pericarditis. In this disease,

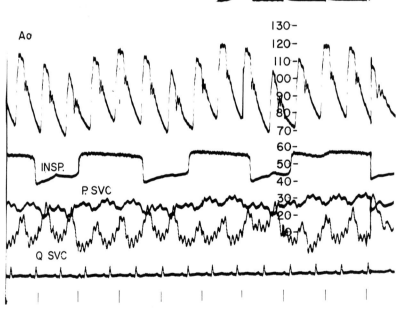

Figure 8. Arterial and venous pressures in a patient with severe cardiac tamponade (pericardial pressure equal to 27 mm. Hg). From top: aortic pressure, respiration, superior vena caval pressure, and superior vena caval blood flow velocity. Note the pulsus paradoxus (aortic systolic pressure falls 15 mm. Hg during inspiration). During inspiration, pressure falls and blood flow velocity is increased in the superior vena cava. The superior vena caval velocity record is monophasic, the peak corresponding to the x descent. (Reproduced from Shabetai et al.[1] with permission.)

intrapericardial pressure cannot be measured but cardiac filling is limited by the constriction. Immediately following end systole, the heart is at its minimal volume and there is no impediment to filling which indeed occcurs more rapidly then normal. Once the limit set by the constricting pericardium has been reached, no further cardiac filling is possible. Thus, the normal X and Y descents which occur respectively in systole and early diastole are preserved and indeed are exaggerated.[1] Thereafter the central venous pressure rapidly achieves an elevated value which is maintained throughout the remainder of diastole. The X and Y descents of venous pressure are accompanied by systolic and diastolic peaks of flow respectively.[1, 15] Thus in constrictive pericarditis, as opposed to cardiac tamponade, the normal biphasic pattern of venous return is preserved. Another important difference between constrictive pericarditis and cardiac tamponade is that whereas in cardiac tamponade inspiratory decline in venous pressure and increase in venous return are maintained, in constrictive pericarditis respiratory variation in both venous pressure and return are abolished.[1] Venous pressure does not increase during inspiration, rather, respiratory variation in venous pressure is absent, representing a forme fruste of Kussmaul's sign (Fig. 9).

These abnormalities of the central venous pressure and pulsations can be precisely documented and quantified in the cardiac catheterization laboratory. At the bedside, the clinician may achieve almost the same results by careful examination of the jugular venous system. Both in constrictive pericarditis and cardiac tamponade the venous pressure is elevated, frequently to extreme values. In the presence of hypovolemia, which may result from vigorous diuretic therapy for constrictive pericarditis or from hemorrhage in traumatic tamponade, the elevation in venous pressure may be amelio-

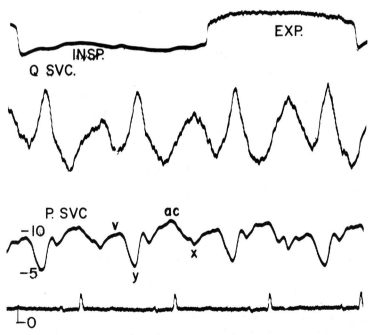

Figure 9. Superior vena caval pressure and flow velocity in a mild case of chronic constrictive pericarditis. From top: respiration, superior vena caval blood flow velocity (Q SVC), superior vena caval pressure (P SVC), and electrocardiogram. Note the absence of respiratory variation in the superior vena cava pressure and velocity records. The velocity pattern is biphasic. The flow velocity peaks correspond to the x and y pressure troughs. (Reproduced from Shabetai et al.[1] with permission.)

rated (see Fig. 6). When the venous pressure exceeds 15 to 20 mm. Hg, venous pulsations may not be visible because of overdistention of the veins. Frequently, the pulsations reappear when the patient is examined in the upright posture.

In constrictive pericarditis the X and Y descents are the dominant features of the jugular venous pulsations, so that the clinician appreciates the collapsing rather than the expanding motion of the deep jugular pulse and of the column in the superficial jugular veins. Respiratory variation is absent.

In cardiac tamponade, the venous pressure is also greatly elevated, but does not show two sharply collapsing waves with each cardiac cycle. Furthermore, inspiration is associated with a decrease in the venous pressure.

Arterial Blood Pressure

The normal arterial blood pressure is 120/80. The central aortic pressure displays a slightly lower peak systolic value, a slightly higher diastolic value, and a slightly higher mean value than are found in peripheral pulses such as that of the brachial artery. The upstroke should be sharp and brisk and the downstroke should show a clearly identifiable dicrotic notch or incisura. These criteria for a satisfactory pressure pulse in the arterial system are seldom met by conventional catheter-transducer systems because these are seldom critically damped. With great attention to detail, such pulses can be obtained with conventional instrumentation and they can be obtained quite easily with micromanometer catheter tip transducers. The latter possess the additional advantage of obviating delay caused by transmission through a long fluid-filled system. During inspiration a slight fall occurs in the arterial blood pressure. This decline is approximately equal for systolic pressure, mean pressure, and diastolic pressure with the result that there is little if any change in arterial pulse pressure during the respiratory cycle. During normal quiet breathing in a healthy individual, inspiratory decrease in arterial pressure does not exceed 10 mm. Hg and more commonly averages 3 to 5 mm. Hg. If at the time of study the patient is hyperventilating because of anxiety, or has labored breathing because of cardiac or pulmonary disease, considerable exaggeration in the amount of respiratory variation in arterial pressures results. This should not be confused with the pulsus paradoxus associated with pericardial disease and some cases of restrictive cardiomyopathy. Measurement of blood flow velocity in the aorta and in the peripheral arteries demonstrates that a small decline accompanies inspiration. In the aorta this does not exceed 15 percent of the stroke volume during quiet respiration. Many factors combine to produce the normal inspiratory decline in arterial blood pressure.[4] These include transmission of the inspiratory decline in intrathoracic pressure to the heart and aorta, and a transit delay in the lungs of the normal inspiratory increase in right ventricular stroke volume. The augmented right ventricular output associated with inspiration is not manifest in the aorta until the succeeding expiration and therefore arterial pressure appears to fall slightly during inspiration. Changes in heart rate and in ventricular transmural pressures as well as other autonomic reflex activity during the respiratory cycle also contribute to the net respiratory change in arterial pressure.

Several changes in arterial blood pressure may be associated with cardiac tamponade. First, it must be emphasized that considerable cardiac tamponade may be present without any obvious change in the arterial blood pressure. More severe cardiac tamponade, however, is usually associated with abnormalities of the arterial blood pressure. The arterial pulse pressure is sometimes decreased, reflecting a reduction in cardiac output and stroke volume. In addition, pulsus paradoxus is apt to appear. This is defined as an abnormal inspiratory decline in arterial blood pressure, and from the foregoing this means an inspiratory decline greater than 10 mm. Hg in the absence of dyspnea or labored breathing. The inspiratory decline in systolic arterial pressure is considerably greater than that in the arterial diastolic pressure so that there results a striking inspiratory decrease in the arterial pulse pressure. This implies that during inspiration there is a major decrease in aortic stroke flow. That this in fact is so has been amply confirmed by means of measurements of blood flow velocity in the aorta, both in experimental cardiac tamponade in the dog and in clinical cardiac tamponade in patients with pericardial disorders (see Fig. 8).[12, 14]

When cardiac tamponade is extreme and severe hypotension present, pulsus paradoxus may decrease or even disappear.

Two other abnormalities of the arterial blood pressure in severe cardiac tamponade should be mentioned. Mechanical pulsus alternans, with or without electrical alternans, may occur when the intrapericardial pressure is extremely high. In the experimental preparation, cardiac tamponade sufficiently severe to produce sustained mechanical alternans proves fatal unless a portion of the pericardial fluid is removed. The second abnormality is the dicrotic pulse. This is a pulse associated with extreme reduction of the stroke volume in which the dicrotic wave which follows the incisura is greatly exaggerated, imparting a second (dicrotic) peak to the pulse. This dicrotic peak is greater in the peripheral pulses than in the aorta but it can be recorded quite easily in the latter location.

Pulsus paradoxus can be measured by means of an indwelling arterial catheter or needle. This sign may also be easily appreciated at the bedside. The examiner palpates a peripheral pulse while observing the patient's respirations. During inspiration the pulse weakens, or in more severe cases disappears altogether. If doubt exists, pulsus paradoxus can be brought out by having the patient breathe more deeply, but it should be recalled that this maneuver will cause a slight decrease even in a normal pulse. When the patient has hypotension and or a small volume pulse, pulsus paradoxus may not be appreciated in the radial pulse but is obvious in larger pulses such as the femorals.

When the clinician wishes to *measure* pulsus paradoxus he takes the blood pressure without asking the patient to alter his respirations. The cuff is deflated slowly while the examiner observes or palpates the rise and fall of the chest. Pulsus paradoxus is measured by the pressure at which systolic sounds are heard only in expiration minus the pressure at which they are heard throughout the cardiac cycle.

Frequent and painstaking observations of the venous pressure, the venous pulsations, and of the degree of pulsus paradoxus constitute the most useful tools available to the clinician whose duty it is to watch a patient for increasing tamponade or the development of cardiac constriction.

Considerable speculation and a lot of experimental work has attended the question of the mechanism of pulsus paradoxus in cardiac tamponade. It has been suggested that pulsus paradoxus is caused by inspiratory traction by the diaphragm upon an already taut and stretched pericardium.[15] Others have proposed that pericardial fluid under tension creates an inspiratory pressure gradient between the pulmonary veins and the left atrium[16, 17, 18] and between the venae cavae and the right atrium.[18] Yet another hypothesis was that during inspiration the intraventricular septum is displaced from the right ventricle toward the left ventricle to accommodate the inspiratory increase in right ventricular filling.[19] In fact, there is probably no simple single explanation for the occurrence of pulsus paradoxus in cardiac tamponade. Rather, pulsus paradoxus results from the complex interplay of a large variety of factors. Based upon experimental studies in the cardiac catheterization laboratory and in the experimental animal laboratory, the following can be considered as firm data. In cardiac tamponade with pulsus paradoxus, the stroke volume is reduced and a further reduction occurs during inspiration.[2] At the beginning of inspiration, venous return to the right atrium through the superior and inferior vena cava increases. This augmentation in venous return is promptly followed by an increase in right ventricular stroke volume. When, in the experimental animal respiratory variation in venous return is abolished by means of a right heart bypass, cardiac tamponade, of whatever severity, never produces pulsus paradoxus.[2] In the control situation, inspiration is associated with little if any change in the transmural pericardial pressure (pericardial pressure minus pleural pressure). In the presence of cardiac tamponade, inspiration produces a small but definite increase in transmural pericardial pressure. Furthermore, the sudden addition of a small volume of blood to the pulmonary circulation in an animal with cardiac tamponade produces a prompt increase in pulmonary arterial and intrapericardial pressure and a simultaneous decrease in aortic pressure. Over the next three or four cardiac cycles the aortic pressure climbs to a value which exceeds the control and then returns to the control value.[2]

From these data it may be concluded that several factors combine to reduce the arterial pressure during inspiration. The stroke volume is reduced and a further reduction caused by inspiration has a profound effect on blood pressure. Further inspiratory expansion of right ventricular volume and increased stretch of the pericardium combine to increase an already elevated intrapericardial pressure. Superimposed upon these abnormal mechanisms are the mechanisms responsible for the normal inspiratory decline in arterial pressure. The result is a great exaggeration of this phenomenon, that is, pulsus paradoxus.

The Pulmonary Arterial Pressure

A moderate or mild degree of pulmonary hypertension is an inevitable feature of cardiac tamponade. In general, the pulmonary arterial pressure in cardiac tamponade is equal to the normal pulmonary arterial pressure plus the intrapericardial pressure. This usually results in a pulmonary arterial systolic pressure which approximates 40 mm. Hg. Pulmonary arterial hypertension which is significantly in excess of this suggests

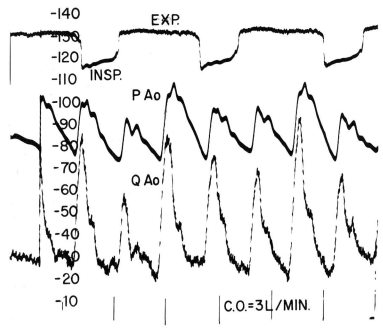

Figure 10. Pulsus paradoxus in constrictive pericarditis. From top: respiration, aortic pressure (P Ao), and aortic blood flow velocity (Q Ao). Time lines = 1 second. During inspiration, aortic systolic and pulse pressures decline and aortic blood velocity drops sharply. (Reproduced from Shabetai et al.[1] with permission.)

complicating cardiac or pulmonary disease or both.[20] Since pericardial effusion involves all the cardiac chambers and the pulmonary artery, one of the hemodynamic hallmarks of this condition is the equilibration between the central venous pressure, the right atrial pressure, the left atrial pressure, the right and left ventricular diastolic pressures, and the pulmonary wedge pressure.[21] These are usually more or less identical to the intrapericardial pressure. There is no other condition except constrictive pericarditis in which this equalization of pressure is found. Fortunately, the wave form of the ventricular diastolic and atrial pressures is so different in constrictive pericarditis that it should not be possible to confuse this condition with cardiac tamponade (see Figs. 7, 9, 11, and 20).

When there is severe pre-existing disease of the left ventricle, left ventricular diastolic and left atrial or pulmonary wedge pressures may be significantly higher than the pericardial pressure. In such cases, right ventricular diastolic and right atrial pressures equilibrate with pericardial pressure. This combination is quite characteristic of cardiac tamponade complicating end stage renal disease, e.g., that occurring during hemodialysis.

Arterial blood pressure changes are less striking on the average in constrictive pericarditis than they are in cardiac tamponade. As in cardiac tamponade the arterial blood pressure may be normal. In chronic constrictive pericarditis, atrial fibrillation is apt to supervene and the variations in pulse amplitude associated with varying R – R intervals may obscure small degrees of pulsus paradoxus or pulsus alternans. As in cardiac tamponade the more severe cases are associated with hypotension and small pulse pres-

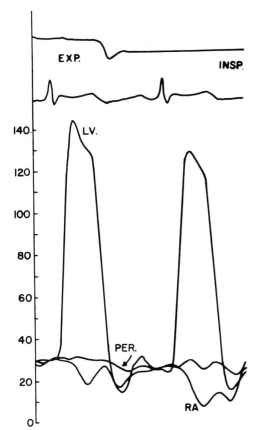

Figure 11. Hemodynamic data from an 18-year-old boy with cardiac tamponade and acute constrictive pericarditis studied two weeks after the clinical onset of infection. From above down: Respiration (exp, insp), ECG, left ventricular pressure (LV), pericardial pressure (PER), and right atrial pressure (RA). Intrapericardial pressure is elevated to 30 mm. Hg and in diastole is equal to the right atrial and left ventricular pressures. Ventricular and atrial pressures have already assumed the dip and plateau configuration. Note 20 mm. Hg of pulsus paradoxus. Pericardectomy was performed 24 hours after the study.

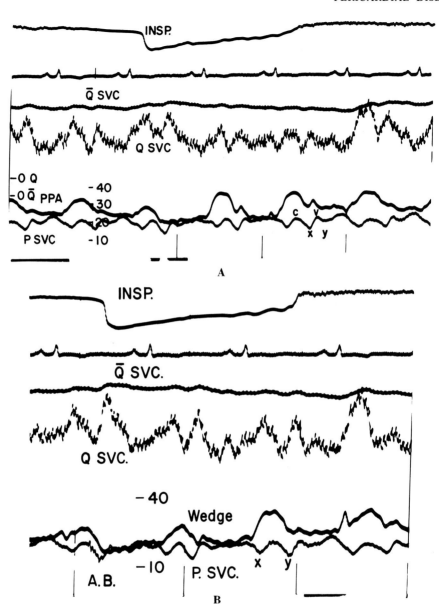

Figure 12. Data obtained during cardiac catheterization of a patient with subacute constrictive pericarditis. A, From above down: respiration, ECG, mean blood flow velocity in the superior vena cava (Q SVC), phasic blood flow velocity in the superior vena cava, pulmonary arterial pressure (PPA) and superior vena cava pressure (PSVC). B, Same as A except pulmonary wedge pressure replaces pulmonary arterial pressure. Note (1) equilibration of pressures during diastole, (2) prominent x and y descents of superior vena caval pressure with corresponding peaks of blood flow velocity, (3) minimal respiratory variation in venous pressure.

sure. Pulsus paradoxus is much less common in constrictive pericarditis than in cardiac tamponade and occurs only in about a third of the patients.[22] Pulsus paradoxus is more common in subacute and acute noncalcific constrictive pericarditis than in chronic calcific constrictive pericarditis (Fig. 10).[21]

The mechanism of pulsus paradoxus in constrictive pericarditis must differ in some respects from the mechanism responsible for this phenomenon in cardiac tamponade. In constrictive pericarditis without effusion, it is not possible for increased transmural pericardial pressure or additional stretching to occur during inspiration because the pericardial space is obliterated and the epicardium, myocardium, and frequently the parietal pericardium are firmly bound together as a single layer. Furthermore, constrictive pericarditis is not associated with an inspiratory increase in venous return to the right heart. A superimposition of normal inspiratory decline in arterial pressure and the effects of low stroke volume and possible intraventricular septal motion during inspiration may account for pulsus paradoxus in constrictive pericarditis. In other cases such as subacute constrictive pericarditis, pericardial effusion under a degree of pressure is present in addition to the constricting pericardium (subacute effusive constrictive pericarditis).[23] In these cases the mechanism of pulsus paradoxus is probably the same as in cardiac tamponade (Fig. 11). Pulmonary arterial pressure is elevated in constrictive pericarditis. As in cardiac tamponade, pulmonary hypertension is not severe. Characteristically the systolic pressure lies between 40 and 50 mm. Hg. Also as in cardiac tamponade there is equilibration between pressures in the left and right atria, the ventricular diastolic pressures, the pulmonary arterial diastolic pressure, and the pulmonary wedge pressure (Fig. 12).[1]

Ventricular Function

In cardiac tamponade the left ventricular diastolic pressure is elevated throughout diastole and is essentially equal to the intrapericardial pressure. The elevated ventricular diastolic pressure is not a manifestation of ventricular failure but simply represents

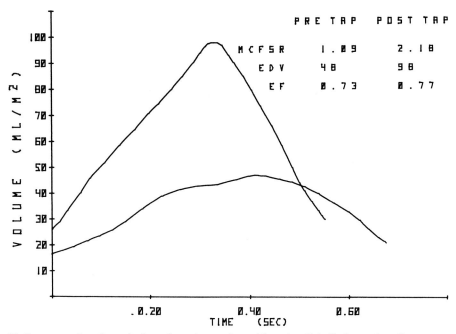

Figure 13. Computer plot of ventricular volume in a patient with pericardial effusion and cardiac tamponade secondary to a primary myocardial malignancy. Following pericardiocentesis, ventricular diastolic volume is double and the rate of ventricular filling is increased. During tamponade, the ejection fraction and mean circumferential fiber shortening rate are normal but they increase following pericardiocentesis.

the transmission of increased intrapericardial pressure to the left and right ventricles. Transmural left and right ventricular diastolic pressures are normal, or sometimes slightly below normal. The ventricular end diastolic volume is reduced in proportion to the degree of compression exerted by the pericardial effusion, that is, to the intrapericardial tension. The left ventricular end systolic volume is normal or less than normal and therefore the ejection fraction is normal, and indeed commonly is supranormal. Likewise, the mean circumferential fiber shortening rate is normal or higher than normal. Following pericardiocentesis the left ventricular diastolic pressure decreases and left ventricular end diastolic volume increases (Fig. 13). We have seen a case of subacute cardiac tamponade in which left ventricular volume doubled following the removal of 900 ml. of bloody pericardial fluid. The abrupt checking of ventricular volume expansion causes a loud third heart sound, sometimes spoken of as the pericardial knock (Fig. 14). Little if any change occurs in left ventricular end systolic volume and therefore the stroke volume increases. The isovolumic parameters of left ventricular performance are normal or high. Thus until almost the end, the left ventricle which is embarassed by cardiac tamponade and suffers impairment of ventricular diastolic filling, empties in a normal or supranormal manner.[24] During left ventriculography the small vigorously contracting opaque-filled left ventricular cavity presents a startling contrast with the stationary density of the pericardial effusion. When contrast agent is injected into the superior vena cava and followed through the circulation it is observed that all four car-

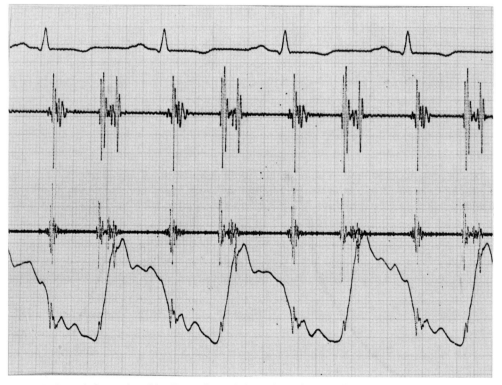

Figure 14. Constrictive pericarditis. From above down: ECG, phonocardiogram lower left sternal border, phonocardiogram upper left sternal border, and apexcardiogram. Note inverted T wave and loud third heart sound (pericardial knock). This sound occurs when rapid ventricular filling is abruptly checked by the constricting pericardium. The apexcardiogram appears inverted because of systolic precordial retraction.

diac chambers are small, hyperdynamic and empty more completely than normal within the nonpulsatile pericardial effusion.

A pericardial effusion under tension presents an obstacle to cardiac filling throughout the cardiac cycle, and therefore rapid filling during protodiastole is abolished and the ventricle fills slowly and incompletely throughout diastole. As will be seen later, this pathophysiologic alteration is in sharp contrast to that which is found in constrictive pericarditis in which the impediment to ventricular diastolic filling is limited to the latter two thirds of diastole.[25] The abolition of rapid ventricular filling during protodiastole accounts for the absence of an early diastolic dip in the left and right ventricular diastolic pressure tracings. In turn, the absence of a diastolic dip of pressure in early diastole in the ventricles accounts for the absence of a Y descent in the atrial pressure tracings in cardiac tamponade.

In constrictive pericarditis the heart is surrounded by a rigid pericardial box which totally limits the diastolic size of the heart. During systole, cardiac volume shrinks and the heart falls away from its restraining pericardial box. During early diastole, the ventricle fills with great rapidity until it reaches the absolute limit of cardiac volume imposed by the constricting pericardial wall. Thereafter, no further cardiac filling is possible. This accounts for the early diastolic dip of pressure found in the left and right ventricular pressure tracings and for the subsequent plateau of pressure during mid and late diastole.[26] Characteristically, in the right ventricle the ventricular diastolic plateau achieves an amplitude of one third or more of the right ventricular systolic pressure. The early diastolic dip pattern tends to be exaggerated by conventional fluid-filled catheter manometer systems. However, an unmistakable early diastolic ventricular pressure dip can be recorded from both ventricles by means of micromanometers (Fig. 15).

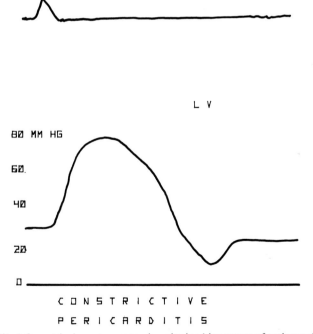

Figure 15. High fidelity left ventricular pressure tracing obtained by means of catheter tip micromanometer from a patient with chronic constrictive pericarditis. Note the early diastolic dip followed by plateau.

Furthermore when left and right ventricular pressures are recorded simultaneously on carefully calibrated equisensitive pressure measuring systems, left and right ventricular pressures are equal to each other throughout diastole. The right and left atrial pressures are equal to each other throughout diastole. The right and left atrial pressures are equal to each other and to the ventricular diastolic pressures. Thus the early diastolic dip in the right and left ventricles and the Y descent in the left and right atria are superimposed upon each other and in the period of diastole following the completion of ventricular filling. The pressures in all four chambers remain equal and at a constant elevated level until end diastole (Fig. 16). Restrictive cardiomyopathy is a rare form of idiopathic or secondary myocardial disease which mimics the hemodynamics of constrictive pericarditis and in which the characteristic early diastolic dip and mid to late diastolic plateau of pressure is recorded from the left and right ventricles. However, in this disorder left ventricular diastolic pressure is characteristically higher than right ventricular diastolic pressure (Fig. 17).[20] If fortuitously left and right ventricular diastolic pressures are approximately equal to each other in restrictive cardiomyopathy, exercise will increase left ventricular diastolic pressure more than right. In constrictive pericarditis, left and right ventricular diastolic pressures remain equal to each other during muscular exercise (Fig. 18). Contrary to what might reasonably have been anticipated, the iso-

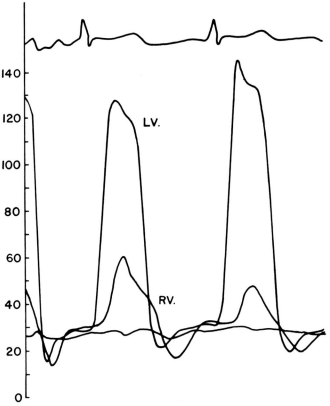

Figure 16. From the same patient as Figure 11. Right ventricular pressure now replaces right atrial. Note pulsus paradoxus is "out of phase" between the left and the right ventricles. End diastolic pressures are equal in the two ventricles which both display the dip and plateau sign of diastolic pressure. Right ventricular systolic is shortened and right ventricular diastolic pressure is >⅓ of right ventricular systolic pressure.

84

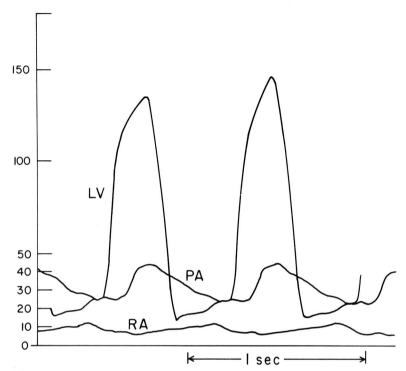

Figure 17. Patient with restrictive myocardial disease. Note that the right atrial pressure is elevated but is lower than the left ventricular diastolic pressure.

volumic and ejection phase indices of myocardial contractility fail to differentiate between restrictive cardiomyopathy and constrictive pericarditis. In both they are usually normal, but occasionally may be impaired. In our laboratory dp/dt max, V_{max}, V_{pm}, V_{40}, the ejection fraction, and the mean circumferential fiber shortening rate have been normal or supranormal in all cases of constrictive pericarditis and all cases of cardiac tamponade. In the latter, contractility indices may become enhanced immediately following pericardiocentesis.

In constrictive pericarditis, left ventricular diastolic pressure is high and rises precipitously from its lowest point at the nadir of the early diastolic dip. It is therefore not surprising to find that calculated ventricular diastolic compliance is severely reduced. This is demonstrated by the steep slope of the graph of diastolic pressure change versus volume change (see Fig. 3) and by the greatly increased value for the calculated stiffness of the left ventricle.

Clinically, cardiac tamponade and constrictive pericarditis simulate congestive heart failure.[27] Common features include dyspnea, edema, raised venous pressure, pulmonary congestion, reduced cardiac output, and arrhythmia. When the pump function of the heart is measured it is found to be decreased. However, raised filling pressure is caused by the pericardial disorder and reduced cardiac output by the small end diastolic volume and by the withdrawal of the Frank Starling mechanism in a ventricle in which expansion is prevented by the pericardial constraint.[27] We have encountered cases in which the ventricular end diastolic volume was lower than the normal stroke volume. It is not surprising that the contractility indices remain normal in cardiac tamponade because usually the underlying myocardium is normal. This is frequently true also in con-

85

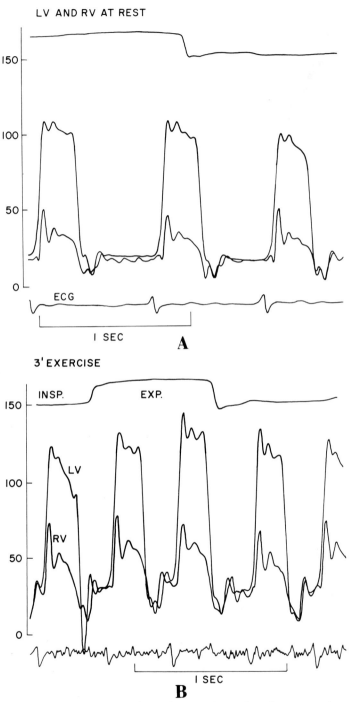

Figure 18. The effects of bicycle exercise on left and right ventricular diastolic pressures in a patient with constrictive pericarditis (A). The diastolic pressures in the two ventricles increase slightly but remain equal to each other (B). Note that tachycardia shortens or abolishes the plateau which may be absent for the same reason in the absence of exercise, particularly in infants and young children with acute or subacute constrictive pericarditis.

strictive pericarditis, but in some cases of chronic calcific constrictive pericarditis the myocardium may be involved and the contractility parameters are then impaired.[28]

Ventricular Filling by Diastolic Suction

It has long been speculated that the early diastolic dip of ventricular pressure may be a manifestation of ventricular filling by means of active suction. Experimental work has shown that ventricular diastolic suction can be demonstrated when ventricular diastolic filling is impeded by hemorrhage, occlusion of the mitral or tricuspid orifice,[29] or by cardiac tamponade.[30] Filling by diastolic suction is most likely to occur when the ventricular end systolic volume is small.[31]

In constrictive pericarditis the left ventricular end diastolic volume may be enlarged, normal, or small. In uncomplicated cases it is usually small. The ejection fraction is normal and therefore the end systolic volume is greatly reduced. Ventricular filling is impeded by the constrictive pericarditis and therefore the conditions for ventricular diastolic filling by suction are met. When a cardiac work loop is constructed by plotting left ventricular volume on the abscissa and left ventricular pressure on the ordinate for an entire cardiac cycle, it is found that in patients with constrictive pericarditis and a small left ventricle, the period of rapid filling during early diastole is accompanied by decreasing left ventricular pressure (Fig. 19). This association can best be explained by the occurrence of ventricular diastolic suction. Ventricular diastolic suction has been demonstrated in the dog with severe cardiac tamponade by means of subatmospheric transmural ventricular diastolic pressures. We have observed the same phenomenon in our laboratory in at least one patient in whom we measured transmural ventricular pressures by means of a differential transformer which measured and subtracted from each other left ventricular and intrapericardial pressures (Fig. 20).

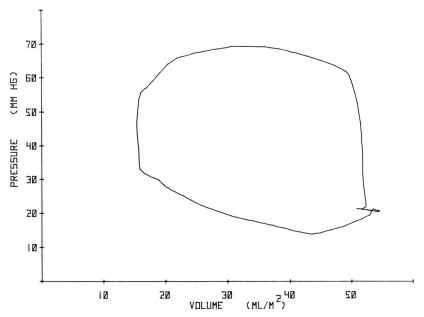

Figure 19. Left ventricular pressure volume loop obtained from a patient with severe chronic constrictive pericarditis. Note that in early diastole, pressure is falling while volume is expanding. For the left ventricular pressure wave form in this patient, see Figure 15. Diastolic expansion during a period of pressure decline is taken as evidence that the ventricle is filling by suction.

87

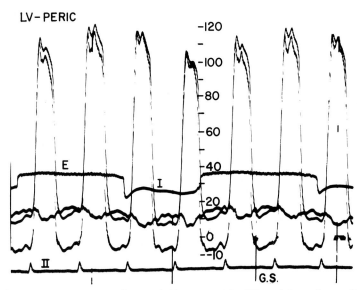

Figure 20. Cardiac Tamponade. Pressure is recorded by means of a differential transformer from the left ventricle and the intrapericardial sac. The roughly square shaped wave running along the lower third of the tracing marks the respiratory cycle. E = expiration; I = inspiration. The differential pressure gauge records left ventricular pressure, minus intrapericardial pressure. The intrapericardial pressure is approximately 18 mm. Hg. During diastole, the intrapericardial and the ventricular diastolic pressures form a box with the intrapericardial pressure above and the ventricular diastolic pressure below. The bottom of the tracing where the ventricular tracing becomes single represents the transmural ventricular diastolic pressure. This pressure is subatmospheric, indicating left ventricular filling by diastolic suction. Note that the diastolic pressure in the ventricle does not display the early diastolic dip and mid to late diastolic plateau characteristic of constrictive pericarditis.

REFERENCES

1. SHABETAI, R., FOWLER, N. O., AND GUNTHEROTH, W. G.: *The hemodynamics of cardiac tamponade and constrictive pericarditis*. Am. J. Cardiol. 26:480, 1970.

2. SHABETAI, R., FOWLER, N. O., AND FENTON, J. C.: *Pulsus paradoxus*. J. Clin. Invest. 44:1882, 1965.

3. MORGAN, B. C., GUNTHEROTH, W. G., AND DILLARD, D. H.: *Relationship of pericardial to pleural pressure during quiet respiration and cardiac tamponade*. Circ. Res. 16:493, 1965.

4. SHABETAI, R., FOWLER, N. O., AND GUERON, M.: *The effects of respiration on aortic pressure and flow*. Am. Heart J. 65:525, 1963.

5. DODGE, H. T., SANDLER, H., BALLEW, D. W., ET AL.: *The use of biplane angiocardiography for the measurement of left ventricular volume in man*. Am. Heart J. 60:762, 1960.

6. KARLINER, J. S., GAULT, J. H., ECKBERG, D., ET AL: *Mean velocity of fiber shortening. A simplified measure of left ventricular myocardial contractility*. Circulation 44:323, 1971.

7. PETERSON, K. L., SKLOVEN, D., LUDBOOK, P., ET AL: *Comparison of isovolumic and ejection phase indices of myocardial performance in man*. Circulation 49:1088, 1974.

8. DIAMOND, G., FORRESTER, J. S., HARGIS, J., ET AL.: *Diastolic pressure-volume relationship of the canine left ventricle*. Circ. Res. 29:267, 1971.

9. MIRSKY, I., COHN, P. F., LEVINE, J. A., ET AL.: *Assessment of left ventricular stiffness in primary myocardial disease and coronary artery disease*. Circulation 50:128, 1974.

10. HOLT, J. P.: *The normal pericardium*. Am. J. Cardiol. 26:455, 1970.

11. WETLER, L., BERGEL, D. H., GABE, J. T., ET AL.: *Velocity of blood flow in normal human venae cavae*. Circ. Res. 23:349, 1968.

12. DEGRISTOFARO, D., AND LIV, C. K.: *The hemodynamics of tamponade and blood volume overload in dogs*. Cardiovasc. Res. 3:292, 1969.

13. GUNTHEROTH, W. G., MORGAN, B. C., AND MULLINS, G. L.: *Effect of respiration on venous return and stroke volume in cardiac tamponade.* Circ. Res. 20:381, 1967.

14. GABE, I. T., GAULT, J. H., ROSS, J., JR., ET AL.: *Measurement of instantaneous blood flow velocity and pressure in conscious man with a catheter tip velocity probe.* Circulation 40:603, 1969.

15. DOCK, W.: *Inspiratory traction on the pericardium. The cause of pulsus paradoxus in pericardial disease.* Arch. Intern. Med. 108:837, 1961.

16. SHARP, J. T., BUNNEL, I. L., HOLLAND, J. F., ET AL.: *Hemodynamics during induced cardiac tamponade in man.* Am. J. Med. 29:640, 1960.

17. GOLINKO, R. J., KAPLAN, N., AND RUDOLPH, A. M.: *The mechanism of pulsus paradoxus during acute pericardial tamponade.* J. Clin. Invest. 42:249, 1963.

18. KATZ, L. N., AND GAUCHAT, H. W.: *Pulsus paradoxus (with special reference to pericardial effusion).* Arch. Intern. Med. 33:350, 1924.

19. DORNHORST, A. L., HOWARD, P., AND LEATHART, G. L.: *Pulsus paradoxus.* Lancet 1:746, 1952.

20. SHABETAI, R., FOWLER, N. O., AND FENTON, J. C.: *Restrictive cardiac disease. Pericarditis and the myocardiopathies.* Am. Heart J. 69:271, 1965.

21. SHABETAI, R.: *Hemodynamics of pericardial disease,* in Grossman, W. (ed.): *Cardiac Catheterization and Angiography.* Lea & Febiger, Philadelphia, 1974.

22. WOOD, P.: *Chronic constrictive pericarditis.* Am. J. Cardiol. 7:48, 1961.

23. HANCOCK, E. W.: *Subacute effusive-constrictive pericarditis.* Circulation 43:183, 1971.

24. SHABETAI, R.: *Cardiac catheterization,* in Fowler, N.: *Cardiac Diagnosis and Treatment.* Harper & Row, New York (in press).

25. MOSCOVITZ, H. L.: *Pericardial constriction versus cardiac tamponade.* Am. J. Cardiol. 26:546, 1970.

26. HANSEN, A. T., ESKILDSEN, P., AND GOTZSCHE, H.: *Pressure curves from the right auricle and the right ventricle in chronic constrictive pericarditis.* Circulation 3:881, 1951.

27. GAASCH, W. H., SHABETAI, R., AND PETERSON, K. L.: *Left ventricular function in constrictive pericarditis.* Am. J. Cardiol. 34:107, 1974.

28. VOGEL, J. H. K., HORGAN, J. A., AND STRAHL, C. L.: *Left ventricular dysfunction in chronic constrictive pericarditis.* Chest 59:486, 1971.

29. FOWLER, N. O., COUVES, C., AND BEWICH, J.: *Effect of inflow obstruction and rapid bleeding on ventricular diastolic pressure.* J. Thorac. Surg. 35:532, 1958.

30. SHABETAI, R., FOWLER, N. O., BAUNSTEIN, J. R., ET AL.: *Transmural ventricular pressures and pulsus paradoxus in experimental cardiac tamponade.* Dis. Chest 39:557, 1961.

31. BRECHER, G. A.: *Critical review of recent work on ventricular diastolic suction.* Circ. Res. 6:556, 1958.

The Radiology of Pericardial Disease

Florencio A. Hipona, M.D., and Santiago Paredes, M.D.

Radiology has offered important techniques in the diagnostic evaluation of patients with pericardial disease. These radiologic examinations can be divided into noninvasive and invasive procedures. They are presented in a comprehensive fashion with an emphasis on the diagnostic clues including an essential discussion of the technical aspects, indications, advantages and limitations of the different modalities. We have chosen this approach rather than going by individual pathology to give the reader an overview of the radiologic investigations for pericardial disease.

Through the years, the types and sequence of radiologic examinations for pericardial disease have changed. The current and conventional practice is to perform chest roentgenography with or without fluoroscopy followed by echocardiography. Pericardiocentesis is usually done with ultrasonic guidance. The other modalities are occasionally used and mainly for confirmatory purposes.

ANATOMIC CONSIDERATIONS

A review of pertinent anatomic considerations is necessary for better understanding of the radiologic signs used in the diagnosis of pericardial disease.

The *parietal pericardium* separates the heart and proximal segments of the main vessels from the surrounding mediastinal structures. At the same time, it gives a certain degree of fixation to the heart by several points of attachment. Superiorly, the pericardium extends into portions of the superior vena cava, the ascending aorta, and the main pulmonary trunk. The fibrous portion of the parietal pericardium continues with the external coat of the great vessels. Inferiorly, most of the parietal pericardium is loosely connected to the diaphragm by fibroareolar tissue except in a small segment where the central tendon of the diaphram is fused to the pericardium. Posteriorly, the pericardium separates the heart from other mediastinal structures. The pulmonary veins are covered by the pericardium before entering into the left atrium. Anteriorly, it is separated from the thoracic wall by the pleura except at the level of the left fourth and fifth costal cartilages where it is in direct contact with the anterior chest wall. Laterally, it is separated by the pleura from the external surface of the lungs. From each side, the phrenic nerve runs in a vertical direction in between the pleural and pericardial membranes (Fig. 1).[24]

The *visceral pericardium* after covering the external surface of the heart and part of the great vessels, reflects to continue covering the inner surface of the parietal portion. The visceral layer of pericardium is continuous with the interstitial tissue of the myocardium. It contains fat tissue mainly along the ventricular border of the coronary sul-

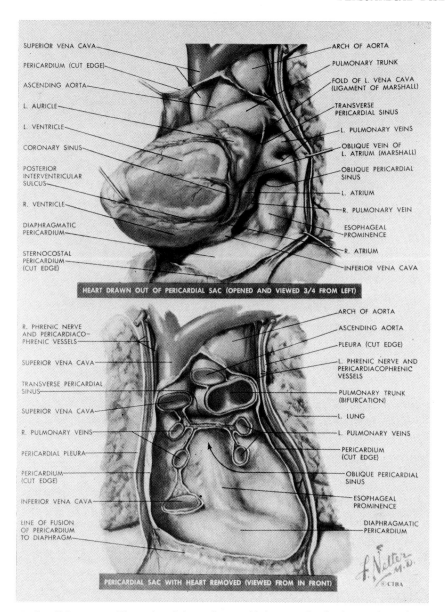

Figure 1. Pericardial anatomy. The pericardial membrane with its normal reflections and attachments are illustrated with the heart drawn out of the opened pericardial sac and with the heart removed to view the posterior aspect of the pericardium. © Copyright 1969 CIBA Pharmaceutical Company, Division of CIBA-GEIGY' Corporation. Reproduced, with permission, from *The CIBA Collection of Medical Illustrations* by Frank H. Netter, M.D. All rights reserved.

cus, the inferior border of the heart, and the interventricular grooves. With optimal radiographic technique, this epicardial fat can be identified on chest roentgenograms and fluoroscopy.

It is also important from the anatomic point of view to remember that certain normal or abnormal *extracardiac structures* are localized next to the pericardium. Most of them contain soft tissues with radiographic density similar to that of the cardiac silhouette. Thus, the thymus is in contact with the anterior aspect of the upper portion of the pericardium. The enlargement of this gland usually overlaps and produces apparent enlargement of the cardiac silhouette. Anterior mediastinal tumors may produce a similar effect. Pleuropericardial adhesions can produce localized areas of abnormal bulging or irregularities which makes one consider possible cardiac or pericardial pathology.

Normal pericardial fat usually shows as a triangular shaped soft tissue density which blends with the shadow of the right or left heart border and the corresponding diaphragmatic surface. Sometimes, this familiar density presents a different shape or is excessive in amount, as observed in certain patients receiving prolonged steroid therapy. Usually congenital, and rarely acquired, defects of the right hemidiaphragm allow herniation of part of the liver, mesentery, or kidney into the thoracic cavity. Radiographically, it shows as a rounded soft tissue mass which blends with the density of the right atrium in the frontal view of the chest.[28]

NONINVASIVE INVESTIGATIONS

Chest Roentgenography

This is the most common type of examination requested for the diagnosis of pericardial disease. When analyzing any chest roentgenogram, one should be alert for pericardial pathology based on the knowledge of the radiographic signs thereof even in patients with unsuspected pericardial disease. The roentgenographic manifestations to be looked for may be divided into cardiac and extracardiac signs.

Cardiac Signs

SIZE OF THE CARDIAC SILHOUETTE. At this point, there is a need for clarification of common terminology employed when dealing with the radiology of pericardial prob-

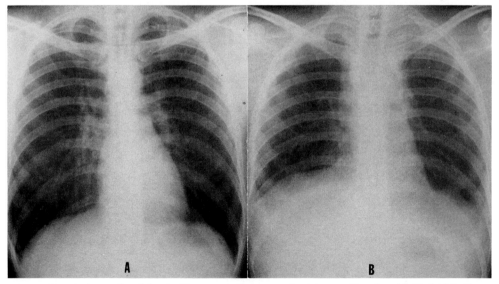

Figure 2. Restrictive pericarditis. A, Chest roentgenogram of a 24-year-old male with Hodgkin's disease shows an essentially normal chest. There is residual contrast material in normal Virchow's node superimposed on the left apex from a previous lymphangiogram. B, Followup chest x-ray 6 months after mantle radiation therapy to the neck and mediastinum demonstrated a smaller heart with widening of superior mediastinum and bilateral apical pleural thickening secondary to radiation fibrosis. The high diaphragm also indicates restrictive changes.

lems. The word "heart" is generally used when referring to the radiographic image of the heart including the pericardium in plain chest roentgenograms. For practical purposes, since the space between parietal and visceral pericardium is almost nonexistent, it is an acceptable term. However, when the same radiographic outline becomes enlarged due to true cardiomegaly, pericardial effusion without cardiomegaly, or a combination of both, the term "cardiac silhouette" is better.

Normal Cardiac Silhouette. A normal size of the cardiac outline does not rule out pericardial disease. This may be seen in constrictive pericarditis, postradiation pericarditis, or in patients with relatively small sized heart due to advanced chronic pulmonary emphysema or other causes of microcardia (Fig. 2).

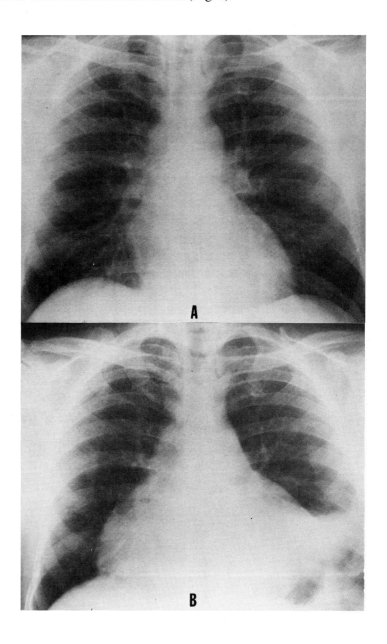

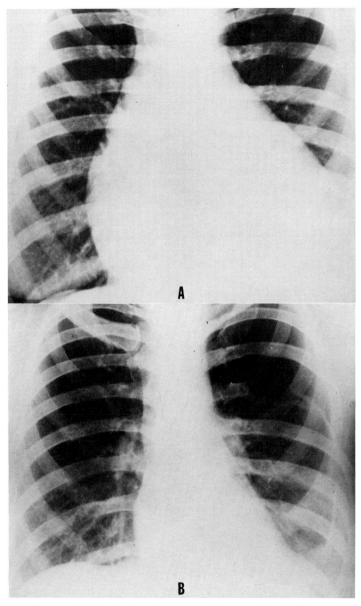

Figure 4. Mediastinal lipoma. A, Plain chest roentgenogram of an asymptomatic 21-year-old female shows an apparent enlargement of the cardiac silhouette mimicking pericardial effusion or cardiomegaly. B, Postoperative chest examination demonstrates a normal cardiovascular silhouette after surgical removal of the anterior mediastinal lipoma.

◀ **Figure 3.** Dressler's syndrome. A, Initial chest roentgenogram of a 54-year-old man with an acute myocardial infarction demonstrates an essentially normal chest. B, Examination 3 weeks later shows an enlarged cardiovascular silhouette suggestive of pericardial effusion which was confirmed by angiocardiography.

Enlarged Cardiac Silhouette. This is the classic and best known radiographic manifestion of fluid within the pericardial sac. In early stages or questionably borderline cases, comparison with a previous chest roentgenogram is very helpful to make the observation valid. In doing so, one should carefully consider the patient's position, degree of inspiration, and presence of congestive failure. This becomes very important in evaluating patients after cardiovascular surgery for early detection of hemopericardium or the development of effusion as a manifestation of the post-pericardiotomy syndrome.

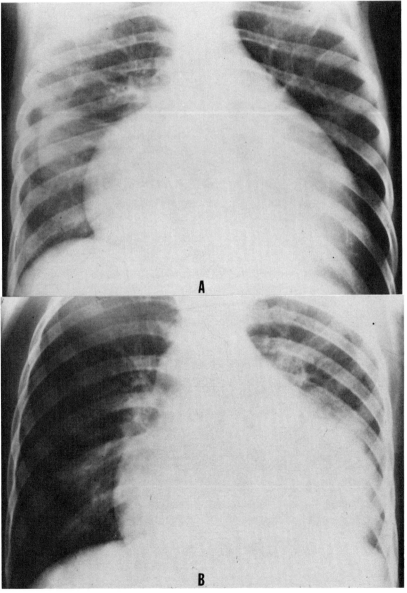

Figure 5. Positional chest roentgenography for pericaricardial effusion. A, Upright examination of a young adult female demonstrates an enlarged cardiac silhouette with a flask configuration. B, Recumbent examination under identical conditions shows widening of the cardiac base and an altered cardiac configuration. This phenomenon can also be observed during fluoroscopy.

CONFIGURATION OF THE CARDIAC SILHOUETTE. As fluid accumulates within the pericardial space, the cardiac outline increases in size and loses its normal configuration. The sharp angulation between two contiguous surfaces such as the left and right cardiophrenic angles, the pulmonary artery and left atrial appendage, the right atrium and superior vena cava as well as the aortic knob and the pulmonary artery disappear progressively. At this point, the classic "bottle shape" configuration is characteristic of massive pericardial effusion (Fig. 3).

One should be aware, however, that some patients with longstanding cardiac disease may present with a markedly enlarged heart which mimicks massive pericardial effusion. Occasionally, an anterior mediastinal mass mainly of thymic origin may attain a large size and may resemble the configuration of pericardial effusion (Fig. 4).

Under normal conditions, certain limited changes are observed in the configuration of the heart in chest roentgenograms taken in the recumbent and upright positions. In most cases of pericardial effusion, the recumbent position view shows widening of the base of the heart as compared to the upright view. In patients with constrictive pericarditis, adhesions between the pericardium and surrounding structures may produce absence of positional shift of the heart with changes in position of the patient (Fig. 5).

Besides the already described characteristic configuration of the cardiac silhouette due to pericardial effusion, other abnormal shapes are seen in the following conditions: pericardial defect, pericardial cyst, pleuropericarditis, and tumors.

Pericardial defects of the parietal pericardium may involve only a segment (partial) or the entire pericardium (complete). It may be congenital or acquired in origin.[6, 13, 14] About 30 percent of cases of congenital pericardial defects are associated with congenital cardiac, pulmonary, or peritoneal abnormalities. The acquired forms are usually related to resection of part of the pericardium during corrective surgery for cardiac lesions, recurrent intractable effusion, or constriction.

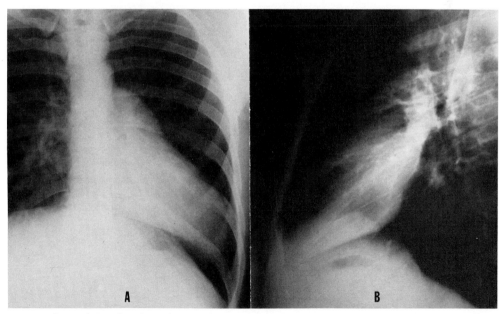

Figure 6. Congenital pericardial defect. A, Chest roentgenogram in the frontal projection of a young adult male shows sharp delineation of the left heart margin from the pulmonary artery segment to the apex and inferiorly. The heart is partially shifted and rotated to the left assuming a right anterior oblique view. B, The lateral projection demonstrates a sharp inferior margin of the heart which is separated from the left hemidiaphragm due to interposition of part of the left lower lobe. These findings indicate a complete left sided congenital pericardial defect.

Congenital defect of the left pericardium occurs more often than in the right. If only a small segment of the left pericardium is absent, it usually occurs at the level of the left atrium and main pulmonary artery. In the frontal chest roentgenogram, there is an unusual sharply outlined left atrial appendage which is bulging and may resemble left atrial enlargement or a mediastinal mass.

If the entire left portion of the pericardium is absent, there is a characteristic shift of the heart to the left hemithorax without deviation of the trachea or any other thoracic pathology that may account for such a shift.[32] There is associated minimal to moderate rotation of the heart to the left. The entire left heart border from the pulmonary trunk down to cardiac apex is sharp in outline. Very often, the inferior border of the heart can be seen clearly separated from the diaphragm in the frontal and lateral projections (Fig. 6).

Congenital pericardial cysts and diverticula are the result of abnormal fusion of mesenchymal lacunae. Acquired pericardial cyst may be related to neoplastic, traumatic, or parasitic disease.[21, 22] Certain diverticula are the result of inflammatory disease producing encapsulated effusions.

On chest roentgenograms, the most common location is the right cardiophrenic angle, but it may develop also in the left cardiophrenic angle and superior mediastinum. They have a rounded or oval shape with a well demarcated free border while the rest of the mass blends in with the cardiac silhouette. Calcification may occur in the wall which is a helpful sign in considering this diagnosis. The differential diagnosis should include omental, renal, or hepatic herniation through a diaphragmatic defect, pericardial fat and certain mediastinal masses (Fig. 7).

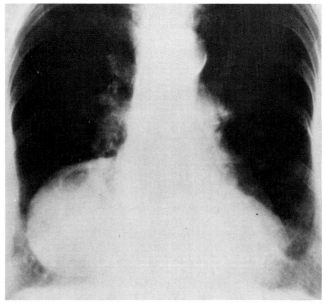

Figure 7. Congenital pericardial cyst. Chest x-ray of a 62-year-old male demonstrates a mass density located at the right cardiophrenic angle. The mass merges medially with the right heart margin, has a rounded superolateral margin, and is separated from the diaphragm.

Pleuropericardial adhesions occasionally occur with healing of an inflammatory or a traumatic process primarily of the pleura which may involve secondarily the adjacent pericardium. This results in an abnormal configuration of the cardiac contour which should be distinguished from primary cardiac pathology such as pericardial mass or ventricular aneurysm.

PERICARDIAL CALCIFICATION. Calcification of the pericardium has been found to be related to multiple causes, although inflammatory diseases are among the most common. When pericardial calcification is present, signs of constrictive pericarditis should be looked for. However, many cases of constrictive pericarditis show no evidence of pericardial calcification at all.

The configuration of the calcification is usually that of a homogeneous or irregularly mottled curvilinear density along the borders of the heart. Although it is possible to be recognized in any projection of the chest, optimal visualization is obtained when the x-rays are tangenital to the calcification.[27] Since the anterior pericardium is most commonly involved, the lateral chest roentgenogram shows this finding to a better advantage. Localized calcification of the left atrial pericardium is rare, but it is important to recognize since constrictive effects upon the left atrium can produce a clinical picture similar to that of mitral stenosis (Fig. 8).

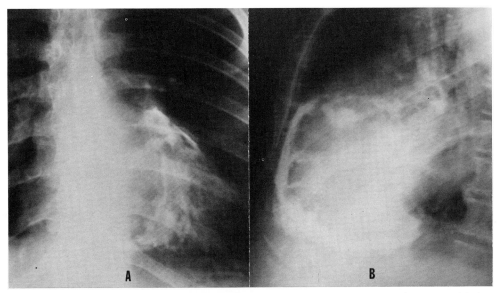

Figure 8. Pericardial calcification. A, Posteroanterior and B, lateral roentgenograms of a young adult male who had an episode of acute viral pericarditis a few years earlier demonstrate diffuse calcifications in the thickened pericardium enveloping the right ventricle and the diaphragmatic surfaces of the right atrium and left ventricle.

THE EPICARDIAL FAT SIGN. In the normal heart, there is a certain amount of adipose tissue underneath the visceral pericardium, which is commonly called the epicardial fat. The external surface of the parietal pericardium is also surrounded by adipose tissue called the pericardial fat. Thus, the visceral and parietal pericardium are sandwiched between two layers of fat. For this reason, by centering the x-rays tangential to these tissue planes, the radiographic appearance is that of a radiolucent band (the fat planes) containing more or less central radiopaque band (pericardium) of about 2 mm. in thickness. This is best demonstrated in a straight lateral view of the chest with the tube centered on the anterior chest wall.[20] According to the degree of thickening of the pericardial band, the diagnosis of pericardial thickening or effusion can be entertained (Figs. 9 and 10).

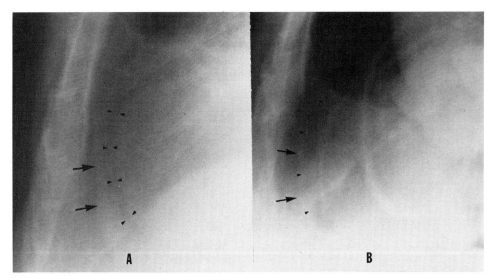

Figure 9. Normal epicardial fat. A, Lateral roentgenogram of a young adult male shows a curvilinear radiolucent stripe (marked by small arrowheads) in the retrosternal area just posterior to the right ventricular border. This represents the epicardial fat at the interventricular groove. B, The supravalvar aortogram demonstrates conical deformity of the aortic valve indicative of aortic valvar stenosis. There is opacification of the left anterior descending coronary artery coursing at the posterior border of the epicardial fat.

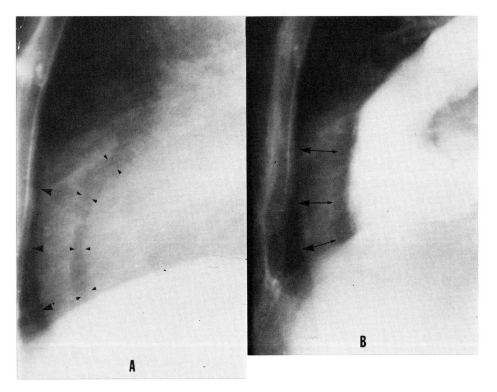

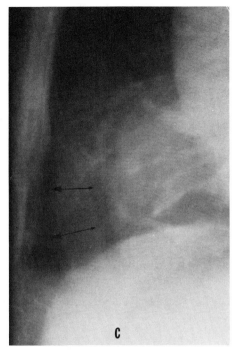

Figure 10. Epicardial fat sign indicative of pericardial effusion. A, Lateral roentgenogram of a middle-aged female with hypothroid heart disease shows a widened epicardial fat which is displaced posteriorly from the anterior margin of the cardiac silhouette. This sign is indicative of pericardial effusion. B, Right ventriculogram in the lateral view demonstrates the position of the epicardial fat just posterior to the anterior pericardial effusion (space between arrows). C, Levoangiocardiographic phase confirms the position of the epicardial fat at the interventricular groove just in front of the faintly opacified left ventricle.

LUCENCIES IN THE CARDIAC SILHOUETTE. Normally, there are no radiolucencies within the cardiac silhouette except for the epicardial fat. The presence of lucencies therefore indicates abnormalities. Such intracardiac lucencies are due to fat or air. The fat is due to lipoma or liposarcoma and air is due to pneumocardium which indicates air embolism. Air in the pericardial space usually indicates penetrating trauma of the chest, communication with a hollow viscus, or pericarditis with air forming organisms.[5] Chest roentgenograms in different positions, especially the left lateral decubitus position, will help differentiate the aforementioned conditions as well as mediastinal emphysema (Figs. 11 and 12).[16]

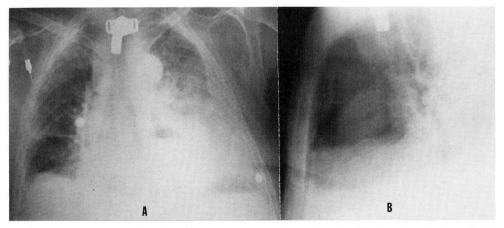

Figure 11. Hydropneumopericardium. Chest roentgenogram in A, frontal and B, lateral projections of a 79-year-old female in intractable congestive failure shows appearance of hydropneumopericardium 10 days after insertion of a nasogastric tube. Postmortem examination a few days later demonstrated a necrotic ulcer in the distal esophagus communicating with the pericardial cavity.

101

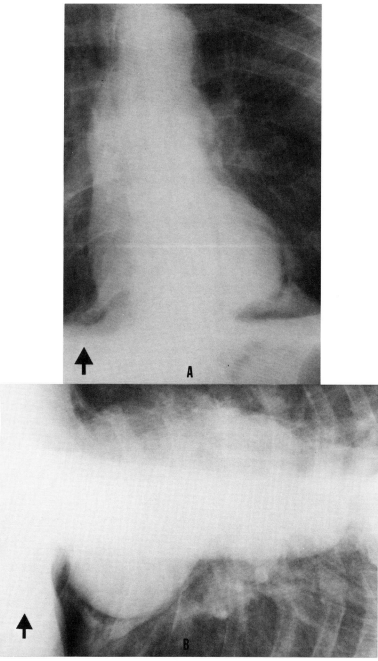

Figure 12. Mediastinal emphysema. A, Chest roentgenogram in the upright position of a young male who was stabbed in the left chest demonstrates a curvilinear radiolucency at the cardiac apex. This finding can be mistaken for pneumopericardium although air in the pericardial space should be trapped in the superior-most portion of the pericardial space which is at the pulmonary artery attachment of the pericardium. If still in doubt, a left lateral decubitus projection, B, should be taken, and with mediastinal emphysema will show persistence of the radiolucency in the same position whereas a pneumopericardium will show a shift of air to the pericardial space above the right atrium. Radiolucent stripes may also be seen in the left chest wall indicating subcutaneous emphysema.

Extracardiac Observations

Widening of the mediastinum should be carefully analyzed since it may be due to vascular structures that could be related to a pericardial problem.

SUPERIOR VENA CAVA. Distension of the superior vena cava is often present with pericardial effusion. Also, the azygos vein which is a density projecting on the right aspect of the tracheobronchial angle may be dilated in the frontal chest roentgenogram. Dilatation of superior vena cava and azygos vein with minimal pericardial effusion is most commonly seen in right heart failure. Its recognition becomes significant in the differentiation of constrictive pericarditis without cardiac enlargement or pericardial effusion with cardiac tamponade (Fig. 13).

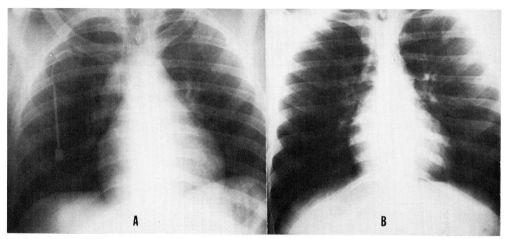

Figure 13. Cardiac tamponade. It is not necessary to have enlargement of the cardiac silhouette. A, Chest x-ray of a 22-year-old male who had a stab wound in the precordium. The findings are within normal except for dilatation of the azygos vein indicative of cardiac tamponade. B, It is helpful to compare with previous films when these are immediately available: the previous examination 4 months earlier shows a normal azygos vein.

THORACIC AORTA. Widening of the ascending aorta and/or the arch in a patient with chest trauma or a known disease of the aorta could be related to the sudden onset of cardiac tamponade following rupture of the proximal aorta into the pericardial sac.

NONVASCULAR ELEMENTS. Certain mediastinal tumors and pseudotumors may simulate cardiac enlargement or masses. Dilatation of the esophagus, as seen in cases of achalasia or a hiatal hernia, can produce confusing diagnostic problems as well (Fig. 14).

PULMONARY VASCULATURE. The absence of radiographic signs for left sided failure as manifested by redistribution of the pulmonary vasculature and/or pulmonary edema in the presence of a rapid increase in size of the cardiac silhouette should be considered strongly suggestive of pericardial effusion.

In some instances, pulmonary congestion due to left sided failure and pericardial effusion may coexist. In such a case it will be difficult to entertain the possibility of pericardial effusion due to the overlapping of signs. In such instances, other diagnostic modalities such as ultrasonography are necessary.

In the unusual cases of constrictive pericarditis affecting mainly the pulmonary veins – left atrium area, one may see a pulmonary vascular pattern similar to that of pulmonary venous hypertension due to mitral stenosis.

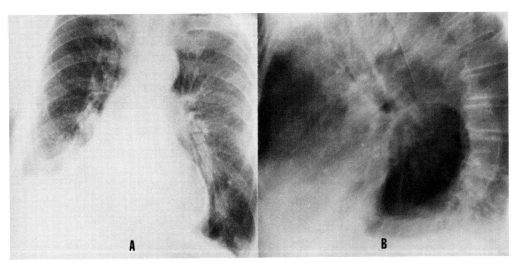

Figure 14. Apparent hydropneumopericardium due to hiatal hernia. A, The frontal roentgenogram of an elderly female shows a radiolucency with a fluid level superimposed on the heart resembling hydropneumopericardium. The upper margins of the air do not follow the normal pericardial reflections. B, For confirmation, the lateral examination reveals the gaseous distention of the herniated gastric fundus posterior to the heart.

Fluoroscopy

Cardiac fluoroscopy with an image intensifier can provide contributory information regarding pericardial disease.[18] Fluoroscopy is used as a standard noninvasive procedure or as part of special procedures such as angiography and pericardiocentesis.

As a standard procedure, fluoroscopic findings may be considered doubtful due to the subjectivity involved. For this reason, it is recommended that the fluoroscopic examination be recorded by means of video tape, cine, or spot filming techniques. Three major findings should be looked for: character of cardiac pulsations, localization of the epicardial fat, and pericardial calcification.

Cardiac Pulsations

It has been taught through the years, that when fluoroscopy shows an enlarged cardiac contour which pulsates poorly, the so-called "large quiet heart," pericardial effusion should be suspected. Such finding, however, is not specific since it may be observed in patients with marked cardiomegaly associated with limited myocardial contractility or in the presence of arrhythmias such as atrial fibrillation.

In cases of constrictive pericarditis, diminished pulsations will be present in association with a normal sized cardiac contour.

Fluoroscopic observation should not be limited to the heart alone, but it should include observations in the changes of size of the superior vena cava and the azygos vein from the upright to the supine positions. Similar changes should be observed by comparison during inspiration and expiration, as well as with the Valsalva maneuver.[33]

The Epicardial Fat

With optimal positioning of the patient and with the help of collimation, the epicardial fat should be seen in most patients. The increased distance of the epicardial fat from the pericardial fat plane and the active motion of the epicardial fat against a motionless pericardial margin strongly suggest pericardial effusion. When the coronary arteries are calcified, it is also possible to see the corresponding branch running along the plane of the epicardial fat, which is a helpful observation.

Pericardial Calcification

There are two main situations in which fluoroscopy becomes very important. First, a small area of calcification in the heart in general and in particular in the pericardium may not be demonstrated on plain chest roentgenograms. Consequently, the presence of pericardial calcification can not be excluded until fluoroscopy is performed.[17] Second, when the distribution of the pericardial calcification is rather atypical, such as in

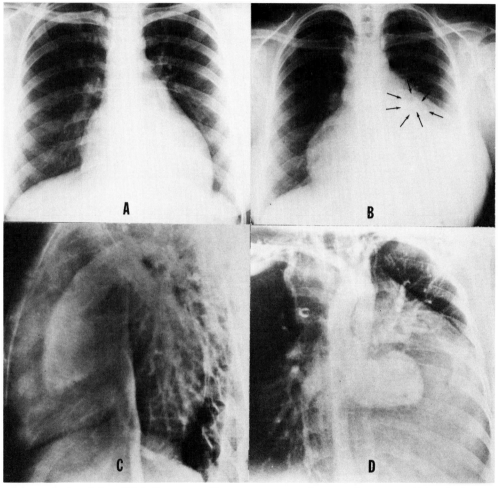

Figure 15. Pericardial ossifying fibroma. A, Chest roentgenogram in 1959 of a 20-year-old female shows a minimally enlarged cardiac silhouette. B, Followup examination in 1962 reveals massive enlargement of the cardiac silhouette indicating pericardial effusion. The arrows point to an irregular triangular area of calcification which moves with cardiac pulsations on fluoroscopy. C, Lateral view of the dextroangiocardiographic phase demonstrates pericardial effusion. D, Frontal view in the levoangiocardiographic phase confirms the massive pericardial effusion. Note that the calcification is located in the vicinity of the insertion of the left lower lobe vein to the left atrium. At surgery, the pericardial fluid was a transudate; and the irregular calcification, which was found to be partially adherent to the epicardial surface of the left atrium and the adventitial layer of the left lower lobe pulmonary vein, was an ossifying fibroma.

cases of calcification around the left atrium, or there is difficulty localizing an area of calcification that may be intramyocardial or at any other plane, fluoroscopy is essential. By placing the patient in different angles in relation to the x-ray beam during fluoroscopy, it is possible to determine the localization of such calcification (Fig. 15).

Laminography

Radiographic sectional studies of the heart may be used in order to confirm the presence, localization and distribution of calcification.[4]

In spite of recent technical improvement in the use of laminography in other areas of the body, it is generally not a practical procedure in cardiac radiology. It is a time consuming examination, lacking of any dynamic information, and may lead to erroneous interpretation when improperly performed. For these reasons and because of the recent development of more reliable studies, laminography for pericardial problems has a limited role in modern radiology (Fig. 16).

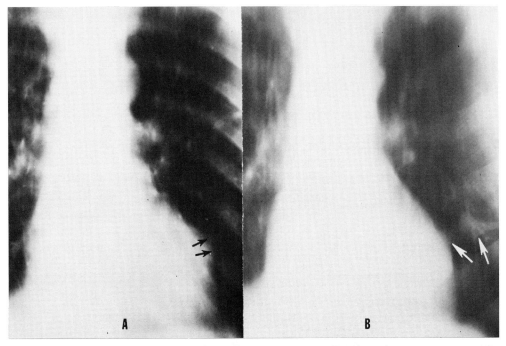

Figure 16. Pleuropericarditis simulating left ventricular aneurysm. A, Previous chest roentgenogram of a middle aged male as well as a laminographic study demonstrate an unusual bulge of the left ventricular aneurysm (black arrows) without clinical or electrocardiographic confirmation of a myocardial infarction. Cardiac fluoroscopy showed no abnormality in cardiac pulsations but there was retraction of the pericardium at the area of abnormality with respiratory maneuvers. B, Further laminographic examination demonstrates tenting of the pericardium merging with patchy fibrosis of the adjacent pleura (white arrows).

Kymography

This is not a widely used radiographic technique at the present time, but it offers certain advantages in recording pulsations of the heart and great vessels. Thus, a permanent film recording of diminished or absent cardiac pulsations in cases of pericardial effusion and constrictive pericarditis can be obtained for future comparative studies. Also, the cardiac pulsations can be analyzed and compared in better detail than with fluoroscopy (Fig. 17).

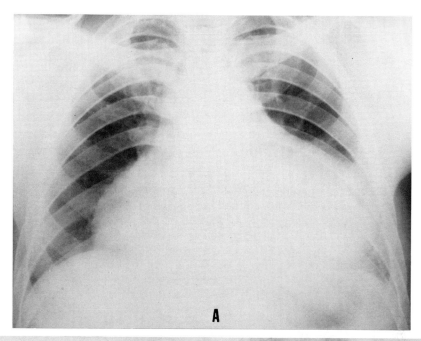

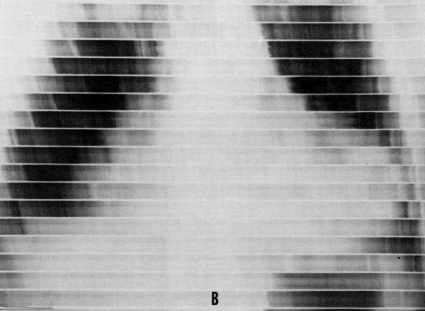

Figure 17. Kymography for pericardial effusion. A, Chest roentgenogram of a 28-year-old male demonstrates massive enlarged cardiac silhouette with a flask configuration. B, Kymography demonstrates absence of pulsations at the borders of the enlarged cardiac silhouette.

Intercalative Chest Roentgenograms

This is another radiographic method to study the pulsations of the heart and great arteries which also has been replaced by other diagnostic examinations.

Two separate radiographic exposures of the patient's chest are done in the frontal projection with the aid of electrocardiographic gating: one is taken during ventricular systole and the other during diastole. By superimposition of both films, a third film is obtained. By analyzing the cardiac contour in this intercalative roentgenogram, it is possible to evaluate the changes in configuration and size of the cardiac silhouette during the cardiac cycle.[15] In the presence of pericardial effusion, very little or no change at all will be registered. Once again, this is not a specific sign by itself.

Echocardiography

One of the most common requests in our department for echocardiography is the evaluation of patients with the clinical suspicion of pericardial effusion. The ultrasound evaluation of cardiac patients is noninvasive and can be readily performed in the department as well as at the bedside. The study can be repeated for the analytic progress of the pericardial effusion. The echocardiographic diagnosis of pericardial effusion is dependent on the visualization of a sonolucent space separating the ventricular wall motions from a nonmoving pericardial echo.[7]

The technique of examination is done by positioning the ultrasound transducer at the left parasternal fourth interspace to localize the mitral valve. The transducer is then angled laterally and slightly inferiorly in the direction of the left ventricular apex.

The posterior border of the heart is the moving echo of the left ventricular wall. It is characterized by a weak internal echo (the endocardium) and a stronger echo (the epicardium). These echoes move together anteriorly in systole and posteriorly in diastole. The diffuse lung echoes are seen directly behind the heart in normal patients.

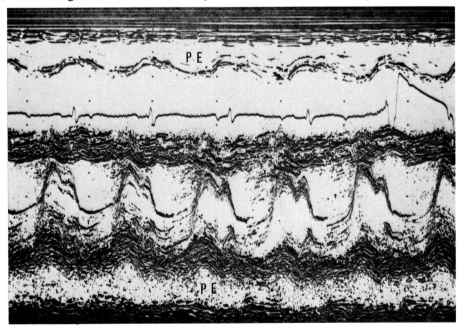

Figure 18. Echocardiography. M-mode examination at the left parasternal fourth interspace with the ultrasound transducer directed through the mitral valve demonstrates an echo-free space anterior to the right ventricle and similar findings posterior to the left ventricle indicative of moderate pericardial effusion.

108

When pericardial effusion exists, the fluid splits the moving echo of the left ventricle from the lung as the pericardial fluid gravitates behind the left ventricle in the supine position when the patient is examined. Gross quantification of pericardial effusion is possible but accurate determination is not feasible. Minimal effusion occurs when a sonolucent space is seen behind the left ventricle in ventricular systole. As the fluid increases, the sonolucent space widens and is seen both in systole and diastole. The moderate pericardial effusion envelopes the entire heart so that a sonolucent space is also seen anteriorly separating the anterior chest wall and the frontal surface of the right ventricle. Severe pericardial effusion provides a further extension of the aforementioned findings (Fig. 18).

It has been proven in animal experimentation that the diagnostic accuracy of the ultrasonic method is better than the intracardiac carbon dioxide or nuclear medicine examinations.[3] However, the accuracy in clinical studies is less certain as there are false positives to reckon with such as pulmonary infiltrates and masses, left pleural effusion, and poor technique.[10, 11, 23, 29]

Hence, refinements in the diagnosis of pericardial effusion have come into clinical use with the accumulation of experience in the usage of echocardiography. One such method is to reduce the sensitivity of the ultrasound by 7 to 10 decibels after delineation of the left ventricular wall. This is a method to better show the strong epicardial echo of the left ventricle through an anechoic fluid with demonstration of the parietal pericardium in front of the lung.

One of the better ways to demonstrate pericardial effusion is by obtaining a continuous recording from the left ventricular apex through the mitral valve to the aortic root, the so-called mitral-aortic trace. This will enable detection of pericardial effusion behind the left ventricle and stopping short at the left atrial wall. This confirms the anatomic pericardial attachments discussed earlier (Fig. 19).

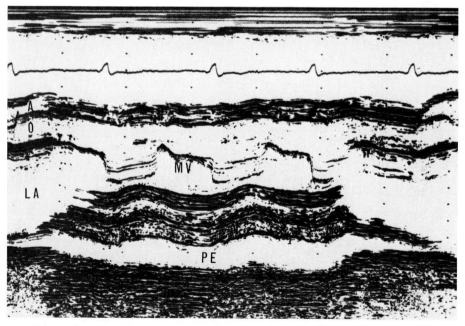

Figure 19. Echocardiography. Ultrasound examination at the left parasternal fourth interspace with the transducer directed for an aorto-mitral-aortic continuous recording demonstrates an echo-free space posterior to the left ventricle disappearing towards the left atrium indicative of minimal pericardial effusion. The dilated left atrium and right ventricle are due to congestive failure.

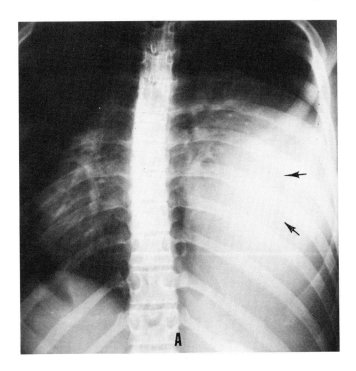

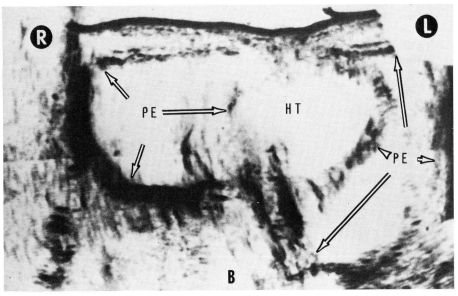

Figure 20. Echocardiography. B-scan of the heart. A, Chest roentgenogram of a 15-year-old female demonstrates a mass density in the lower two-thirds of the left chest which merges with the heart. There is also a rounded density in the right chest similarly merging with the heart. Note a curved band of lucency indicating the position of the epicardial fat at the interventricular groove. B, B-scan of the chest shows a fluid density surrounding the heart including a wide separation of the heart from the diaphragm. Because of the bizarre presentation, exploratory thoracotomy was performed and revealed massive pericardial effusion of undetermined etiology.

Another method is an unorthodox technique. This is accomplished by placing the transducer in the right supraclavicular or sternal notch with the ultrasound beam directly inferiorly to study the diaphragmatic surface of the heart.[12]

The previously described methods of echocardiographic detection of pericardial effusion were undertaken previously by A-mode and are currently practiced by the M-mode recording. B-scanning of the heart has gained some acceptance in the larger medical centers. In most instances, this latter method requires cardiac gating to obviate the blurring motion of the heart. With further advancement in electronics, a few centers are using real time ultrasound utilizing multielement transducers in the evaluation of cardiac patients (Fig. 20).

Pericardiocentesis was previously done at the bedside or occasionally with fluoroscopic guidance. Now, the pericardial puncture is done with ultrasound guidance by using a special doughnut transducer where a needle can be inserted through the center. In this manner, the appropriate depth of needle insertion can be ascertained as well as the determination of recession of the pericardial fluid so that the needle may be withdrawn appropriately (Fig. 21).

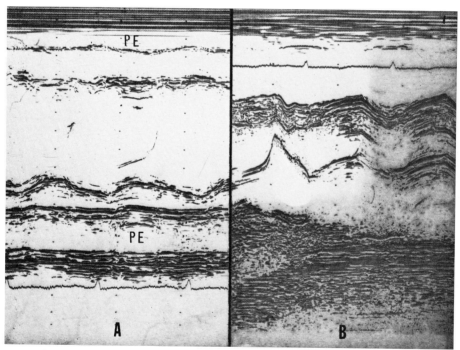

Figure 21. Echocardiography. A, Ultrasound detection of moderate pericardial effusion is evidenced by anterior and posterior echo-free spaces. B, Followup examination with a mitral-aortic trace shows regression to normal after pericardiocentesis performed by ultrasound guidance.

INVASIVE INVESTIGATIONS

Radioisotopic Examination

For almost two decades, radiopharmaceutical substances have been used for the diagnosis of pericardial effusion. In the early years, serum albumin labeled radioactive iodide was used. Then, indium-113m bound to transferrin in vivo was employed in some centers. In recent years, technetium-99m bound to serum albumin or techne-tium-99m pertechnetate are the radioactive substances more commonly used by intravenous injection. The two basic modalities of examination depend on the isotopic determination of the intracardiac blood pool.

Blood Pool Scan

The most commonly used type of examination utilizes the graphic summation of the isotopic image of the intracardiac blood pool which is compared to or approximately superimposed on the cardiac silhouette as demonstrated on a chest roentgenogram.[1, 25] Other major points of observation are the "cold area" between the inferior surface of the intracardiac blood pool and the superior margin of the blood pool of the liver, as well as the lateral borders of the intracardiac blood pool and the pericardial margins of the pulmonary blood pool (Fig. 22).

By this technique, pericardial effusion can be diagnosed when the intracardiac blood pool is less than 80 percent of the roentgenographic area of the cardiac silhouette and a clear separation is observed between the intracardiac blood pool and the superior margin of the liver.[2]

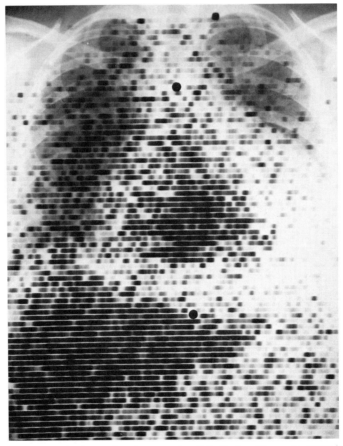

Figure 22. Radioisotopic scan for free and moderate pericardial effusion. The nuclear scan is superimposed on a chest roentgenogram. Note the "cold area" surrounding the "hot" blood pool within the cardiac chambers; the distribution of pericardial fluid is similar to the illustration of pericardiography and angiocardiography. The increased thickness between the liver and heart is one criterion for pericardial effusion.

The diagnostic accuracy of this technique has been questioned. Small amounts of minimal pericardial effusion are hardly diagnosed. Many false positive and false negative interpretations have been made because of suboptimal quality of studies which are related to technical difficulties in most instances.

Radioisotopic Angiocardiography

More favorable results are obtained with the use of a gamma camera with a special scintiphotography system.[19] This modality allows sequential serial documentation of the cardiac events. Although the signs of pericardial effusion are similar to those obtained with the aforementioned method, this technique offers several advantages in the evaluation of pericardial effusion with the use of technetium-99m pertechnetate. The images are sharper as the problem of respiratory and cardiac movements are minimized. The findings of pericardial effusion are confirmed in the left heart phase and the circulation time can also be determined (Fig. 23).

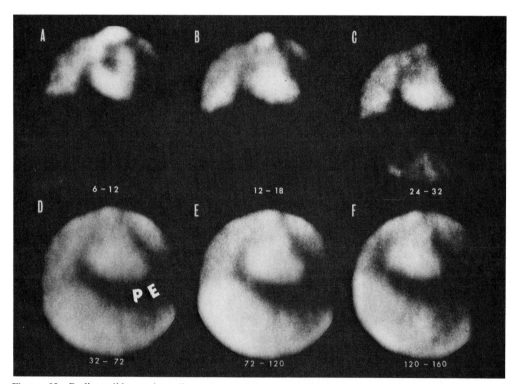

Figure 23. Radionuclide angiocardiography. Serial scans after intravenous injection of 10 mc. of technetium-99m pertechnetate show pericardial effusion.

Angiocardiography

The basic principle of angiocardiography is to determine the distance between the endocardial surface of a cardiac chamber (as demonstrated by injecting a radionegative or radiopaque contrast material) and its adjacent pericardial-pleural lung interface.

The right atrial wall has a normal measurement of 2 to 3 mm. A demonstration of 5 to 10 mm. thickness is usually due to pericardial thickening and/or minimal pericardial

113

effusion. Any increase beyond 10 mm. is certainly due to pericardial fluid inasmuch as pericardial thickening of 10 mm. or more is a rare occurrence. Obviously, there are cases with borderline figures which are exceptions to the rule.

Pericardial disease can also be confirmed in the levophase of the frontal angiocardiogram. Proper allowance must be made for the normal thickness of the left ventricle (10 mm.) or for left ventricular hypertrophy resulting from known underlying pathology. If a lateral angiocardiogram is done, similar observations may be made on the posterior aspect of the left ventricle. In addition, one may refer to the normal retrosternal right ventricular thickness of 6 mm. All ventricular measurements must be made only in ventricular diastole.

Capnoangiocardiography

During the rapid intravenous injection of 60 to 100 ml. of pure carbon dioxide gas into the left antecubital vein of the patient, the right heart border is radiographed by rapid serial filming in the left lateral decubitus position (the patient's right side is up) using a horizontal x-ray beam.[26]

There are some important features of this procedure. Possible complications inherent to iodinated contrast material are avoided. The examination is accomplished in a relatively short time by a simple injection through a vein puncture without additional discomfort to the patient (Figs. 24 and 25).

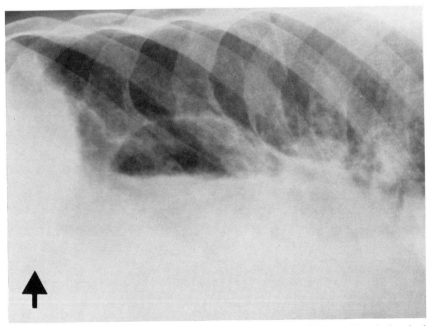

Figure 24. Normal capnoangiocardiogram. Examination in left lateral decubitus position during the injection of pure carbon dioxide gas into a left antecubital vein demonstrates the radiolucent superior vena cava leading into the right atrium which shows the blood fluid level. The "right atrial thickness" is normal (less than 5 mm.) and is comprised of the combined thickness of the right atrial wall (endocardium, myocardium, epicardium), parietal pericardium, and pericardial pleura.

One of the most common causes of *false-positive* studies is related to the failure of recognition of a right pleural effusion overlying the right border during filming. For this reason, the presence of right pleural effusion should be determined by careful analysis

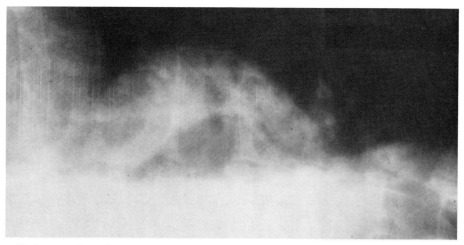

Figure 25. Capnoangiocardiogram. A moderate degree of pericardial effusion is demonstrated by injection of 60 cc. of pure carbon dioxide gas into a left antecubital vein and x-rays taken with the patient in left lateral decubitus position.

of the preliminary films. Other less common sources of false-positive results have been the use of the pericardial fat around the right cardiophrenic angle or the margin of an enlarged left atrium as the outer point of measurement. The presence of right atrial thrombi and mediastinal masses have been reported to produce similar wrong interpretations (Figs. 26 and 27).

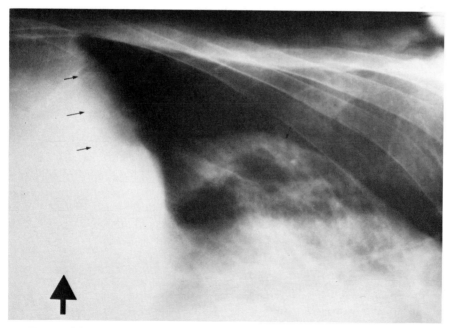

Figure 26. False-positive capnoangiocardiogram. The study can be quickly mistaken as a positive study for pericardial effusion. On closer inspection the effusion is pleural in nature (note the arrows showing the "fluid meniscus" seen through the diaphragm which makes an angled direction indicating free fluid trapped in the area of the pericardial pleura adjacent to the right atrial border). The peak of free pericardial effusion should parallel the dome of the right atrium.

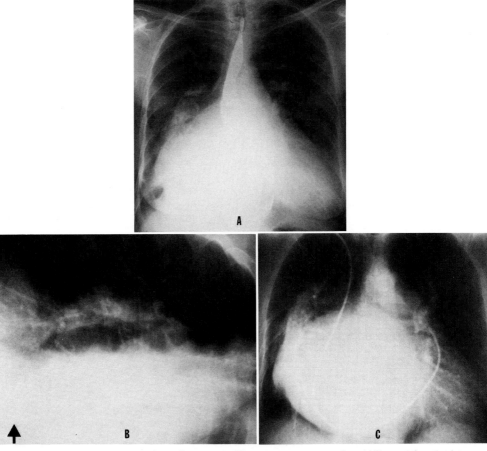

Figure 27. False-positive capnoangiocardiogram. A, Chest roentgenogram of a middle aged female shows an enlarged cardiac silhouette due to rheumatic mitral valvar insufficiency. B, Capnoangiocardiogram was performed to rule out pericardial effusion. Note the apparent "thick right atrial wall" which usually indicates pericardial effusion. However, the lateral margin of the heart is the left atrium. C, The problem is solved by the catheter position in the right atrium and contrast angiocardiography which delineates the left atrium.

False-negative results are less frequently observed and are most likely related to improper technique. There is also the possibility of missing a small effusion with fluid accumulation in the dependent portions of the pericardial cavity attributable to the patient's position at the time of examination.

Standard Angiocardiography

The conventional examination is performed by the rapid injection of 50 to 60 ml. of radioiodinated contrast material into a systemic vein through a large bore needle or into the right atrial cavity through a multiple hole transvenous catheter. Corresponding dosage adjustment should be made for pediatric patients. Sequential opacification of the right cardiac chambers, pulmonary vasculature, left chambers, and the aorta is made by single or biplane rapid filming.

This approach offers an immediate advantage. During fluoroscopy, the catheter tip is placed against the lateral aspect of the right atrial endocardial surface. The distance between the catheter tip and the adjacent pericardial pleura is evaluated by simple fluoroscopic observation or film recording.

On angiocardiography, the degree, extension and distribution of the pericardial fluid can be evaluated by criteria previously mentioned.[31] Moreover, the diagnosis of clinically unsuspected pericardial effusion can be made, as was experienced by the authors in two patients undergoing angiocardiography for pulmonary embolism.

In addition to the determination of the presence or absence of pericardial fluid, careful attention should be given to the configuration of the opacified right atrial cavity.[30] In the supine position, the normal outer convex margin of the right atrium is preserved in both ventricular systole and diastole. However, in cases of effusion with mild cardiac tamponade there may be straightening of the right atrial margin in ventricular diastole, and with severe cardiac tamponade there is inward concavity of this outer margin in both systole and diastole. Furthermore, there is dilatation of the superior vena cava superior to the pericardial attachment with reflux into the azygos vein. There may be active opacification of the inferior vena cava and hepatic veins similar to that of tricuspid insufficiency, except that the opacification is seen during ventricular systole with tricuspid insufficiency. The overall transit of contrast material through the heart may be delayed (Figs. 28 and 29).

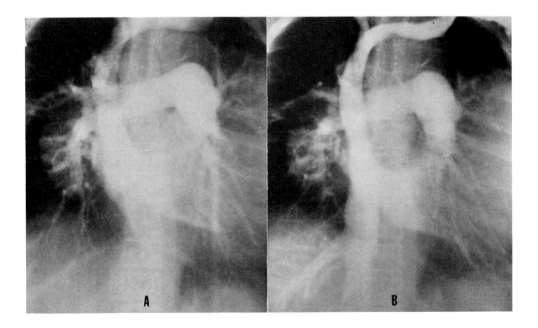

Figure 28. Angiocardiography for minimal cardiac tamponade. A, Dextroangiocardiographic phase in *atrial diastole* from a venous injection shows pericardial effusion. The contour of the right atrium shows normal convexity which parallels that of pericardial effusion. B, In *atrial systole*, the right atrial contour is flattened and the blood is driven to the inferior vena cava and hepatic veins. The progression of blood flow through the cardiac chambers is minimally delayed.

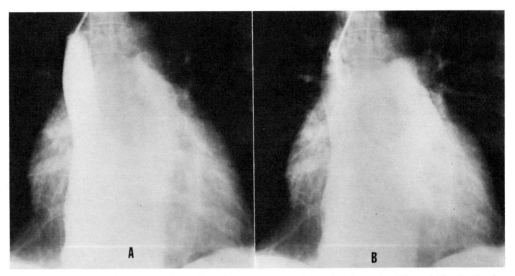

Figure 29. Severe cardiac tamponade. A, Superior vena cava angiography shows the right atrial border having a concavity instead of the normal convexity seen during ventricular systole due to pericardial effusion under tension. B, In ventricular diastole, the right atrial concavity does not change which is contrary to normal physiology.

In constrictive pericarditis, the extraluminal distance adjacent to the opacified right atrial cavity due to pericardial thickening usually measures no more than 10 mm. There is straightening of the lateral margin of the right atrial cavity and the superior vena cava which does not angiographically change in multiple films.[8]

In certain difficult cases, capnoangiocardiography and standard angiocardiography have been used as complementary procedures in order to establish the difference between simple pericardial thickening and effusion. If the abnormally increased pericardial space changes in contour and size as seen in several films in both examinations, pericardial fluid rather than thickening should be considered (Fig. 30).

Diagnostic Pericardiography

Pericardial aspiration is performed as a therapeutic life-saving procedure in cases of cardiac tamponade. Pericardiocentesis is also a diagnostic adjunct in the diagnosis of pericarditis or pericardial effusion by the physical evaluation and laboratory analysis of the pericardial aspirate.

Just before the needle is withdrawn, it is the opportune time to inject contrast material into the pericardial cavity. By pericardiography one is able to analyze the thickness and smoothness of the pericardium. The presence of adhesions, irregularities, or masses can be demonstrated.[9] Furthermore, the true cardiac size can be evaluated.

Thus, pericardiography offers important information related to abnormalities of the pericardium such as furnishing clues toward the possible etiology of the process, the degree and extent of pericardial involvement and compromise of the cardiac status. Such information together with the laboratory results of the aspirated fluid should afford an accurate pathophysiologic evaluation and diagnosis of the pericardial disorder.

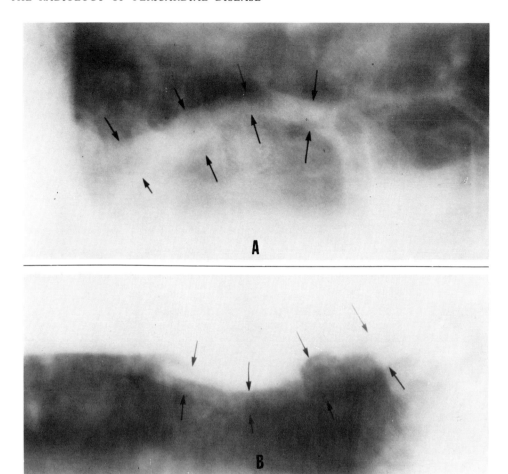

Figure 30. Angiocardiographic diagnosis of pericardial thickening. A, Capnoangiocardiogram in left lateral decubitus position demonstrates increased thickness of the "right atrial wall" which may signify minimal pericardial effusion or pericardial thickening. B, Complementary angiocardiography with radiopaque contrast medium in right lateral decubitus position shows essentially similar findings. The change in position of the patient usually shifts the free fluid by gravitational action within the pericardial cavity whereas pericardial thickening as illustrated in this case is not altered by positional change of the patient.

Pneumopericardiography

Whenever possible, pericardiocentesis should be performed where radiologic facilities are available. It affords the advantages offered by fluoroscopic and/or ultrasound guided needle insertion. In this way, roentgenograms can be immediately obtained after the pneumopericardium has been completed (Figs. 31 and 32).

Utilizing the physical principle of buoyancy of gases, the patient is placed in different body positions interplayed with vertical and horizontal roentgenographic filming. The injected air (½ to ⅔ of the volume withdrawn from the pericardial cavity) should move within the pericardial space allowing radiographic investigation of multiple areas of the pericardium.

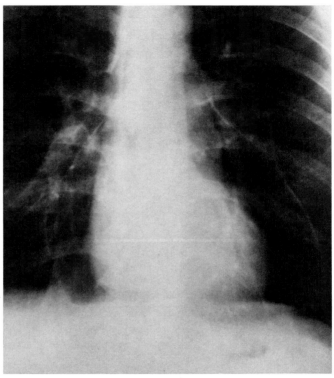

Figure 31. Diagnostic pneumopericardium for chylothorax. Pericardiocentesis for pericardial effusion revealed chylous fluid. Air should be introduced after extraction of pericardial fluid in order to analyze the nature of the pericardium. In this case, the pericardium is uniformly thin, revealing an enlarged pericardial sac with minimal fluid at the diaphragmatic area. Note the normal heart size and shape. A successful outcome followed pericardiectomy for treatment of the chylothorax after an unsuccessful medical regimen.

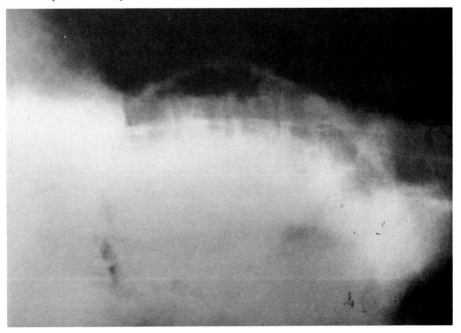

Radiopaque Pericardiography

Similar to angiocardiography, liquid radioiodinated contrast material can be injected into the pericardial sac. After pericardiocentesis, a small volume (up to 30 cc.) of Renografin 60 is injected which becomes diluted with residual pericardial fluid and allows visualization of the pericardial sac by roentgenographic examination. The contrast medium is heavier than pericardial fluid and one must therefore utilize this gravitational property to distinct advantage by positional radiography with horizontal and vertical x-ray exposures (Fig. 33).

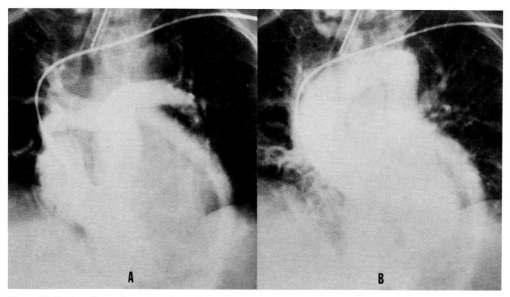

Figure 33. Pericardiography and angiocardiography. A, Dextroangiocardiographic phase demonstrates a thin layer of pericardial fluid with contrast medium surrounding the normal contour of the right atrium. There is more fluid at the diaphragmatic surface of the right ventricle. B, Levoangiocardiographic phase shows most of the pericardial effusion just lateral to the left ventricle. The thickness of the right atrium, right ventricle, and left ventricle are shown as a radiolucency in normal increasing proportion between the intracardiac and pericardial contrast. The contours and motions of the cardiac chambers as well as the normal timing of progression of blood flow indicated no evidence of cardiac tamponade.

One of the drawbacks of conventional pericardiography is the recurrence of cardiac tamponade. Pericardial effusion with cardiac tamponade is only transiently relieved with pericardiocentesis but it recurs because the volume of pericardial fluid withdrawn has been replaced by a similar volume of soluble contrast material. One must therefore be careful that the volume of injectate is considerably less than that of the pericardial aspirate. In addition, the injectate is hyperosmolar and will tend to increase fluid accumulation by diffusion and permeation of tissue fluids through the pericardial membranes. Although unproven, the direct chemical irritation of the contrast material and hypersensitivity reaction may be additional factors.

◄ **Figure 32.** Diagnostic pneumopericardium. The examination of the chest in left lateral decubitus position with injection of air after a pericardiocentesis demonstrates a thickened parietal pericardium. The margins of epicardial surface of the right atrium is hazy and shaggy with minimal similar changes of the parietal surface. *Staphylococcus aureus* was cultured from the purulent pericardial exudate. (Courtesy of Dr. Otoniel R. Sullesta)

Double Contrast Pericardiography

On occasion, it is worthwhile to inject a small amount of radioiodinated water soluble contrast material followed by injection of room air into the pericardial sac. This is particularly helpful in instances of combined pericardial effusion and adhesions.

Diagnostic Pneumothorax

This procedure may be performed to confirm the diagnosis of congenital pericardial defects. After injecting a large volume of air into the pleural space, the patient is placed in lateral decubitus position with the injected side on the table surface and roentgenograms are taken with a horizontal beam. The air will distribute toward the pericardial pleura and produce a pneumopericardium with the air trapped in the contralateral pericardium since there is a defect of the ipsilateral parietal pericardium. The inability to produce a pneumopericardium by this examination, however, does not rule out the diagnosis of congenital pericardial defect as adhesions may have occurred to seal off the defect (Fig. 34).

An uncommon indication for this procedure is pericardial cyst. The performance of a diagnostic pneumothorax helps in distinguishing whether the mass lesion is pleural or pericardial in nature.

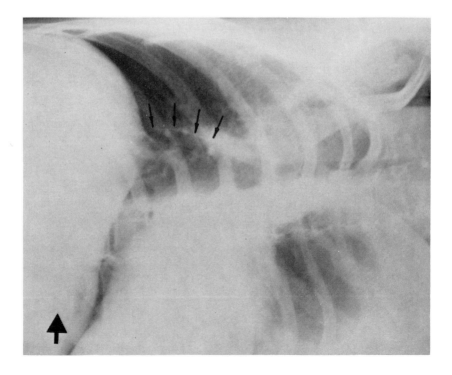

Figure 34. Diagnostic pneumothorax. Chest x-ray taken in the left lateral decubitus position after a diagnostic pneumothorax demonstrates a pneumopericardium which is diagnostic of a left sided congenital pericardial defect. The air is trapped by an intact and normal right pericardium. If there is a defect on the right, a right pneumothorax will be seen as well. (Courtesy of Dr. John P. Tampas)

REFERENCES

1. BONTE, F. J., AND CURRY, T. S.: *The radioisotope blood pool scan.* Am. J. Roentgenol. 96:690, 1966.

2. BURCH, G. E., AND PHILLIPS, J. H.: *Methods in the diagnostic differentiation of myocardial dilatation from pericardial effusion.* Am. Heart J. 64:266, 1962.

3. CHRISTENSEN, E. E., AND BONTE, F. J.: *The relative accuracy of echocardiography, intravenous CO_2 studies and blood pool scanning in detecting pericardial effusion in dogs.* Radiology 9:265, 1968.

4. DAVIES, P., AND BUCKY, N. L.: *Tomography of calcified aortic and mitral valves.* Br. Heart J. 21:17, 1959.

5. DICKSON, D. S. P., AND GIRLING-BUTCHER, M.: *Spontaneous pneumopericardium.* N. Z. Med. J. 59:250, 1960.

6. DIMICH, I., GROSSMAN, H., BOWMAN, F. O., JR., ET AL.: *Congenital absence of the left pericardium.* Am. J. Dis. Child. 110:309, 1965.

7. FEIGENBAUM, H.: *Echocardiographic diagnosis of pericardial effusion.* Circulation 35:358, 1967.

8. FIGLEY, M. M., AND BAGSHAW, M. A.: *Angiocardiographic aspects of constrictive pericarditis.* Radiology 69:46, 1957.

9. FUSON, R. L., SEIM, D. E., AND LESTER, R. G.: *Intrapericardial mesothelioma: interesting radiologic findings on pneumopericardium. Report of a case.* Dis. Chest 51:554, 1967.

10. GOLDBERG, B. B., OSTRUM, B. J., AND ISARD, H. J.: *Ultrasonic determination of pericardial effusion.* J.A.M.A. 202:103, 1967.

11. GOLDSCHLAGER, A. W., FREEMAN, L. M., AND DAVIS, P. J.: *Pericardial effusions and echocardiography: false results with ultrasound reflection method.* N. Y. State J. Med. 67:1854, 1967.

12. GRAMIAK, R., AND SHAH, P. M.: *Cardiac ultrasonography. A review of current applications.* Radiol. Clin. N. Am. 9:469, 1971.

13. HERING, A. C., WILSON, J. S., AND BALL, R. E., JR.: *Congenital deficiency of the pericardium.* J. Thorac. Cardiovasc. Surg. 40:49, 1960.

14. HIPONA, F. A., AND CRUMMY, A. B., JR.: *Congenital pericardial defect associated with tetralogy of Fallot: herniation of normal lung into the pericardial cavity.* Circulation 29:132, 1964.

15. HIPONA, F. A., AND GREENSPAN, R. H.: *Intercalative chest roentgenography.* Radiology 82:304, 1964.

16. HIPONA, F. A., AND PAREDES, S.: *The radiology evaluation of patients with chest trauma: cardiovascular system.* Med. Clin. N. Am. 59:65, 1975.

17. JORGENS, J., BLANK, N., AND WILCOX, W. A.: *Cinefluorographic detection of calcifications in heart.* Radiology 74:550, 1960.

18. JORGENS, J., KUNDEL, R., AND LIEBER, A.: *The cinefluorographic approach to the diagnosis of pericardial effusion.* Am. J. Roentgenol. 87:911, 1962.

19. KRISS, J. P.: *Diagnosis of pericardial effusion by radioisotopic angiocardiography.* J. Nucl. Med. 10:233, 1969.

20. LANE, E. J., JR., AND CARSKY, E. W.: *Epicardial fat: Lateral plain film analysis in normals and in pericardial effusion.* Radiology 91:1, 1968.

21. LULL, G. F., JR.: *Pericardial celomic cyst. A reevaluation.* Radiology 71:534, 1958.

22. MAIER, H. C.: *Diverticulum of the pericardium with observations on mode of development.* Circulation 16:1040, 1957.

23. MOSS, A. J., AND BRUHN, B. L.: *The echocardiogram: an ultrasound technique for the detection of pericardial effusion.* N. Engl. J. Med. 274:380, 1966.

24. NETTER, F. H.: *The Ciba collection of medical illustrations: Heart.* 5:4, 1969.

25. O'MALLIE, L. P., LOVE, W. D., AND BURCH, G. E.: *Differentiation of massive pericardial effusion from cardiac dilatation using I ^{131} albumin.* Am. Heart J. 62:453, 1961.

26. PAUL, R. E., DURANT, T. M., OPPENHEIMER, M. J., ET AL.: *Intravenous carbon dioxide for intracardiac gas contrast in roentgen diagnosis of pericardial effusion and thickening.* Am. J. Roentgenol. 78:224, 1957.

27. PLUM, G. E., BRUWER, A. J., AND CLAGETT, D. T.: *Chronic constrictive pericarditis. Roentgenologic findings in 35 surgically proved cases.* Proc. Staff Meet. Mayo Clin. 32:555, 1957.

28. ROGERS, J. V., JR., AND LEIGH, T. F.: *Differential diagnosis of right cardiophrenic angle masses.* Radiology 61:871, 1953.

29. ROTHMAN, J., CHASE, N. E., KRISCHEFF, J. J., ET AL: *Ultrasonic diagnosis of pericardial effusion.* Circulation 35:358, 1967.

30. SPITZ, H. B., AND HOLMES, J. C.: *Right atrial contour in cardiac tamponade.* Radiology 103:69, 1972.

31. STEINBERG, I., VON GAL, H., AND FINBY, N.: *Roentgen diagnosis of pericardial effusion.* Am. J. Roentgen. 79:321, 1958.

32. TABAKIN, B. S., HANSON, J. S., TAMPAS, J. P., ET AL: *Congenital absence of the left pericardium.* Am. J. Roentgenol. 94:122, 1965.

33. WHITLEY, J. E., AND MARTIN, J. F.: *The Valsalva maneuver in roentgenologic diagnosis.* Am. J. Roentgenol. 91:291, 1964.

Echocardiography in the Diagnosis of Pericardial Effusion

Pravin M. Shah, M.D., and Navin C. Nanda, M.D.

Clinical syndromes associated with pericardial effusion are varied. A large effusion may be present in a relatively asymptomatic patient, whereas a smaller collection of fluid may be associated with severe cardiac restriction and low output state. A major determinant of clinical presentation is rate of fluid accumulation. Once the steep portion of pressure volume curve in the pericardial sac is reached, a small further addition of fluid is often life threatening. Treatment, generally under emergency conditions, consists of pericardiocentesis. This is, however, not a benign procedure; hence the need for a quick and accurate diagnosis.

Rapid developments in the diagnostic applications of echocardiography have supplanted other methods such as intravenous injection of carbon dioxide or intra-atrial injection of contrast material. Edler, who is responsible for much of the pioneering work in diagnostic ultrasound, appreciated its potential application in diagnosis of pericardial effusion.[1] However, it remained for Feigenbaum to demonstrate by a systematic study the usefulness of echocardiography in this condition.[2] Several studies then followed confirming this role.[3-6]

ECHOCARDIOGRAPHIC PRINCIPLES AND TECHNIQUES

For a detailed consideration of the principles of diagnostic ultrasound, the reader is referred to a text on the subject. Briefly, the method consists of short pulses of sound waves in frequency range of 2 to 2.5 MHz entering the precordium and being reflected at altered acoustic interfaces. A single piezoelective crystal acts as both transmitter and receiver of ultrasound in the pulse reflection technique. The electrical impulse generated by the transducer in response to returning echoes is displayed on the oscilloscope in the conventional A-mode echography display. The A-mode display presents information on depth of the returning echoes on X axis and the amplitude of the echoes reflected by their height. Intensity modulation of the echo signal is swept across an oscilloscope screen or on a physiologic recorder, providing an M-mode representation of a moving echo. In this mode, time is represented on the X axis and depth of returning echoes on the Y axis whereas intensity of the dots represents their amplitudes. Most current diagnostic ultrasound work in cardiac applications includes M-mode display and recordings.

A 2 to 2.5 MHz transducer is placed in the third, fourth, or fifth intercostal space along the left sternal border. Patient is positioned so his chest is either in supine or left lateral decubitus with an elevation of approximately 30 degrees from the horizontal.

125

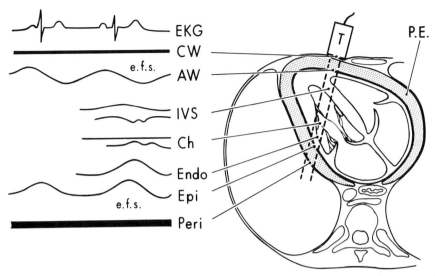

Figure 1. Schematic diagram to demonstrate echographic technique of increasing gain to show anatomic landmarks presented to the transducer beam. Abbreviations: EKG = electrocardiograms; CW = chest wall; AW anterior wall; IVS = interventricular septum; Ch = chordae tendinae; Endo = endocardium; Epi = epicardium; Peri = pericardium; T = transducer; P. E. = pericardial effusion.

The mitral valve echo is identified by its characteristic movement pattern. Inferolateral angulation of the transducer from this position allows recording of the echoes from the ventricular structures. Simultaneous recordings of echoes from the anterior heart wall, interventricular septum, mitral chordae, left ventricular posterior wall endocardium, epicardium, and pericardium constitute a technically satisfactory study (Fig. 1). The damping (attenuation) control is then abruptly increased after the optimal gain setting for the ventricular structures has been achieved. This helps to locate the strong pericardial echo. Continuous reading over several cardiac cycles with maximal damping enables clear observation of isolated pericardial movement. A slight reduction in damping then brings out the epicardium and occasionally a small separation between the posterior epicardium and pericardium may be observed. Further reduction in damping obscures this separation and allows identification of all ventricular structures. Anterior heart wall is noted to move toward and away from the chest wall with near apposition of the two in diastole.

Added modifications of the recording technique consist of lateral angulation and movement of the transducer to demonstrate separation of the lateral cardiac border from the left lung in presence of a large effusion.

CRITERIA FOR DIAGNOSIS OF PERICARDIAL EFFUSION

Accumulation of considerable free fluid in the pericardial sac results in consistent separation of the strong pericardial from the epicardial echoes creating a sonolucent space throughout cardiac cycle. Cardiac movements are dampened by the fluid and the posterior pericardium is "flat" or poorly moving (Figs. 2 and 3). This classic pattern is considered unequivocally positive for effusion. The diagnosis of pericardial effusion should not, however, generally be made without further angulation of transducer to demonstrate echo-free spaces around the cardiac chambers that are covered by pericardial reflection. Thus, an echo-free space, presumably from fluid filled transverse sinus, may also be seen between aortic root and left atrium.[7] Such an approach would

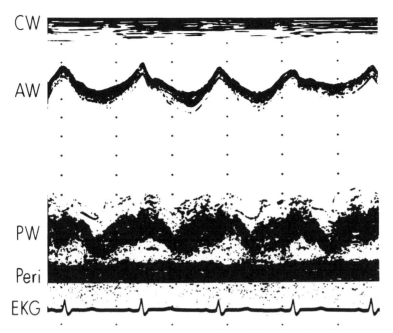

Figure 2. Anterior and posterior echo-free spaces in a patient with confirmed pericardial effusion (vertical dots denote 1 cm.). A 3 cm. space is seen between chest wall (CW) and anterior wall (AW), and a smaller space between posterior wall (PW) and non-moving pericardium (Peri).

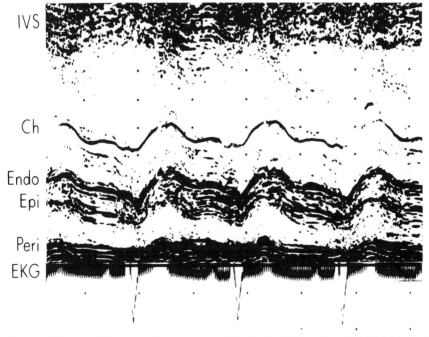

Figure 3. Echocardiogram of left ventricular structures with chordae (Ch), endocardial (Endo) and epicardial (Epi) layers of the posterior wall. An echo-free space separates the epicardium from a poorly moving pericardium (Peri).

127

avoid false positive diagnosis when other structures are responsible for localized sono-lucent areas. Horowitz and others noted this pattern of sonolucent space between epicardium and flat posterior pericardium generally in association with fluid in excess of 20 ml. measured at surgery.[8] Often the total pericardial fluid exceeded well over 100 ml. In presence of a large posterior echo-free space, an anterior separation is associated with moderate to large pericardial effusion. On the other hand an anterior echo-free space in and of itself is not diagnostic. Such a space may result from epicardial fat or some other tissue such as fibrous tissue being interposed between the heart and the chest.

Although diagnosis of pericardial effusion can be firmly made from the changes described, its quantitation is imprecise. Horowitz and others calculated the difference between cubed diameters of the pericardium and the epicardium at end diastole.[8] Subtracting volume of the heart from the total pericardial volume gave an estimate of the pericardial fluid volume: The correlation between calculated and actual measured volume at surgery was good (r = 0.98) and the standard error of the estimate was 43.7 ml. The correlation coefficient dropped to 0.41 on excluding two cases with more than 100 ml. of fluid. It was concluded that small increments in pericardial volume are poorly quantitated by this method, although gross quantitation upward of 50 ml. increments may be valid. Their findings agree with our general experience that accurate quantitation of fluid is not possible.[7]

In cases where pericardial separation from the epicardial echo was seen only in systole, no significant effusion was noted. When this extended well into, but not throughout, diastole small effusion was generally present. Complete separation with attenuated pericardial movements denotes larger effusions.

FALSE-POSITIVE DIAGNOSIS

When the criterion of clear separation of epicardium and pericardial echo is demonstrated throughout the cardiac cycle with flat or attenuated pericardial movement, false-positive diagnosis is rare. Difficulty may be observed in some patients with left pleural effusion, especially in the posterior recess. Here a moving pericardial echo may be mistaken for epicardial, and the echo-free space behind it as pericardial effusion. In some instances, a correct diagnostic clue may be provided by absence of anterior echo-free space in presence of a large posterior effusion. A repeat examination after placing a patient in left lateral decubitus may drain the fluid from retrocardiac space and provide correct diagnosis. When pleural and pericardial effusions coexist, parietal pericardium may be seen to separate the two sonolucent spaces behind the posterior left ventricular wall. As previously pointed out, a false positive diagnosis from anterior echo free space is more frequent. Similarly, posterior echo-free space has also been noted with pulmonary infiltrates or a giant left atrium.[9] Also, a medial transducer angulation may demonstrate a false-positive echo-free space.

FALSE-NEGATIVE DIAGNOSIS

It has been estimated on the basis of animal studies as well as more recent studies in man that false-negative diagnosis of pericardial effusion is extremely rare by echocardiography.[6, 8] A likely situation may be pericardial adhesions, where despite obliteration of pericardial space in some areas significant fluid accumulation may occur in others.

OTHER ECHOCARDIOGRAPHIC FEATURES

ELECTRICAL ALTERNANS. In presence of large effusions the heart may swing back and forth every alternate beat. Thus, the heart is physically nearer to the chest wall

128

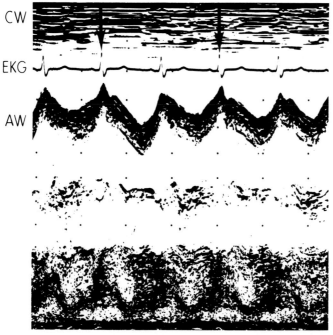

Figure 4. Electrical alternans in a patient with large pericardial effusion. The beats denoted by black arrows demonstrate a taller QRS and more anterior location of the anterior heart wall (AW) as compared to the other three beats.

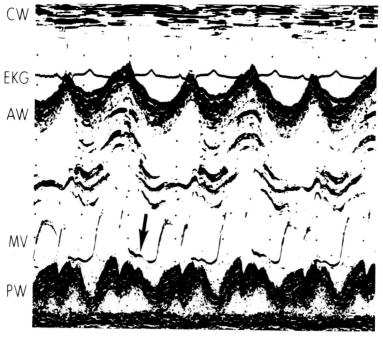

Figure 5. Simulation of mitral valve (MV) prolapse with posterior displacement of mitral valve in systole as denoted by arrow. Posterior wall (PW) has motion pattern of atrial wall resulting from transducer angulation to record mitral motion. Note extension of pericardial fluid behind the left atrial posterior wall.

129

with every other beat. This may be associated with a taller R wave as compared to beats when the heart is further from anterior chest wall. Electrical alternans generally indicates large effusions and is abolished after pericardiocentesis. Figure 4 shows an example of mild electrical alternans in a patient with large pericardial effusion.

VALVE MOVEMENTS. Since the normal motion of the heart is considerably exaggerated in presence of an effusion, this is reflected in echo display of valve motion.[10] Thus, in late systole as the heart moves posteriorly away from the transducer, mitral valve prolapse may be simulated (Fig. 5). A similar motion artefact is observed on tricuspid valve as well. Similarly, a vigorously forward moving annulus and posterior wall in early systole may simulate abnormal systolic anterior movement (SAM) of hypertrophic subaortic stenosis. Also, the semilunar valves may demonstrate motion simulating midsystolic closure. All those movement artifacts resulting from excessive motion of the heart within fluid filled pericardial sac are reversed after pericardiocentesis.

ECHOCARDIOGRAPHIC AID TO PERICARDIOCENTESIS. A recent report describes use of an echo transducer specially constructed with a hole in the center to allow passage of a needle.[11] The needle is advanced under ultrasonic guidance such that the tip can be seen to enter the anterior echo-free space. This potentially useful method may significantly reduce the risks of this procedure.

SUMMARY

Echocardiography is perhaps the most useful and accurate method of diagnosis of pericardial effusion. Its noninvasive nature and the ease with which it may be repeated make it doubly attractive. In the hands of a skilled echocardiographer, its accuracy is unequaled by other methods such as carbon dioxide injections, radionuclide angiography, and intra-atrial angiography.[12] In addition, echocardiography as an aid to safe pericardiocentesis may become widely applicable.

REFERENCES

1. EDLER, I.: *The diagnostic use of ultrasound in heart disease.* Acta Med. Scand. Suppl. 308:32, 1955.
2. FEIGENBAUM, H., WALDHAUSEN, J. A., AND HYDE, L. P.: *Ultrasound diagnosis of pericardial effusion.* J.A.M.A. 191:107, 1965.
3. MOSS, A. J., AND BRUHN, F.: *The echocardiogram. An ultrasound technic for the detection of pericardial effusion.* N. Engl. J. Med. 274:380, 1966.
4. GOLDBERG, B. B., OSTRUM, B. J., AND ISARD, J. J.: *Ultrasonic determination of pericardial effusion.* J.A.M.A. 202:103, 1967.
5. ROTHMAN, J., CHASE, N. E., KRICHEFF, I. I., ET AL.: *Ultrasonic diagnosis of pericardial effusion.* Circulation 35:358, 1967.
6. CHRISTENSEN, E., AND BONTE, F.: *The relative accuracy of echocardiography, intravenous CO_2 studies, and bloodpool scanning in detecting pericardial effusion in dogs.* Radiology 91:265, 1968.
7. GRAMIAK, R., AND SHAH, P. M.: *Cardiac ultrasonography. A review of current applications.* Radiol. Clin. N. Am. 9:469, 1971.
8. HOROWITZ, M. S., SCHULTZ, C. S., STINSON, E. B., ET AL.: *Sensitivity and specificity of echocardiographic diagnosis of pericardial effusion.* Circulation 50:239, 1974.
9. RATSHIN, R. A., SMITH, MC. K., AND HOOD, W. P., JR.: *Possible false positive diagnosis of pericardial effusion by echocardiography in the presence of large left atrium.* Chest 65:112, 1974.
10. NANDA, N. C., GRAMIAK, R., AND GROSS, C. J.: *Altered motion of cardiac valves in pericardial effusion.* Circulation 52 (Suppl. II): 528, 1975.
11. GOLDBERG, B. B., AND POLLACK, H. M.: *Ultrasonically guided pericardiocentesis.* Am. J. Cardiol. 31: 490, 1973.
12. ELLIS, K., AND KING, D. L.: *Pericarditis and pericardial effusion.* Radiol. Clin. N. Am. 11:393, 1973.

Clinical Aspects of Acute Pericarditis

Marvin Dunn, M.D., and Robert L. Rinkenberger, M.D.

INCIDENCE

It is difficult to assess the actual incidence of pericarditis because it is frequently a self-limited or an unrecognized part of a systemic disease or infection. Wartman and Hellerstein found an autopsy incidence of 2 to 6 per cent, reporting on 32 cases of acute fibrinous and 20 cases of healed pericarditis in 2000 consecutive autopsies; but this did not include uremic pericarditis or pericarditis secondary to acute myocardial infarction.[1] Other studies have reported a similar incidence,[2, 3] but clinically recognized pericarditis occurs in only about 1 in 1,000 hospital admissions.[4, 5]

The incidence of specific types of pericarditis will vary from one hospital to another depending on the patient population. For example, in hospitals with a large renal dialysis program, uremia may be the most common cause of pericarditis, whereas in small community hospitals, myocardial infarction may be the most common cause of pericarditis. Economic and geographic factors influence the incidence of rheumatic, tuberculous, and echinococcal pericarditis.[6]

Frequently, pericarditis is not recognized clinically; for example, there is a high incidence of unrecognized pericarditis associated with rheumatoid arthritis and scleroderma.[7, 8] Pericarditis complicating acute myocardial infarction is common, but often clinically unrecognized. For example, Wartman and Hellerstein found evidence of acute pericarditis in 28 percent of 111 autopsied cases, but Toole and Silverman recognized acute pericarditis in only 7.2 percent of 554 patients studied clinically.[1, 9]

Even though the incidence of bacterial pericarditis declined with the use of antibiotics, it is still seen as a consequence of septicemia, as an extension of a mediastinal or pulmonary infection, as a complication of thoracic surgery, and as a complication of impaired immune responses. Although the incidence of tuberculosis has decreased, tuberculous pericarditis still occurs in 5 to 10 percent of these patients.[10]

Common causes of acute pericarditis are acute idiopathic (23 percent), uremic (17 percent), pyogenic (16 percent), myocardial infarction (11 percent), tuberculosis (7 percent), neoplastic (8 percent), rheumatic (11 percent), traumatic (3 percent), and pericarditis associated with collagen disease (3 percent).[11] Acute idiopathic pericarditis, which is the most common cause, is probably not a single disease entity but a clinical syndrome due to viral and autoimmune mechanisms. All etiologic types of pericarditis are more common in males than in females (ratio 3:2) and less frequent in children.[12] Rheumatic and bacterial pericarditis are the most common causes of pericarditis in children, and acute bacterial pericarditis is the most common cause of cardiac tamponade in children.[13]

Acute pericarditis may be associated with a variety of acquired medical and surgical

131

diseases.[14] Since only a few disease processes affect the pericardium alone, pericarditis may be the first clue to a systemic illness.

Systemic Lupus Erythematosus

Nearly 50 percent of patients with systemic lupus erythematosus have clinical manifestations of pericarditis during the course of the disease, but at autopsy pericarditis may be present in 60 to 80 percent of cases.[15] It may be the initial sign of systemic lupus erythematosus in 2 to 4 percent of patients.

Rheumatoid Arthritis

In an autopsy series of patients with rheumatoid arthritis, 50 percent had some form of cardiac involvement.[16] Often this was not clinically apparent and until recent years remained undiagnosed during life. Using echocardiography as a diagnostic tool, pericardial effusion or thickening was found in 14 of 30 patients with rheumatoid arthritis.[8] Pericardial effusion is usually transient and generally disappears spontaneously or with steroid therapy. Acute tamponade is a rare complication of rheumatoid arthritis. There were only 20 documented cases and the majority of these had severe rheumatoid arthritis.[17] Pericarditis is rarely an initial manifestation of rheumatoid arthritis.

Scleroderma

Pericarditis is a frequent complication of scleroderma, and in one autopsy series, it was present in 70 percent.[18] Pericardial disease may be present as acute pericarditis with manifestations similar to idiopathic pericarditis or as a chronic pericardial effusion.[7]

Uremic Pericarditis

Acute pericarditis is a common complication of acute and chronic renal failure. Clinical pericarditis is present in 40 to 50 percent of patients with chronic renal failure and in approximately 18 percent with acute renal failure.[19] In a more recent study, 25 of 125 patients on chronic dialysis had uremic pericarditis.[20] The etiology of uremic pericarditis is unknown, but it occurs more frequently in young women and is associated with inadequate dialysis, infections, or hyperparathyroidism.

Neoplastic Pericarditis

Primary tumors of the pericardium such as mesotheliomas are quite rare. Pericardial metastasis may occur by direct extension or by hematogenous or lymphatic spread. These implants can be an incidental finding at autopsy, or they can be present with all the manifestations of acute pericarditis or cardiac tamponade. In a series of 13,314 routine autopsies performed at the Mayo Clinic between 1942 and 1958, there were 189 cases of metastatic pericardial disease (1.4 percent).[21] The heart was involved in approximately 20 percent of patients with disseminated malignant tumors, especially in acute leukemia (69 percent), malignant melanoma (64 percent), and lymphoma (24 percent). When the heart was involved, the pericardium was the most common site. The overall incidence of metastatic carcinoma to the pericardium alone is only 3 percent.[22] Pericardial metastases most commonly arose from carcinoma of the lung or breast or lymphomas and leukemias. Metastases to the pericardium without metastases to other thoracic structures are rare.[21] Pericardial metastasis should be suspected in patients with known malignancies who have a persistent effusion, precipitous onset of atrial arrhythmias, or nonspecific electrocardiographic change. Pericardial effusion results from lymphatic obstruction or metastases to serosal surfaces.

Acute pericarditis may follow radiation therapy for malignant disease of the chest and mediastinum. Pericardial damage may result when the total accumulated dose to the anterior surface of the heart reaches 4000 to 5000 rads.[23] Frequently there is a slowly accumulating pericardial effusion in the postradiation period, and diagnosis of acute pericarditis may be difficult unless baseline electrocardiograms and chest x-rays are obtained. In a recent study of patients with Hodgkin's disease, radiation related pericardial effusion was found in 25 of 81 patients studied.[24] In 13 patients the effusion resolved spontaneously; however, 11 others had persistent pericardial effusion with symptoms, but only four had signs and symptoms of acute pericarditis. Dyspnea on exertion was the most common symptom (40 percent) and tachycardia the most frequent clinical sign (48 percent). Twenty-two of these patients developed effusion within one year of completing upper mantle radiotherapy. In this particular series, there was no difference in total-dose or time-dose relationship between the patients who developed effusion and those who did not. Therefore, pericardial lymphatic obstruction by extensive mediastinal adenopathy, viral infection, or some type of immune mechanism may be responsible for the pericarditis. Occult radiation injury may progress to clinically significant pericarditis when steroids are suddenly withdrawn.[25]

Infectious Pericarditis

In an isolated case of pericarditis, it may be difficult to prove a viral etiology; however, epidemics of pericarditis have been related to coxsackie A and B virus and to influenza A and B virus.[26] The primary diseases predisposing to purulent pericarditis are pneumonia, osteomyelitis, septicemia, skin and soft tissue infections, and penetrating wounds of the chest.[27]

Traumatic Pericarditis

Acute pericarditis may result from penetrating or nonpenetrating chest injuries. Nonpenetrating injury to the heart and pericardium is usually due to blunt trauma and is more commonly seen in hospitals caring for automobile accident victims. Acute pericarditis can occur as a complication of cardiopulmonary resuscitation, and there are reports of pericarditis following cardioversion.[28]

Infarction Pericarditis

Pericarditis may occur as an early or late complication of acute myocardial infarction. The early form occurs two to four days after the infarction and is due to the inflammatory process of the acute infarction.[1, 7] The late form is termed the postmyocardial infarction syndrome or Dressler's syndrome and occurs 2 to 12 weeks after the infarction.[29] It is associated with pericardial and pleural effusions. The etiology is unknown but may be due to an autoimmune mechanism.

Miscellaneous Pericarditis

Patients with familial Mediterranean anemia have an increased incidence of pericarditis.[30] The reason for this is unknown. Although it has been suggested that pericarditis occurs more frequently in patients with congenital heart disease, this is more likely due to chance occurrence.[31]

Certain medications can cause acute pericarditis with or without effusion. This is due to a hypersensitivity reaction much like that described with penicillin allergies. Pericarditis has developed with the use of hydralazine and procainamide as part of a drug-induced lupus syndrome.[32, 33]

Acute rheumatic fever continues to be the most common cause of pericarditis in children. It occurs in about 10 percent of patients with acute rheumatic fever and is generally associated with significant valvulitis. However, rheumatic fever may cause pericarditis in adults without producing significant valvulitis and rarely produces ST segment change in the electrocardiogram.[34]

CLINICAL FEATURES

Pericardial Pain

The severity, location, and radiation of pain in acute pericarditis is extremely variable. Pain has always been considered one of the most important clinical features of acute pericarditis but can also be one of its most confusing and misleading manifestations.[12] The quality and location of this pain is quite variable. It is usually abrupt, sharp and severe, with a wide area of radiation to the neck, back, left shoulder, and occasionally to the arm. It may be epigastric in location, particularly in young patients, and may resemble an acute abdomen. Occasionally, pain is located at the cardiac apex and felt synchronously with each heart beat. The pain can be localized as follows: trapezius ridge, nuchal, precordial, substernal, epigastric, right upper quadrant abdominal, right chest, dorsal, generalized abdominal, or left nipple.

Only the outer layer of the lower parietal pericardium is pain sensitive.[35] This is an area below the fifth or sixth intercostal space supplied by the left phrenic nerve as it courses toward the diaphragm. Stimulation of the area produces pain which is then referred to the neck and trapezius ridge. Since only a relatively small portion of the pericardium appears to be pain sensitive, most of the pain in acute pericarditis arises from inflammatory involvement of surrounding structures, particularly the pleura. This accounts for the sharp pleuritic pain during respiration. The dull, oppressive precordial sensation in acute pericarditis probably stems from stretching of the pericardial sac. Weissbein and Heller demonstrated that pericardial pain could be relieved by left stellate ganglion block, challenging the concept that the phrenic nerve is the only afferent pathway.[36] In general, the pain of acute pericarditis can be classified as sharp, dull, aching, burning, constricting, pressure, or throbbing with heart beat.

One confusing aspect of pericarditis is that pain may be trivial or completely absent. There are several possible explanations for this. The inflammatory process may be confined to the large nonsensitive surface of the pericardium, or the pain threshold may not be reached either because the inflammation is mild or slowly progressing. Pain may be absent in 50 percent of all acute pericarditis,[37] particularly in uremic and tuberculous pericarditis, but is usually present (90 percent) and quite striking in idiopathic pericarditis. Postinfarction patients infrequently have transient rubs without pain.

The pain is commonly increased by maneuvers that have no effect on pain of myocardial infarction (deep breathing, rotation of the trunk, elevation of the arms, swallowing, coughing, or perhaps yawning). The discomfort is often worse in recumbency and may be eased by sitting up and leaning forward. Pericardial pain should be differentiated from pain due to other thoracic disease such as myocardial infarction, dissecting aneursym, pulmonary embolism, esophageal rupture, volvulus of a thoracic stomach, Prinzmetal's angina, and pneumothorax.

Signs and Symptoms

DYSPNEA. A complaint of dyspnea at rest or with exertion is common; however, its pathogenesis is not entirely clear. Patients may feel dyspneic with the onset of pain and

134

adopt a rapid, shallow breathing pattern which helps relieve the pain by splinting the chest.

COUGH. A nonproductive cough is extremely common and may be an initial symptom. Hiccup can occur, though rare, and suggests involvement of the diaphragmatic pleura.

MISCELLANEOUS. Dysphagia may appear either as a primary symptom of inflammatory esophageal disease that has secondarily caused pericarditis or from impingement of the posterior parietal pericardium against the esophagus. Many other symptoms may be present including generalized malaise, dizziness, nausea, vomiting, and palpitations. These are self-limiting and resolve within 24 to 48 hours after onset. Weakness may be a nonspecific complaint. Weight loss is uncommon in idiopathic forms but may be an important feature of either tuberculous or neoplastic pericarditis. Anorexia may occur in idiopathic and viral forms but rarely persists long enough to account for weight loss. Anxiety, particularly during the early onset of chest discomfort, may be a pronounced feature, and the patient occasionally sits or leans forward to relieve the pain.

FEVER. Fever is extremely common but not invariable and depends upon the primary disease. When present it is usually less than 39 C and chills may follow spiking fevers.

PERICARDIAL FRICTION RUB. Pericardial friction rub is a distinctive and diagnostic finding of pericarditis. In acute pericarditis an audible rub may be transient or may persist intermittently or continuously for weeks. Although often changing in character from minute to minute, friction rubs classically have a superficial quality that is grating or scratchy. Rubs tend to be migratory and shift in a matter of hours. If one is entertaining the diagnosis of pericarditis, a diligent examination must be made with the patient lying, sitting, and leaning forward. Repeated observations are important until the diagnosis is excluded. Rubs may be louder during either respiratory phase; however, more often they are louder during inspiration. In Spodick's evaluation of 100 patients, 41 had rubs louder during inspiration, 24 during expiration, and 34 had no respirational change.[38] Pericardial friction rubs may be present with scant or large pericardial effusions. It is incorrect to assume that pericardial friction rubs disappear with the accumulation of effusion. Loud rubs may be heard even in the presence of massive effusions.

The sound of the rub apparently originates from the grating of epicardial and pericardial surfaces roughened by serofibrinous exudate as myocardial motion occurs within the pericardial sac. Although there are three components of the pericardial friction rub, the number of components present and the intensity of each relates to the force of the cardiac motion responsible for that component. The presystolic component is synchronous with atrial contraction and heard in approximately 70 percent of cases.[38] The ventricular systolic component is the loudest, longest, and best heard. It occurs in virtually all cases. This sound may extend through systole and be confused with systolic murmurs. The protodiastolic phase is the least constant of the three and is synchronous with the rapid diastolic filling. It occurs in approximately 60 percent of cases. Often the protodiastolic and presystolic phases cannot be separated, resulting in the apparent biphasic "to and fro" quality so frequently described. In Spodick's study, the true biphasic rub occurred in only 24 of 100 patients.[38] Triphasic rubs are heard approximately 50 percent of the time and are best heard at the lower left midsternal border. Auscultation is facilitated by listening during inspiration and full expiration while the patient sits upright and leans forward. Sometimes the rub may be accentuated by applying pressure with the stethoscope. More capricious rubs may be heard by placing the patient on his abdomen, propping him up on his elbows, and listening during deep inspiration. Another useful maneuver is to examine the patient while he is lying supine with his arms extended above his head during the peak of inspiration (Fig. 1).

A monophasic rub may represent an early finding. In Spodick's series, only 12 out of 100 patients had a monophasic rub with regular sinus rhythm. Two patients with atrial

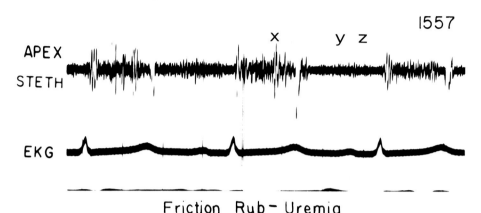

APEX
STETH

EKG

Friction Rub - Uremia

Figure 1. Phonocardiogram showing triphasic pericardial friction rub. In this tracing, x represents systolic rub, y the mid- or early-diastolic rub, and z the presystolic rub.

fibrillation had monophasic rubs, but more commonly patients with atrial arrhythmias have biphasic rubs.

Rubs must be differentiated from heart murmurs, skin scratches, the apical rub of left ventricular hypertrophy, the conus rub of dilatation of the pulmonary artery, a precordial crunch, and mediastinal emphysema. The following characteristics help make this differentiation possible:[14]

1. Rubs do not change in a consistent manner with respiration as is characteristic of murmurs.
2. Rubs do not radiate in a consistent fashion as is characteristic of murmurs.
3. Rubs are loudest at the mid- and low-sternal areas rather than at valve areas which is characteristic of murmurs.
4. Rubs change in character and intensity from one examination to another, unlike murmurs.
5. Rubs are frequently seen with the other manifestations of an acute illness (pain, fever, etc) whereas murmurs are not.
6. Rubs may be confirmed by typical electrocardiographic changes of pericarditis.

Electrocardiogram

Typical changes in the electrocardiogram are often diagnostic of acute pericarditis. The electrocardiographic abnormalities occur within a few hours or days after the onset of chest pain. The diagnosis is based primarily on the presence of sequential changes in the ST segments and T waves in multiple leads generally evolving through four stages.[12] The ST segment elevation reflects a current of injury secondary to the inflammatory reaction in the subepicardial muscle fibers; however, injury is not sufficient to produce abnormal Q waves as seen in myocardial infarction. The electrocardiogram is abnormal in most cases of pericarditis (90 percent) and can be diagnostic even in the absence of other manifestations.[39]

Stage one generally occurs with the onset of pain and may last several days. It is recognized by upward ST segment displacement with loss of the normal concave configuration of the ST segment. The ST segment vector points toward the injured area and is usually oriented downward, to the left, and anterior. Displacement is generally less pronounced than that seen in myocardial infarction and is seldom over 5 mm. in height.[38] Electrocardiograms commonly show elevation in all three standard limb leads, in aVL,

136

aVF, and in all precordial leads with the possible exception of V_1. ST segment elevation rarely persists more than a few days and can be transient (Fig. 2).

The second stage occurs after several days and represents return of the ST segment to the baseline. The T wave generally diminishes in size and flattens. ST segments characteristically return to the baseline before T wave inversion occurs, whereas in myocardial infarction, T waves become inverted before ST segments reach the baseline. Occasionally the T waves remain normal with return of the ST segment to the baseline (Fig. 3).

In the third stage, T waves become inverted and reach maximum negativity. The pathogenesis of T wave inversion relates to delay in repolarization of the subepicardial myocardium. T wave inversion generally occurs in more leads than it does in myocardial infarction and is usually less inverted (Fig. 4).

Stage four represents return of the electrocardiogram to normal. However, T wave inversion may remain for several months or may be permanent.

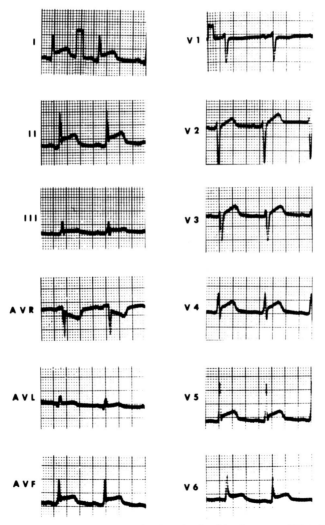

Figure 2. This electrocardiogram shows ST segment elevation in all leads except aVR and V_1. These findings are characteristic of stage 1.

137

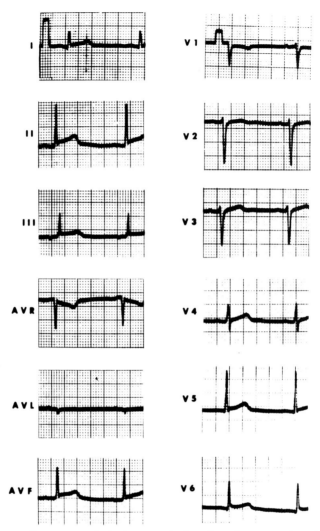

Figure 3. This electrocardiogram was obtained two weeks later from the same patient shown in Figure 2. It shows the ST segments returning to baseline without T wave inversion. These findings are characteristic of stage 2.

Unfortunately, changes from stage 1 to stage 4 cannot be documented in all patients with acute pericarditis, but can be demonstrated in approximately 50 percent of patients. Electrocardiographic changes evolve quickly in some instances and can be missed. The typical ST segment elevation is diagnostic. Other stages are nonspecific and only suggest the presence of pericarditis.

Other electrocardiographic changes can occur during acute pericarditis. PR segment shift is now recognized as an important feature of acute pericarditis, and occurs in approximately 80 percent of patients.[40, 41] This change may be due to atrial inflammation and abnormal atrial repolarization which produces an atrial current of injury from the epicardial surface. The net vector points toward aVR (right shoulder). This would result in ST segment elevation in aVR and depression in other leads.

Sinus tachycardia may occur during some phase of pericarditis but is not necessarily

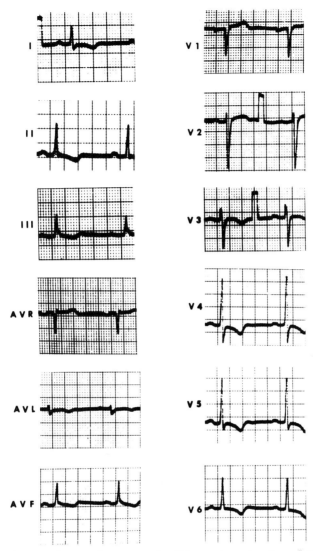

Figure 4. This electrocardiogram shows generalized T wave inversion characteristic of stage 3.

related to fever or to other cardiac problems.[42] In our experience, tachycardia lasts only a few days in the presence of uncomplicated acute pericarditis but has been reported to persist for months. Transient episodes of atrial fibrillation have been reported in 13 percent of patients.[43] Paroxysmal supraventricular tachycardia and atrial flutter also occur.[44] The etiology of these atrial arrhythmias is unclear. They may be due to sinus node involvement or to atrial inflammation or irritation. Ventricular ectopic beats occur frequently, but ventricular tachycardia and fibrillation are rare. Heart block is also uncommon except in acute rheumatic fever.

Chest X-Ray

The conventional chest roentgenograms are of no diagnostic value in uncomplicated pericarditis. However, they may be helpful if there is a pericardial effusion or if associated pulmonary pathology can help establish an etiology such as tuberculosis or carcinoma.

Laboratory Data

Laboratory studies reflect systemic reaction to pericardial inflammation and may suggest the presence of a primary underlying disease. Anemia occurs frequently in pericarditis, primarily as a reflection of systemic illness or infection. Leukocytosis occurs during the height of inflammation, usually as a neutrophilia followed by lymphocytosis. Leukopenia can occur with systemic disease (such as lupus erythematosus), drug therapy, and radiation therapy. The sedimentation rate is invariably elevated during the acute inflammation. Myocardial enzymes are usually normal but may be slightly elevated.

Therapy

Specific treatment for acute pericarditis depends on the establishment of a specific etiology. For example, hemodialysis is the specific treatment for uremic pericarditis and antituberculous medication for tuberculous pericarditis. General supportive measures are extremely important and should include bed rest until fever and pain subside and analgesics for control of the pain. Left stellate ganglion block has been used to obtain relief from severe pain.[36] Corticosteroids may produce dramatic clinical improvement.

Rhythm disturbances are treated in the usual fashion; however, procainamide should not be used since it may induce a lupus syndrome. Antibiotics should only be used to treat infections which have been established by appropriate cultures. They have no beneficial effect in the treatment of idiopathic pericarditis.

DEVELOPMENT OF PERICARDIAL EFFUSION

Pericardial effusion may not produce symptoms and may not be recognized clinically, and, for this reason, its incidence is difficult to determine. It occurs with all etiologic forms of acute pericarditis. Symptoms usually develop as a consequence of hemodynamic alterations which are in turn related to the rate and volume of fluid accumulation. If fluid accumulates slowly, the parietal pericardium stretches and may accommodate several liters of fluid without significant elevation of intrapericardial pressure.[45] When the pericardium is stretched to its maximum size, an additional volume of fluid may cause cardiac tamponade. Conversely, if a small amount of fluid (usually less than 200 ml.) accumulates quickly, cardiac tamponade may occur. As the fluid accumulates, the initial 80 to 120 ml. are accommodated in the pericardial sac without an increase in pressure, but additional fluid will cause a rapid rise of intrapericardial pressure.

Symptoms

Patients who develop effusion may complain of an extremely disagreeable precordial oppression. This probably stems from the actual stretch of the pericardial sac and is frequently eased by leaning forward. Dyspnea may be quite prominent and has several possible etiologies including associated pain and apprehension, decreased cardiac output secondary to cardiac tamponade, or decreased vital capacity secondary to pulmonary compression. Tachypnea may arise from chest splinting or be a compensatory mechanism to increase minute volume of ventilation. Syncope can occur from decreased cardiac output. Cough is common and stems from compression of the trachea and bronchi by the expanding pericardial sac. Hoarseness has also been observed secondary to compression of the recurrent laryngeal nerve. Nausea and abdominal pains

140

occur frequently and probably stem from congestion of abdominal viscera. True orthopnea and paroxysmal nocturnal dyspnea are uncommon.

Physical Findings

When the pericardial effusion is small, there are no specific findings. Tachypnea is the earliest and most common physical finding. Other physical findings are due to either cardiac tamponade or the increased size of the pericardial sac.

Patients with cardiac tamponade appear anxious and have peripheral cyanosis, tachypnea, and tachycardia. The blood pressure may be low, and a paradoxical pulse of greater than 10 mm. Hg is usually present. In tamponade the paradoxical pulse may be 15 to 25 mm. Hg. Though invariably present, the paradoxical pulse is not diagnostic of tamponade and may occur in heart failure, chronic obstructive lung disease, and obesity. The venous pressure is elevated, and the neck veins are distended. Kussmaul's sign (an inspiratory rise in venous pressure) is often absent. The heart tones are muffled, and diastolic sounds are unusual. Hepatomegaly, positive hepatojugular reflux, and peripheral edema are common. Beck summarized the physical findings of cardiac tamponade as a triad of rising venous pressure, falling arterial pressure, and a quietly beating heart. Coma and shock may occur, but if the patient is conscious, he will appear anxious or apprehensive. Vasoconstriction and tachypnea are present, and the patient is frequently sitting or leaning forward. Tachycardia is always present. Blood pressure may be normal initially but will show decreasing pulse pressure as tamponade proceeds. Neck vein distention is usually quite prominent due to increased venous pressure. Increased venous pulsations occur even in hypovolemic tamponade and have sharp X descent. The Y descent is not prominent and may be absent.

Chest X-Ray

Chest x-rays are of limited value in the diagnosis of pericardial effusion. Significant enlargement of the cardiac silhouette will not occur until 250 ml. of fluid accumulates. A normal chest roentgenogram does not exclude the diagnosis of acute cardiac tamponade. The sudden onset of a large cardiac silhouette and clear lung fields suggests the

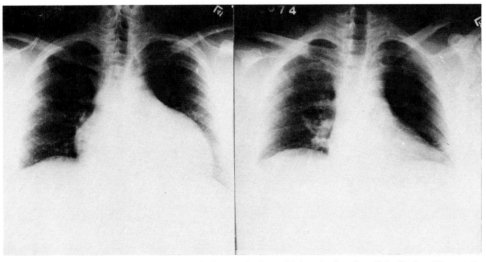

Figure 5. This shows a standard chest x-ray before and after withdrawl of pericardial effusion. The cardiac silhouette is diffusely enlarged but does not show a "water bottle" configuration. The lung fields are not congested.

141

diagnosis (Fig. 5). Pericardial effusion can be demonstrated angiographically by showing a 1.0 cm. separation of the right border of the cardiac silhouette with a catheter against the atrial wall or with a carbon dioxide or dye-filled atrium. Radioisotopes may also be used to show a separation of the cardiac and liver pools indicative of effusion.

Electrocardiogram

The electrocardiogram is of limited value in the diagnosis of pericardial effusion and tamponade. Low voltage may develop as effusion accumulates, but this is a nonspecific finding. We have observed large effusions without any significant change in the size of the QRS complex. Electrical alternation of the QRS size may develop in pericardial effusion with tamponade and reflects an abnormal pendular motion of the myocardium

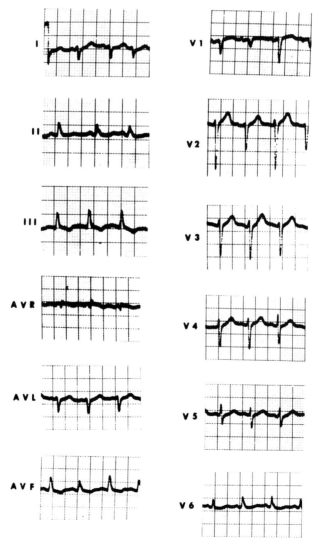

Figure 6. This electrocardiogram shows electrical alternans of the QRS complex. This is best seen in the right precordial leads. There is P wave alternans as well.

142

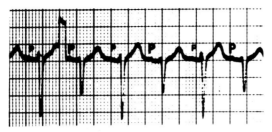

Figure 7. This strip of lead V₂ shows electrical alternans of the QRS complexes. The large and small P waves are designated by P and p respectively.

within the pericardial sac. This has been noted angiographically and echocardiographically. Alternation of both atrial and ventricular complexes is pathognomonic of cardiac tamponade (Figs. 6 and 7).

Echocardiogram

Echocardiography is the most accurate technique for detecting pericardial fluid. The technique is noninvasive, safe, rapid and can be performed at the bedside. Normally the pericardial space is only a potential space and echocardiographically the anterior right ventricular wall is in direct contact with the chest wall, and the posterior left ventricular wall is in contact with the posterior pericardium and pleura. The pericardial motion is the same as the endocardial surface, and no epicardial-pericardial space is present. In the presence of pericardial effusion, this space fills with fluid which does not emit an echo and echocardiographic separation occurs between the anterior right ventricular wall and the chest wall and between the posterior left ventricular wall and the posterior pericardium. It is important to identify intracardiac structures, particularly the mitral valve, so the exact position of the echo beam is known before making a con-

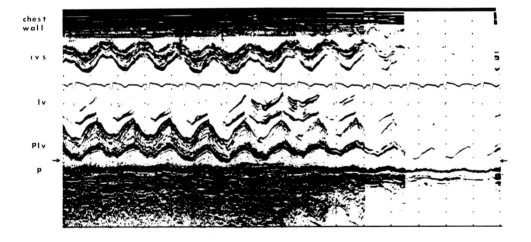

EFFUSION

Figure 8. This echocardiogram shows an echo-free space posteriorly throughout systole and diastole consistent with an effusion of 100 to 300 ml. This space is designated by the arrow. There is a dense pericardial echo designated p. In this echocardiogram, ivs is the interventricular septum; lv is the left ventricular chamber; Plv is the posterior left ventricular wall.

143

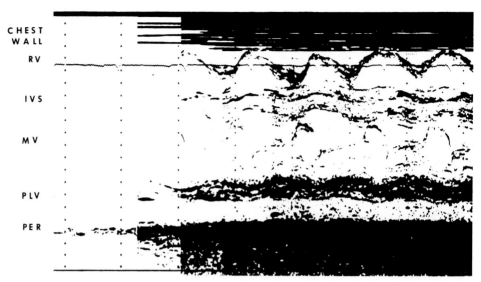

Figure 9. This echocardiogram shows the development of anterior echo-free space consistent with a 300 to 500 ml. effusion. The prominent anterior right ventricular wall echo is the result of scatter of the beam due to the effusion. In this figure MV represents the mitral valve.

clusive diagnosis of pericardial effusion. It is also important to scan from apex to base to demonstrate the absence of echo-free space behind the left atrium.

Small pericardial effusions of 50 ml. or less can be identified echocardiographically by a posterior echo-free space in systole that extends well into but not throughout systole. The pericardial movement is attenuated in relation to epicardial movement. Additional accumulation of fluid will result in echo-free space persisting throughout the cardiac cycle (Fig. 8). Moderate effusion (100 to 300 ml.) can be identified by at least a 1 cm. epicardial-pericardial separation and flat pericardial motion in relation to epicardial movement (Fig. 8). Larger pericardial effusions demonstrate the development of an anterior echo-free space in addition to the posterior echo-free space (Fig. 9).[47]

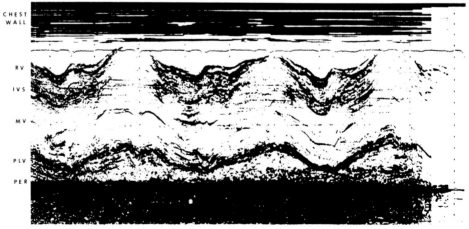

Figure 10. This echocardiogram shows a large effusion with large anterior and posterior echo-free spaces. The echocardiogram also shows electrical alternans characteristic of cardiac tamponade. The ventricular walls move congruently in anterior and posterior directions with alternate cycles. There is also discongruent motion in each cycle. This is characteristic of the "swinging heart" which occurs in cardiac tamponade.

144

Several types of abnormal heart wall motion have been described and are characteristic of larger effusions and cardiac tamponade. Patients with acute small volume tamponade may demonstrate very limited heart wall motion. However, the majority of patients with small to moderate and even large effusions with no evidence of cardiac tamponade demonstrate essentially normal heart wall motion (Fig. 9). Cardiac systole and diastole are represented by reciprocally moving anterior and posterior heart walls. Echocardiograms of large effusions may demonstrate congruently directional motion of the heart walls during some phase of the cardiac cycle (Fig. 10). This finding is consistent with abnormal anteroposterior displacement of the entire heart. This has been noted angiographically and is responsible for electrical alternans in cardiac tamponade. In our experience this has occurred most often in neoplastic effusions greater than 800 ml.

Treatment

Pericardiocentesis is an effective and dramatic treatment for cardiac tamponade and should be done as quickly as possible once the diagnosis is established. Removal of even a small amount of fluid may result in immediate symptomatic improvement with an increase in cardiac output and stroke volume (Fig. 11). We insert a catheter into the pericardial sac, using either an Intra-Cath or a small #6 French catheter inserted by the Seldinger technique.

If a pericardiocentesis cannot be done for technical reasons, one should stabilize the circulation until a pericardiectomy can be done. This can usually be accomplished by expanding venous blood volume with Ringer's lactated solution, Dextran or Plasmanate. Vasopressors and digitalis are usually ineffective in this situation, but isoproterenol may help to increase cardiac output temporarily.

Prognosis

The prognosis is dependent on such factors as the extent of a myocardial infarction, the severity of renal failure, or other associated disease. The prognosis of acute idiopathic pericarditis is usually excellent, but recurrences are common (14 to 30 percent of cases). The critical factors in prognosis are related to complications such as intrapericardial hemorrhage, chronic effusion, pericardial constriction, or residual myocardial impairment. The overall incidence of constrictive pericarditis is less than 1.0 percent; however, in tuberculous pericarditis this may occur in 30 percent of cases.

The physician is justified in anticipating that the majority of patients with acute pericarditis will do well during the acute episode and not develop significant sequelae.

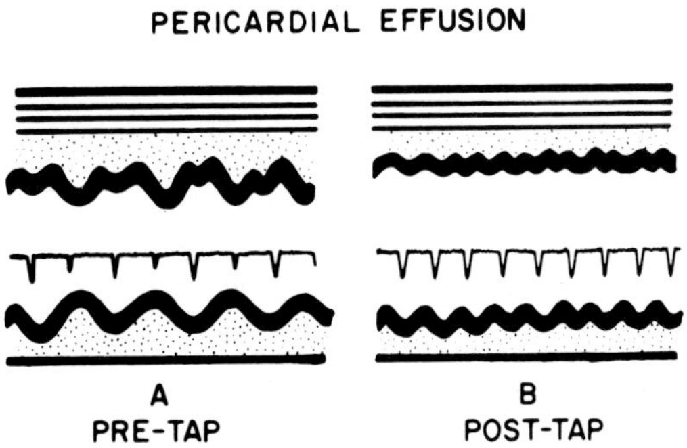

PERICARDIAL EFFUSION

A
PRE-TAP

B
POST-TAP

Figure 11. This diagram depicts the echocardiographic features of the "swinging heart" before and after pericardiocentesis showing both incongruent and congruent motion with each cycle. This motion is corrected by removal of a small amount of fluid.

145

However, he must be aware that complications can arise. These complications include tamponade, acute or subacute constrictive pericarditis, pericardial effusion, and chronic constrictive pericarditis. Development of these complications significantly alters prognosis and treatment.

REFERENCES

1. WARTMAN, W. B., AND HELLERSTEIN, H. K.: *The incidence of heart disease in 2,000 consecutive autopsies.* Ann. Intern. Med. 28:41, 1948.

2. GRIFFITH, G. C., AND WALLACE, L.: *The etiology of pericarditis.* Am. Heart J. 37:636, 1949.

3. LOCKE, E. A.: *The occurrence and diagnosis of pericarditis.* Boston Med. Surg. Soc. J. 175:590, 1916.

4. REEVES, R. L.: *The cause of acute pericarditis.* Am. J. Med. Sci. 225:34, 1953.

5. KEITH, J. D., ROWE, R. D., AND VLAD, P.: *Heart Disease in Infancy and Childhood,* ed. 2. Macmillan Company, New York, 1967.

6. PEREZ-GOMEZ, F., DURAN, H., TAMAMES, S., ET AL.: *Cardiac echinococcosis: Clinical picture and complications.* Br. Heart J. 35:1326, 1973.

7. McWHORTER, I. V., AND LeROY, E. C.: *Pericardial disease in scleroderma.* Am. J. Med. 57:556, 1974.

8. NOMEIR, A. M., TURNER, R., WATTS, E., ET AL.: *Cardiac involvement in rheumatoid arthritis.* Ann. Intern. Med. 79:800, 1973.

9. TOOLE, J., AND SILVERMAN, M. E.: *Pericarditis of acute myocardial infarction.* Chest 67:6, 1975.

10. WOOD, P.: *Chronic constrictive pericarditis.* Am. J. Cardiol. 7:48, 1961.

11. SODEMAN, W. A., AND SMITH, R. H.: *A re-evaluation of the diagnostic criteria for acute pericarditis.* Am. J. Med. Sci. 235:672, 1958.

12. SPODICK, D. H.: *Acute Pericarditis.* Grune & Stratton, New York, 1959.

13. BLACK, I. F. S.: *Pericardial disease in children,* in Cortes, F. M.: *The Pericardium and its Disorders.* Charles C Thomas, Springfield, Ill., 1971.

14. SPODICK, D. H.: *Differential diagnosis of acute pericarditis.* Prog. Cardiovasc. Dis. 14:192, 1971.

15. DUBOIS, E. L. (ED): *Lupus Erythematosus: A Review of the Current Status of Discoid and Systemic Lupus Erythematosus and Their Variants,* ed. 2. Univ. Southern California Press, Los Angeles, 1974.

16. KIRK, J., AND COSH, J.: *The pericarditis of rheumatoid arthritis.* Q. J. Med. 38:397, 1969.

17. THADANI, U., IVESON, J. M. I., AND WRIGHT, V.: *Cardiac tamponade, constrictive pericarditis and pericardial resection in rheumatoid arthritis.* Medicine 54:261, 1975.

18. ORAM, S., AND STOKES, W.: *The heart in scleroderma.* Br. Heart J. 23:243, 1961.

19. WACKER, W., AND MERRILL, J. P.: *Uremic pericarditis in acute and chronic renal failure.* J.A.M.A. 156:764, 1954.

20. COMTY, C. M., COHEN, S. L., AND SHAPIRO, F. L.: *Pericarditis in chronic uremia and its sequels.* Ann. Intern. Med. 75:173, 1971.

21. THURBER, D. L., EDWARDS, J. E., AND ACHOR, R. W. P.: *Secondary malignant tumors of the pericardium.* Circulation 26:228, 1962.

22. LOKICH, J. J.: *The management of malignant pericardial effusions.* J.A.M.A. 224:1401, 1973.

23. COHN, K. E., STEWART, J. R., FAJARDO, L. F. F., ET AL.: *Heart disease following radiation.* Medicine 46:281, 1967.

24. RUCKDESCHEL, J. C., CHANG, P., MARTIN, R. G., ET AL.: *Radiation-related pericardial effusions in patients with Hodgkin's disease.* Medicine 54:245, 1975.

25. CASTELLINO, R. A., GLATSTEIN, E., TURBOW, M. M., ET AL.: *Latent radiation injury of lungs or heart activated by steroid withdrawal.* Ann. Intern. Med. 80:593, 1974.

26. GRIST, N. R., AND BELL, E. J.: *Coxsackie viruses and the heart.* Am. Heart J. 77:295, 1969.

27. BOYLE, J. D., PEARCE, M. L., AND GAGE, L. B.: *Purulent pericarditis: Review of the literature and report of eleven cases.* Medicine 40:119, 1961.

28. STRÖM, S.: *Pericarditis following cardioversion.* Acta Med. Scand. 195:431, 1974.

29. DRESSLER, W.: *The post-myocardial-infarction syndrome: A report on forty-four cases.* Arch. Intern. Med. 103:28, 1959.

30. EHRENFELD, E. N., ELIAKI, M. M., AND RACHMILEWITZ, M.: *Recurrent polyserositis.* Am. J. Med. 31:107, 1961.

31. SEMLER, H. J., BRANDENBURG, R. O., AND KIRLIN, J. W.: *Pericardial disease complicating congenital heart lesions.* Ann. Intern. Med. 53:494, 1960.

32. ALARCÓN-SEGOVIA, D., WORTHINGTON, J. W., WARD, L. E., ET AL.: *Lupus diathesis and the hydralazine syndrome.* N. Engl. J. Med. 272:462, 1965.

33. LADD, A. T.: *Procainamide-induced lupus erythematosus.* N. Engl. J. Med. 267:1357, 1962.

34. PADER, E., AND ELSTER, S. K.: *Studies of acute rheumatic fever in the adult: I. Clinical and laboratory manifestations in thirty patients.* Am. J. Med. 26:424, 1959.

35. CAPPS, J. A., AND COLEMAN, G. H.: *An Experimental and Clinical Study of Pain in the Pleura, Pericardium and Peritoneum.* The Macmillan Company, New York, 1932.

36. WEISSBEIN, A. S., AND HELLER, F. N.: *A method of treatment for pericardial pain.* Circulation 24:607, 1961.

37. EVANS, E.: *Introduction to symposium on pericarditis.* Am. J. Cardiol. 7:1, 1961.

38. SPODICK, D. H.: *Pericardial rub: Prospective, multiple observer investigation of pericardial friction in 100 patients.* Am. J. Cardiol. 35:357, 1975.

39. WARNER, H. F.: *Graphic diagnostic techniques of pericardial disease,* in Cortes, F. M.: *The Pericardium and Its Disorders.* Charles C Thomas, Springfield, Ill., 1971, p. 53.

40. HULL, E.: *The electrocardiogram in pericarditis.* Am. J. Cardiol. 7:21, 1961.

41. SPODICK, D.: *Diagnostic electrocardiographic sequences in acute pericarditis: Significance of PR segment and PR vector changes.* Circulation 48:575, 1973.

42. DRESSLER, W.: *Sinus tachycardia complicating and outlasting pericarditis.* Am. Heart J. 72:422, 1966.

43. SOFFER, A.: *Electrocardiographic abnormalities in acute, convalescent, and recurrent stages of idiopathic pericarditis.* Am. Heart J. 60:729, 1960.

44. JAMES, T. N.: *Pericarditis and the sinus node.* Arch. Intern. Med. 110:305, 1962.

45. MORGAN, B. C., GUNTHEROTH, W. G., AND DILLARD, D. H.: *Relationship of pericardial to pleural pressure during quiet respiration and cardiac tamponade.* Circ. Res. 16:493, 1965.

46. SHABETAI, R., FOWLER, N. O., AND GUNTHEROTH, W. G.: *The hemodynamics of cardiac tamponade and constrictive pericarditis.* Am. J. Cardiol. 26:480, 1970.

47. HOROWITZ, M. S., SCHULTZ, C. S., STINSON, E. B., ET AL.: *Sensitivity and specificity of echocardiographic diagnosis of pericardial effusion.* Circulation 50:239, 1974.

147

Acute Viral Pericarditis*

George E. Burch, M.D.

Viral pericarditis should be considered viral *myopericarditis* for several reasons. For example, experimental production of pericarditis with viruses rarely, if ever, occurs without an associated myocarditis.[1, 2, 3, 4] Furthermore, pericarditis rarely occurs in man without producing electrocardiographic (ECG) changes, but the ECG reflects electric events in the myocardium, not the pericardium. The cardiac manifestations of viral pericarditis include manifestations of myocardial disease, such as arrhythmias, cardiac enlargement, gallop rhythm, and signs of right and/or left ventricular congestive heart failure. That "myopericarditis" is a better term for the disease than "viral pericarditis" is also evident from many publications in the medical literature.[5-13] Therefore, in this presentation viral pericarditis and at least subepicardial myocarditis will be considered interchangeably.

In 1854, Hodges[14] described the first case of idiopathic pericarditis in a 40-year-old woman. The disease received little attention until fairly recently when Lewes and Lane[15] discussed acute benign pericarditis. However, since 1948 when Dalldorf and Sickles[16] isolated the Coxsackie virus from children with paralysis, the Coxsackie viruses have been shown to produce acute myopericarditis in many patients.[5-13, 15, 17-23] The Coxsackie viruses are members of the picornavirus group, all of which are highly cardiotropic. The Coxsackie B group of six viruses more likely produce myopericarditis than do the Coxsackie A group of 26 viruses. Both groups, however, are highly pathogenic and fatal for suckling mammals, including suckling man. These viruses have been isolated from pericardial fluid, throat washings, and feces. Serial changes in neutralizing antibodies in the serum have also been demonstrated in suspected cases.

ETIOLOGY

Viruses

Isolated instances of acute pericarditis have been reported in which most, if not all, viruses have been shown to be involved.[13] The incidence of fully established cases of viral myopericarditis must be considerably greater than the medical literature suggests. Many cases are not detected because of the lack of adequate diagnostic laboratory fa-

*Supported by Grant HL-14789 from the National Heart and Lung Institute of the U.S. Public Health Service, the Rudolph Matas Memorial Fund for the Kate Prewitt Hess Laboratory, the Rowell A. Billups Fund for Research in Heart Disease, and the Feazel Laboratory.

149

cilities for viruses. Furthermore, the physician does not always make an adequate attempt to establish the etiology in patients who have pericarditis. Once he fails to find a bacterial, fungal, or neoplastic agent, the physician is satisfied to discontinue his investigations and considers the disease "idiopathic." "Idiopathic" is a pernicious term. Physicians too often consider the etiologic phase of the clinical study completed when they can state the cause to be idiopathic. Every disease has a cause, and every effort must be made to find it. Were this the general attitude in medical practice, viruses would be identified more frequently as the etiologic agents. Surely, there is a need to provide diagnostic viral laboratories for clinical studies on par with the conventional clinical bacteriologic laboratories found throughout the world.

Conditioning Factors

The role of conditioning factors in the production of any disease, and especially viral cardiac diseases, has not received adequate consideration by physicians. This is certainly true in the case of viral pericarditis. Because viral infections of the upper respiratory tract are so common and pericarditis occurs relatively infrequently, physicians fail to relate the two. However, when conditions are just right, pericarditis will follow an upper respiratory tract infection. Among the accepted conditioning factors are alchol, physical trauma, malnutrition, bacterial infections, age, hypertension, fatigue, and excessive and strenuous physical exertion. Other viral infections, steroids, toxic agents, and drugs must also be considered as conditioning factors. Conditioning factors are of considerable significance to the clinician, for when his patient has an "innocent" upper respiratory infection (URI) but one or more conditioning factors are present he must be extremely careful with his patient to prevent serious viral complications such as myopericarditis. Even more importantly, his patient with a viral, or possibly viral, URI should be advised to avoid factors which "condition" him for serious viral complications. For example, such a patient should be advised to avoid strenuous physical exercise, trauma, alcohol, steroids, toxic agents, fatigue, and so forth even for several days after the URI has subsided. Thus, when the physician has a patient with a URI, he reallizes the infection is not really innocent but potentially dangerous, especially when dangerous conditioning factors are present. Furthermore, he knows that any viral infection such as influenza, mumps, hepatitis, ECHO virus and Rhino virus infections, and many others can produce myopericarditis in man.

PATHOLOGY

The pathology of pericarditis is not diagnostically characteristic as to etiology in many instances. The pathologist always finds inflammatory changes regardless of etiology. He may search for viral crystals or particles with the electron microscope, but the chance of his finding them is extremely remote. The mesothelial cells become necrotic; there is extensive round cell infiltration and fibrinous exudate; there is edema formation; and the pericardium (parietal and visceral) is destroyed and the denuded surfaces exposed. These changes during the acute stages are followed in some instances by the accumulation of fibroblasts with fibrosis and chronic adhesive pericarditis. In most instances the acute pericarditis will heal, with little subendocardial scarring and with re-epithelialization. Unfortunately, the natural history of acute viral myopericarditis is not well known. The detailed aspects of pathogenesis also remain little studied. Coxsackie B_4 virus has received most attention, but there is still a great deal of study yet to be done to learn the pathogenesis and natural history of viral pericarditis. The opportunities are considerable to study the disease in animals and man.

CLINICAL MANIFESTATIONS

Symptoms and Signs

The clinical manifestations of viral pericarditis vary considerably. They may begin with symptoms of the pericarditis itself. Usually, viral pericarditis begins with an upper respiratory tract infection which, as a rule, receives little or no attention. The patient considers the infection as a "cold," episode of "flu," or a "sore throat." He continues his usual daily activities, mild or strenuous. He feels feverish and chilly, with malaise, restlessness at night, and even has nightmares. There may be dyspepsia, headaches, ocular pain, and anorexia. These and other symptoms are noted with careful history taking.

The patient then has vague precordial discomfort advancing to severe excruciating precordial pain at times, initiating the symptoms of pericarditis. He has a sinus tachycardia with or without atrial or ventricular premature contractions. The patient is dyspneic at rest, or at least on mild exertion. The precordial discomfort is constant and is worsened with precordial pressure and at times with deep inspiration. The pain may be referred into the left shoulder, supraclavicular region and/or the left side of the neck. Deep inspiration may exaggerate the pain in the areas of referral as well as in the precordium. Patients, at times, try nitroglycerin sublingually for the pain, but the drug does not produce relief. Fever develops if it has not been present previously. The oral temperature may be as high as 103 F to 104 F, although usually being lower. There is fatigue, weakness, malaise, and a sensation of being rather seriously ill. Unless there is extensive associated myocarditis, the symptoms and signs of congestive heart failure are limited to the dyspnea, if dyspnea is present.

When there is rapid accumulation of pericardial fluid or an accumulation of a large quantity of pericardial fluid, the patient develops the manifestations of cardiac tamponade or restriction of cardiac filling. When this occurs the dyspnea is severe. There may be orthopnea. There may be a cough, some expectoration, pallor, mild peripheral cyanosis, and even distended neck veins. The mass of pericardial fluid produces a sensation of precordial fullness and heaviness. A carefully obtained history can be extremely interesting and informative.

Because of the symptoms the patient consults his physician who notes the pallor, dyspnea, cough, and distended neck veins if cardiac filling is restricted and/or congestive heart failure present. There may be edema of the feet and ankles, a large tender liver, and crepitant rales in the bases of both lungs if congestive heart failure and/or cardiac tamponade are present. The symptoms and signs of congestive heart failure are readily noted by the experienced clinician.

Physical Manifestations

Examination of the heart reveals pericardial fullness if there is associated large pericardial effusion and/or dilatation due to an associated myocarditis. The apex of the heart is difficult, and at times impossible, to palpate when marked effusion is present. The sinus tachycardia is noted, and disturbances in cardiac rhythm should be carefully searched for and noted. Percussion reveals a normal size to large area of cardiac dullness to flatness, depending upon the amount of pericardial effusion and/or cardiac dilatation produced by an associated acute myocarditis. Auscultation will reveal the characteristic to and fro (systolic and diastolic) type friction rub. Unfortunately, the pericardial friction rub is not always classic and may be faint and only systolic in time. Only through experience obtained by hearing a large number of friction rubs will the physician recognize the subtle ones. One of the important diagnostic characteristics of the friction rubs is their tendency to change rapidly from day to day or even within the same day. They change in quality and intensity. The friction rub is the most pathognomonic diagnostic manifestation of pericarditis noted at the bedside. The heart sounds tend to be faint or distant, and a soft, blowing, faint, short to holosystolic mitral murmur may be present. When diffuse myocarditis is present and the ventricles are markedly dilated, the murmur of mitral insufficiency may be more prominent. The pulmonic component of the second sound over the pulmonic area may be loud when left ventricular congestive heart failure is present. The pulmonic second sound may be more prominently split and louder than normal. The auscultatory manifestations tend to change rather rapidly in patients with pericarditis.

When there is marked pericardial effusion with compression of the lung posterior to the heart, compression atelectasis (Ewart's sign) may be present. This unilateral pulmonary manifestation must not be confused with the pulmonary signs of congestive heart failure.

Signs of cardiac tamponade, such as distended neck veins, pulsus paradoxus, and x-ray evidence of considerable pericardial fluid (tamponade can occur with little pericardial effusion, especially when it occurs rapidly), should be carefully considered. Cardiac tamponade should not be confused with congestive heart failure.

Diffuse myocarditis is relatively common in patients with viral pericarditis and relatively rare in patients with bacterial or neoplastic pericarditis. Superficial, subepicardial myocarditis is almost always present to some degree in all patients with viral and bacterial pericarditis, however.

Peripheral Pulsations

The peripheral arterial pulsations, such as the radial pulsations, tend to be weak to feeble, regular, rapid and not as bounding as normal. The change in pulse volume reflects nicely the stroke volume of the left ventricle. Stroke volume tends to be relatively small, not only because of the possible coexistence of congestive heart failure, but, in part, because of the sinus tachycardia and restriction to filling when cardiac tamponade is present. The radial pulse can be extremely informative to the experienced clinician.

SPECIAL STUDIES

Hematology

The leukocyte studies tend to show a higher percentage of lymphocytes than normal. There may be mild leukocytosis, but as a rule the white cells tend to be normal in total number. The fairly characteristic white cell of mononucleosis is present if the pericarditis is due to EB (Epstein-Barr) virus infection; otherwise, there are no characteristic changes in the CBC. From the point of view of differential diagnosis, the absence of leukocytosis tends to rule out a pyogenic bacterial infection. The erythrocytic sedimentation rate is usually increased to a variable degree.

Urinalysis

The urinalysis may reveal a slight proteinuria and a few coarse granular casts with a tendency to a larger number of casts than normal. The offending virus may be isolated from the urine at times, as indicated below.

Roentgenography

As with any type of pericarditis, the presence of pericardial fluid can be suspected from the teleroentgenogram with barium in the esophagus and with four views of the chest. The water-bottle appearance of the cardiac silhouette can be helpful (Fig. 1). Fluoroscopy can be of some value, but large dilated hearts with or without pericardial fluid will manifest small pulsations. Fluoroscopy must be employed cautiously in diagnosis. By means of nuclear scanning, pericardial effusion can be demonstrated at times and usually when the effusion is marked. Intravenous injections of CO_2 may be used to demonstrate pericardial fluid by means of the CO_2 bubble in the right atrium (Fig. 2).[24, 25] Oppenheimer and associates[26, 27] introduced this technique in clinical cardiology. Angiography may be used, but it is better to avoid hazardous procedures unless absolutely necessary.

Paracentesis

Paracentesis of the pericardium is most important. The fluid collected must be studied for fungi, bacteria, viruses, and malignancy cells. It is always advisable to inject

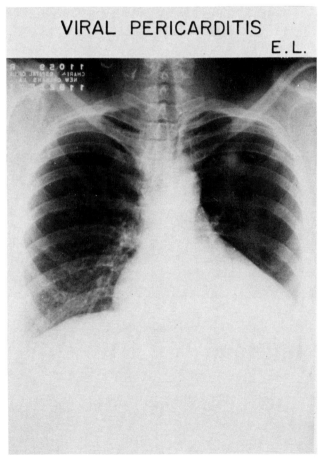

Figure 1. Chest roentgenogram of a patient with viral pericarditis showing "water-bottle" silhouette of the heart.

153

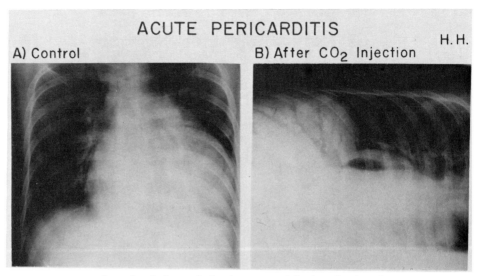

Figure 2. Chest x-rays of a patient before and after intravenous injection of carbon dioxide. Panel A shows the heart before injection, and B shows the bubble of CO_2 in the right atrium with a slight thickening of the pericardial "cap" above the bubble of CO_2 due to slight amount of pericardial fluid.

air or, preferably, CO_2 into the pericardial sac and obtain x-rays of the heart to observe heart size, thickness of the pericardium, and evidence of growths on the epicardium and parietal pericardium. Care in paracentesis cannot be overemphasized. Obviously, absolute care must be taken to avoid injecting air or even CO_2 into the heart.

Electrocardiography

The electrocardiogram in viral pericarditis displays characteristic ST segment elevations and configurations (Fig. 3).

Echocardiography

Echocardiograms (ECHO) can also be extremely useful in diagnosis. Not only does the echocardiogram reveal the presence of pericardial effusion, but it also indicates extremely well the amount of fluid present. Figure 4 shows an ECHO of a patient with pericardial effusion.

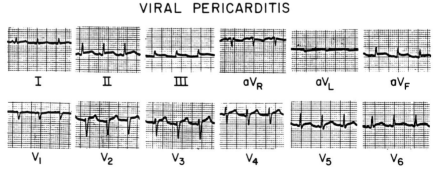

Figure 3. Electrocardiogram showing typical horizontal elevation of ST segment in a patient with viral pericarditis.

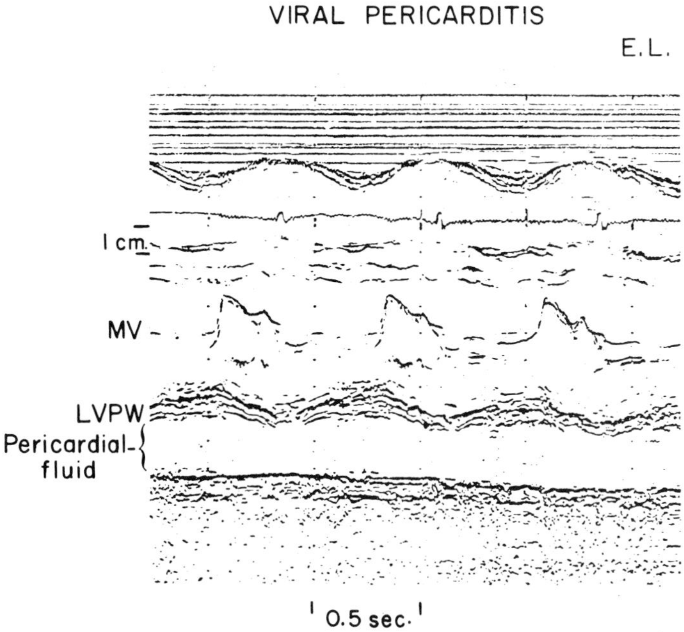

VIRAL PERICARDITIS

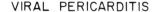

E.L.

I cm.

MV ‑

LVPW
Pericardial‑{
fluid

0.5 sec.

Figure 4. Echocardiogram of a patient with viral pericarditis showing evidence of pericardial fluid.

VIROLOGIC STUDIES

Every attempt should be made to isolate the offending virus. Unfortunately, adequate facilities are not readily available for the study of viral infections in most hospitals and other institutions. The CDC (Center for Disease Control) in Atlanta is overtaxed at present to meet the needs of the entire USA. The CDC may be approached for assistance, however. Cultures of throat washings, blood, urine, and stools should be obtained routinely. Special fluids such as pericardial fluid, when available, should be studied. Changes in viral neutralizing antibody titer in the blood serum should be obtained during the acute stage of illness and at intervals during the illness and convalescence. Such studies are most important. Serial changes in titer of neutralizing antibodies can assist in etiologic diagnosis. At the same time the pericardial fluid should be cultured for all other types of organisms, including bacteria and fungi. To know the cause of the pericarditis is not only most important in therapy and prognosis for the patient's own welfare, but it is essential for learning more about the incidence and natural history of viral pericarditis.

PROGNOSIS

Prognosis is usually favorable if the patient with viral pericarditis is placed at bed rest early. Considerable care in therapy is important. When there is also viral myocarditis and even valvulitis, the prognosis is much worse, and absolute bed rest becomes even more important to prevent occurrence of fatal cardiomyopathy immediately or years later. It is important that the physician follow the patient closely and carefully and guard the prognosis. The cardiac state can change rather rapidly and become worse.

The diet must be soft and bland, and the feedings must be small and frequent and free from salty foods. When congestive heart failure is present, the Karrell diet (800 ml. of

155

milk, only, for 24 hours) may be the best until the acute phases of the illness have subsided.

A cardiologist should be consulted for patients with viral pericarditis in order to outline study and treatment.

CHRONIC ADHESIVE AND CONSTRICTIVE PERICARDITIS

Acute viral pericarditis can ultimately lead to chronic adhesive and constrictive pericarditis. It is not the purpose of this presentation to discuss these and other chronic problems. It is because of the chronic lesions that the patient must be followed carefully and closely for many years. When chronic pericarditis develops, it should be recognized early and treated accordingly.

SUMMARY

Viral infections of the pericardium occur frequently. Unfortunately, the viruses responsible for the infection are rarely isolated or even identified. The clinical manifestations are those of fluid in the pericardium and usually an associated friction rub. There is no specific treatment for a viral agent, but supportive care is important and valuable. The diagnostic and therapeutic principles in the clinical care of patients with viral pericarditis are discussed. Viral pericarditis never occurs without associated subepicardial myocarditis and often occurs in association with diffuse myocarditis. For this reason the disease may be better termed viral myopericarditis.

REFERENCES

1. BURCH, G. E., DEPASQUALE, N. P., SUN, S. C., ET AL.: *Experimental Coxsackievirus endocarditis.* J.A.M.A. 196:349, 1966.
2. SUN, S. C., SOHAL, R. S., BURCH, G. E., ET AL.: *Coxsackie virus B₄ pancarditis in cynomolgus monkeys resembling rheumatic heart lesions.* Br. J. Exp. Pathol. 48:655, 1967.
3. TSUI, C. Y., AND BURCH, G. E.: *Coxsackie virus B₄ pericarditis in mice.* Br. J. Exp. Pathol. 52:47, 1971.
4. BURCH, G. E., AND GILES, T. D.: *The role of viruses in the production of heart disease.* Am. J. Cardiol. 29:231, 1972.
5. FLETCHER, E., AND BRENNAN, C. F.: *Cardiac complications of Coxsackie-virus infection.* Lancet 1:913, 1957.
6. SMITH, W. G.: *Adult heart disease due to the Coxsackie virus Group B.* Br. Heart J. 28:204, 1966.
7. SAINANI, G. S., KROMPOTIC, E., AND SLODKI, S. J.: *Adult heart disease due to the Coxsackie virus B infection.* Medicine 47:133, 1968.
8. SMITH, W. G.: *Coxsackie B myopericarditis in adults.* Am. Heart J. 80:34, 1970.
9. BERGSTRÖM, K., ERIKSON, U., NORDBRING, F., ET AL.: *Acute non-rheumatic myopericarditis: A follow-up study.* Scand. J. Infect. Dis. 2:7, 1970.
10. KAGAN, H., AND BERNKOPF, H.: *Pericarditis caused by Coxsackie virus B.* Ann. Paediat. 189:44, 1957.
11. KOONTZ, C. H., AND RAY, C. G.: *The role of Coxsackie Group B virus infections in sporadic myopericarditis.* Am. Heart J. 82:750, 1971.
12. GARDINER, A. J. S., AND SHORT, D.: *Four faces of acute myopericarditis.* Br. Heart J. 35:433, 1973.
13. HIRSCHMAN, S. Z., AND HAMMER, G. S.: *Coxsackie virus myopericarditis: A microbiological and clinical review.* Am. J. Cardiol. 34:224, 1974.
14. HODGES, R. M.: *Medical cases at Massachusetts General Hospital: Idiopathic pericarditis.* Boston Med. Surg. J. 51:140, 1854.
15. LEWES, D., AND LANE, W. F.: *Acute benign pericarditis due to Coxsackie virus Group B, type 3.* Lancet 2:1385, 1961.
16. DALLDORF, G., AND SICKLES, G. M.: *An unidentified, filtrable agent isolated from feces of children with paralysis.* Science 108:61, 1948.

17. MOVITT, E. R., LENNETTE, E. H., MANGUM, J. F., ET AL.: *Acute benign pericarditis: Report of two cases associated with Group A and Group B Coxsackie viruses.* N. Engl. J. Med. 258:1082, 1958.

18. BELL, J. F., AND MEIS, A.: *Pericarditis in infection due to Coxsackie virus Group B, type 3.* N. Engl. J. Med. 261:126, 1959.

19. KIRK, E. D., MARYMONT, J. H., JR., CROW, E. W., ET AL.: *Acute pericarditis: An outbreak due to Coxsackie viruses B.* J. Kans. Med. Soc. 72:47, 1971.

20. BELL, E. J., AND GRIST, N. R.: *Further studies of enterovirus infections in cardiac disease and pleurodynia.* Scand. J. Infect. Dis. 2:1, 1970.

21. WOODS, J. D., NIMMO, M. J., AND MACKAY-SCOLLAY, E. M.: *Adult heart disease associated with Coxsackie B virus infection.* Med. J. Aust. 2:573, 1973.

22. HACKEL, D. B.: *Diseases of the pericardium.* Cardiovasc. Clin. 4 (2):143, 1972.

23. SPODICK, D. H.: *Acute Pericarditis.* Grune & Stratton, New York, 1959.

24. PHILLIPS, J. H., JR., BURCH, G. E., AND HELLINGER, R.: *The use of intracardiac carbon dioxide in the diagnosis of pericardial disease.* Am. Heart J. 61:748, 1961.

25. BURCH, G. E., AND PHILLIPS, J. H.: *Methods in the diagnostic differentiation of myocardial dilatation from pericardial effusion.* Am. Heart J. 64:266, 1962.

26. OPPENHEIMER, M. J., DURANT, T. M., STAUFFER, H. M., ET AL.: *In vivo visualization of intracardiac structures with gaseous carbon dioxide; cardiovascular-respiratory effects and associated changes in blood chemistry.* Am. J. Physiol. 186:325, 1956.

27. PAUL, R. E., DURANT, T. M., OPPENHEIMER, M. J., ET AL.: *Intravenous carbon dioxide for intracardiac gas contrast in the roentgen diagnosis of pericardial effusion and thickening.* Am. J. Roentgenol. Radium Ther. Nucl. Med. 78:224, 1957.

157

Nonviral Infectious Pericarditis

Richard A. Gleckman, M.D.

Standard textbooks correctly state that virtually every kind of microorganism has been associated with pericarditis. Recent case reports of adults with pericarditis caused by *Neisseria gonorrheae, Hemophilus influenzae, Vibrio fetus, Listeria monocytogenes,* nongroup A beta-hemolytic streptococci and *Nocardia asteroides* underscore the potential variety of responsible bacteria.[1-8] Knowledge of this fact imposes a major burden on the physician responsible for the care of a febrile patient with signs or symptoms consistent with pericardial disease. Not only must infectious pericarditis be separated from the vast array of noninfectious diseases etiologically related to pericarditis, but the availability of definitive antimicrobial therapy forces the clinician to attempt to determine the precise causative agent. The fact that a patient might experience an infectious pericarditis superimposed on another disorder capable of producing pericarditis[9, 10] lends an added dimension of diagnostic difficulty.

For the individual patient, the physican must pursue indirect and sometimes even direct chemical, cytologic, immunologic, and microbiologic studies until he is entirely satisfied that the etiology of pericarditis has been established. Tables listing the most likely infectious etiologies can suggest an initial approach to the diagnostic evaluation, but they can not be relied upon in the individual situation. Recent therapeutic modalities, both medical and surgical, have created totally new forms of pericarditis, and lists of infectious causes of pericarditis compiled in the 1940s to 1950s may no longer be applicable to contemporary practice.[11]

This chapter will offer a commentary on infectious nonviral pericarditis. An attempt will be made to present concepts of pathogenesis, diagnostic approach, and therapy for the most common forms of bacterial and fungal pericarditis experienced by adults in the United States. In order to provide a proper background, however, it will be necessary to discuss some immunologic and microbiologic studies which offer valuable information, particularly when pericardial tissue or effusions are either not available or are not easily accessible for study. Although the clinical features will be stressed, no effort will be made in this chapter to describe angiography, cardiopulmonary radioisotope scanning, and reflected ultrasound, which are so useful to confirm the presence of pericardial effusion. These techniques will be reviewed elsewhere in this volume. In addition, those "clinical clues" used to differentiate the three forms of compressive pericardial disease will not be emphasized since they were the subject of a recent publication.[12]

INDIRECT METHODS OF DIAGNOSIS

Microbiologic Studies

For the febrile patient with pericarditis, culture of the blood is one of the most important procedures that can be performed. If the patient has not received any antimicrobial agent within the week prior to obtaining the blood cultures, four sets of blood cultures obtained over a period of 24 to 48 hours should permit determination of the organism in the great majority of cases.[13] Some experts have suggested that prereduced broth media, containing factors known to favor the growth of anaerobes, will increase the chances for recovery of these agents.[14] In addition, the use of a biphasic blood culture medium, consisting of both broth and agar slant, significantly improves the detection of fungemia.[15] If the patient has recently received penicillin or ampicillin, the addition of penicillinase should be requested.[16] Whether arterial blood culture offers any advantage over venous blood is an unsettled issue.[17, 18] Even more controversial is the need to obtain blood for culture in hypertonic medium to increase the chances of detecting conventional organisms as well as cell wall defective bacterial variants.[19] Nevertheless, this medium is now commercially available. A meticulous search of peripheral blood smears can also be very rewarding.[20] Bone marrow aspirate cultures are occasionally helpful in the attempt to isolate certain organisms,[21, 22] and trephine bone marrow biopsy has been successfully employed to detect evidence of military tuberculosis when liver biopsy was contraindicated.[23, 24]

Additional laboratory studies that have particular relevance to the diagnosis of tuberculous pericarditis would include the following: acid-fast stain of gastric contents;[25] acid-fast stain and culture of spontaneous and aerosol-induced sputum;[26] fluorescence microscopy;[27] animal inoculation;[28] and combined histologic assessment and cultural data obtained from pleural biopsy of exudative pleural effusions.[29, 30] More recently, evidence has become available which appears to demonstrate the fact that thoracoscopy, combined with pleural biopsy, is the most suitable method for diagnosis of a tuberculous pleural effusion.[31, 32]

Immunologic Studies

The tuberculin skin test was formerly regarded as a sensitive measure of tuberculous infection. However, a positive tuberculin test does not signify the presence of active disease, and tuberculin sensitivity may decrease or disappear temporarily due to the influence of the extent of the disease and other illnesses, or following the administration of immunosuppressive drugs or certain live virus vaccines.[33] Although the stabilized antigen is the most reliable testing material, even this improved preparation often fails to detect tuberculin sensitivity in patients with active tuberculosis.[34] It has been suggested that the clinician employ second strength tuberculin test antigen (250TU) when a negative test results from intermediate (5TU) strength PPD. The statement has even been made that a negative second strength test virtually excludes tuberculosis, except in debilitated patients.[35] This sentiment has not been universally accepted, however. A more recently developed immunologic test, the measurement of lymphocyte transformation in vitro, may prove to be of assistance in the diagnosis of tuberculosis in patients who fail to demonstrate tuberculin sensitivity.[36]

The nitroblue tetrazolium dye test determines the ability of phagocytizing polymorphonuclear neutrophils to convert the oxidized form of nitroblue tetrazolium to a blue-black precipitate that can be seen microscopically. The initial enthusiastic reports suggested that the test was capable of distinguishing pyogenic infections from other diseases.[37, 38] The test has subsequently been evaluated as a diagnostic aid in tuberculosis.[39] A more recent detailed review, however, concludes that this test yields inconsistent results in infected patients and is unreliable in the specific diagnosis of infection.[40]

The technique of counterimmunoelectrophoresis has recently been introduced into clinical medicine to detect the presence of disease due to meningococci, pneumococci and *Hemophilus influenzae*.[41] As these organisms have caused acute bacterial pericarditis, this immunologic test, which detects circulating capsular polysaccharide, can be used to significant advantage. The technique is capable of rendering a specific diagnosis in a very brief time and may be particularly valuable when the patient has received prior antimicrobial therapy which has suppressed growth in cultures.

Until recently the ASO (anti-streptolysin O) antibody measurement was regarded as the standard test to detect recent infection caused by group A streptococci. This extracellular hemolysin is also produced by streptococci of groups C and G. The formation of the ASO antibody is suppressed by antibiotic therapy, however, and a rise in titer does not invariably develop in the presence of infection.[42] It is now well established that the anti DNAse B test is the preferred test for serologic documentation of streptococcal pyoderma.[43] In addition, it also appears that antibody responses to DNAse B, one of the four extracellular deoxyribonucleases elaborated by group A streptococci, are generally good regardless of the site of the infection.[44] This test may now represent the best single test for general use in the serologic detection of streptococcal infection.

Immunological tests can be of immense value to confirm the role of additional nonviral infectious agents which have produced pericarditis. It is important to recognize these disorders as they are amenable to therapy. Toxoplasma pericarditis has occurred as an isolated infection[45] or as part of a disseminated disease.[46] Since it has been established that the dye test antibodies may remain elevated for years after initial infection,[47] and encysted organisms can persist for the life of the host,[48] alternative tests had to be found to detect active toxoplasmosis. A recently developed technique, indirect fluorescent antibody test for antitoxoplasma IgM antibodies, appears to have fulfilled the need for a useful indicator of active toxoplasmosis.[49] The hemagglutinin inhibition test, which is available through the division of parasitology, National Communicable Disease Center, Atlanta, Georgia, is very useful in the diagnosis of invasive disease due to *Entamoeba histolytica*.[50]

DIRECT METHODS OF DIAGNOSIS

The insertion of a catheter to decompress the pericardium offers an excellent opportunity to provide fluid for cytologic, chemical, and microbiologic evaluation. Percutaneous catheter drainage of the pericardium has additional advantages compared to needle aspiration: capability of removing larger amounts of fluid and capability of coping with the tendency of effusions to reaccumulate. Although not studied specifically in relationship to infected pericardial fluids, determination of the complement levels,[51] lactic dehydrogenase content,[52] and endotoxin presence[53] have been valuable laboratory studies for definition of the etiologies of other diseased body compartments. Certainly gram stained and acid fast stained smears of pericardial fluid must be performed, as well as inoculation of broths, tissue cultures, and appropriate solid media that will permit the growth of conventional aerobic and anaerobic bacteria, viruses, fungi, and mycobacteria. The quantitative white cell count and the differential count will represent additional helpful diagnostic tools.

When the indirect studies and analysis of the pericardial fluid have failed to divulge the etiology, consideration should be given to pericardial biopsy. The combination of direct microscopic examination of pericardial tissue for organisms, malignant cells, caseating and noncaseating granulomas, and culture of the tissue, can pay significant dividends.[25, 54]

SPECIFIC FORMS OF INFECTIOUS PERICARDITIS

Pneumococcal Pericarditis

Prior to the advent of antibiotics, the pneumococcus was the most common etiologic agent isolated in purulent pericarditis.[55, 56] This situation no longer prevails. A uniform clinical presentation has persisted, however.[57, 58] Virtually all patients have dyspnea, chest pain, fever, tachycardia, peripheral leukocytosis, abnormal electrocardiogram, and evidence of pneumonia. In a moderate number of cases there is concomitant empyema, a manifestation of delayed recognition and therapy of the underlying pneumococcal pneumonia. Pericardial fluid is cloudy, purulent, contains virtually 100 percent polymorphonuclear leukocytes, and demonstrates the organism both by gram stain and culture. The pathogenesis of the pericarditis is probably direct extension from the infected lung.[59] Experiments performed in dogs suggest that the bronchial artery, through its anatomic communications, could also represent a mechanism by which septic processes are delivered to the pericardium.[60] What should be emphasized, however, is the fact that the clinical signs that would direct the clinician's attention to the pericardium, namely increased heart size, muffled heart sounds, pericardial rub, pulsus paradoxus, neck vein distention, and hepatomegaly, can be absent.

Penicillin G remains the drug of choice for disease due to the pneumococcus. A limited number of studies are available,[61, 62] but the evidence appears that penicillin penetrates the pericardium. The optimum dosage has not been established. An acceptable form of therapy would be crystalline penicillin G administered as two million units intravenously every three to four hours. For the penicillin sensitive individual, erythromycin represents an acceptable alternative. Although critical data regarding pericardial penetration are not known, erythromycin has been used successfully for the treatment of pericarditis due to susceptible organisms.[63, 64] What must be underscored is the fact that the cornerstone of therapy for pneumococcal pericarditis is surgical drainage. Pericardiocentesis represents solely a diagnostic maneuver. The risk of repeat pericardial aspiration,[65] as well as the propensity for recurrent tamponade following pericardiocentesis makes adequate surgical drainage mandatory. The important factor is drainage of all purulent material as soon as the diagnosis is established.

Untreated, this disorder has a mortality that approximates 100 percent.[66] If the disorder is recognized early and the patient is treated with adequate surgical drainage and systemic antibiotics, most patients will survive.

Meningococcal Pericarditis

Meningococcal pericarditis represents a metastatic infection. The presumed source of the bacteremia is the nasopharynx. Pericarditis may represent the only complication of meningococcemia,[67-69] but more commonly it occurs in association with meningitis.[70] The manifestations of the pericarditis can represent the dominant symptomatology[71-73] or can be identified as incidental abnormalities.[74] Evidence of pericarditis can occur on the initial examination[75] or may not be present for weeks after the patient is ill.[70] There appears to be a rather consistent clinical presentation, as most patients will experience stabbing substernal chest pain, fever, pericardial rub, electrocardiographic evidence of pericarditis, as well as cardiomegaly detected by conventional chest x-rays. There can be evidence of associated polyserositis, manifested by pleural effusion or arthritis, and metastatic ophthalmitis.[70, 76]

The pericarditis usually occurs between the fourth and sixteenth day after the onset of the illness. The pericardial fluid is usually a serosanguinous exudate which is sterile and contains thousands of white blood cells, virtually all of which are polymorphonuclear leukocytes. The organism has been recovered from the pericardial fluid, however.[73, 77] The explanation for the sterile pericardium has been the fact that patients have invariably received antibiotics for the meningococcemia and/or meningitis that is recognized prior to the pericarditis. Although not documented, the suggestion has been made that the pericarditis which occurs early in the course of the illness represents a consequence of actual bacterial invasion of the pericardium, and the late-onset pericardial inflammation represents a "hypersensitivity reaction" to damaged pericardial tissue. This concept has resulted in the administration of corticosteroid to suppress inflammation and prevent reaccumulation of pericardial effusion.[70, 78] It must be emphasized, however, that this treatment has not always been invariably successful,[79] and its value is questionable.

Penicillin is regarded as the antibiotic of choice for disease due to *Neisseria meningitidis*. Therapy of meningococcal pericarditis would be 24 million units/day of crystalline penicillin G administered intravenously in equally divided doses at two hour intervals. Chloramphenicol would be considered the alternative drug for patients with known hypersensitivity to penicillins. This antibiotic should be administered intravenously as 4 to 6 grams/day in equally divided doses at six hour intervals. There are no adequate data to support the concept that chloramphenicol penetrates pericardial tissue in therapeutic concentrations, but this agent is known to possess excellent capacity for penetration of other tissue.[80]

When the presence of pericardial fluid results in cardiac tamponade, pericardiocentesis must be performed. For those patients who require repeated aspirations, a definitive surgical procedure should be performed, a pericardial window or pericardiectomy. Patients must also be observed for the development of pericardial constriction, as this complication has occurred acutely[81, 82] in spite of proper antibiotic therapy and pericardiocentesis, and necessitates pericardiectomy.

It should be emphasized that in spite of the number of published reports of this entity during the last 10 years, the physician should not assume that meningococcal pericarditis is a common disorder, either as a manifestation of meningococcemia or as a form of bacterial pericarditis. Many of the publications are single case reports and/or descriptions of unusual aspects of the disease.

Staphylococcal Pericarditis

Staphylococcal pericarditis is a grave disorder which must be diagnosed early and treated aggressively. It represents today the most frequent form of purulent pericarditis in children and adults.[83-85] The pathogenesis of this disease is varied, including cardiac trauma from penetrating wounds, cardiotomy,[86] hematogenous dissemination with or without myocardial abscesses,[84, 87-90] and as a complication of endocarditis.[58, 85 91] This disorder can supervene in patients with underlying diseases known to be associated with pericardial inflammation,[9] and, more rarely, staphylococcal pericarditis has developed without a known additional tissue source, in other words, as "primary" pericarditis.[92]

The staphylococcus is a highly invasive organism which produces rapid destruction of tissue and abscess formation. The purulent pericarditis can kill the host by acute cardiac tamponade or acute constriction.[87-89, 91, 93] The pericarditis due to endocarditis is most commonly caused by annular erosion, resulting in a purulent pericarditis from direct extension[91] or hemorrhagic pericarditis, with or without tamponade.[94] Either pathway can result in a fatal outcome.

The staphylococcus produces a grossly purulent pericarditis from which organisms are readily detected by gram stain and culture. The fluid tends to reaccumulate, become tenacious, to loculate, and to form thick adhesions. The patients invariably are very

163

"toxic," febrile, with dyspnea, tachypnea, tachycardia. They have an elevated white blood cell count and may experience hemodynamic embarrassment. When the pericarditis develops as a postoperative intrathoracic infection secondary to a sternal wound infection or mediastinal abscess or as a contiguous spread from endocarditis or myocardial abscess, death is virtually inevitable.[85]

Therapy must be directed at all aspects of the problem: support of the associated illness,[95] removal of infected indwelling intravenous catheters,[96, 97] appropriate antibiotic selection, and surgical drainage.[83] The optimum antibiotic for the therapy of life-threatening disease due to penicillinase producing *Staphylococcus aureus* has never been determined. Clinical experience suggests no significant differences in therapeutic efficacy of the parenteral semisynthetic penicillins (methicillin, oxacillin, nafcillin) used in patients with severe staphylococcal disease.[98] Limited data suggest that methicillin does penetrate the infected pericardium in therapeutic concentrations,[86, 87] as does cephalothin sodium.[62, 99] For the treatment of staphylococcal pericarditis due to penicillinase producing strains, either of these antibiotics should be administered intravenously as 2 grams every four hours[100] for at least four weeks. When the patient is hypersensitive to penicillin or when the organism is resistant to the penicillins or cephalosporins, the drug of choice is vancomycin. This is because it has no cross resistance to other antibiotics, virtually all strains of *Staphylococcus aureus* are susceptible to it, and it exhibits no cross hypersensitivity, for it has no chemical relationship with any other antibiotic. Vancomycin is administered intravenously as 500 mg. every six hours. Vancomycin has a record of proven accomplishment in the management of severe staphylococcal disease,[101] and it penetrates pericardial fluid in therapeutic concentrations.[102] The drug dosage must be monitored very carefully as ototoxicity and nephrotoxicity may occur, particularly in patients with renal insufficiency.

Pericardiocentesis, by needle or catheter, usually is not adequate to effectively and permanently reduce the cardiac compression. Surgical decompression is a vital aspect of the definitive therapy. The most effective surgical treatment has not been determined. Primary pericardiectomy appears to offer many advantages: prompt and effective eradication of the infected space, rapid control of the infection, immediate relief of the mechanical compression, and prevention of subsequent constrictive pericarditis.[103, 104]

Gram-Negative (Non-Hemophilus) Pericarditis

Two recent publications suggest the aerobic gram-negative bacilli are emerging as a more frequent cause of bacterial pericarditis.[58, 85] This disorder appears to develop as either an extension from a contiguous focus (endocardium or colonic fistula) or from hematogenous dissemination from an extrathoracic focus (urinary tract; abdominal organ). Survival of these patients is infrequent and is attributed to the fact that this form of pericarditis is being experienced by patients with severe underlying disorders. The gram-negative bacilli causing pericarditis, as determined by pericardial fluid cultures or blood cultures, include *Pseudomonas aeruginosa*, *Klebsiella pneumoniae* and *Escherichia coli*. Additional gram-negative bacilli, as well as multiple organisms simultaneously, have produced this disorder. Treatment includes antibiotic therapy directed against the organism, measures to manage the tissue source of origin, and adequate surgical drainage of the purulent pericardium, to relieve the circulatory embarrassment.

Correct antibiotic selection presents a formidable problem for the following reasons: the susceptibility patterns of gram-negative bacilli are constantly changing and vary widely from one hospital to another; the drugs employed to treat these organisms have the potential for serious toxicity; there are very limited data available regarding the ability of antibiotics to penetrate the infected pericardium; and there are no controlled studies to compare agents. There are no published studies that detail the therapeutic concentrations of carbenicillin or colistimethate in infected pericardial tissue. Gentamicin, however, does appear to penetrate the pericardium in concentrations that are inhibitory for the majority of gram-negative bacilli.[62, 105]

For the treatment of patients with life threatening infections, such as bacterial pericarditis, gentamicin should be administered initially as 6 mg./kg. per day in three divided doses. After the first day of treatment, the appropriate maintenance dose for the patient without renal insufficiency is 4.5 mg./kg. per day. When azotemia is present, the daily dose should be adjusted according to a published nomogram or, preferably, by sequential determination of serum concentrations.[106, 107] For the treatment of critically ill patients the physician should attempt to insure a peak serum level of 8 to 10 μg./ml. A study has correlated therapeutic efficacy with achievable serum concentrations of gentamicin.[108]

Miscellaneous Forms of Bacterial Pericarditis

Pericarditis — Anaerobes

Anaerobes have the capability of causing endocarditis,[109] myocardial abscesses,[110] and purulent pericarditis.[10, 58] Purulent pericarditis, which results from hematogenous dissemination from a distant focus or by direct extension from pleuropulmonary or esophageal disease, can result in cardiac tamponade. The presence of a foul smell to the pericardial fluid is a strong clinical guide to the presence of anaerobes.

Therapy of anaerobic pericarditis must include drainage of the primary tissue focus of infection and the pericardium, the removal of devitalized tissues, and systemic antibiotics. Surgery is of primary therapeutic consideration.[111] Penicillin G is regarded the drug of choice of all anaerobic infections except those involving *Bacteroides fragilis* and rare strains of *Fusobacterium*. For individuals who have pericarditis due to *Bacteroides fragilis* the most effective antibiotic program would consist of intravenous administration of large doses of clindamycin (900 mg. every six hours), chloramphenicol (1 gm. every four to six hours), or cystalline penicillin G (5 million units every three hours).[112] All these agents have significant defects, and no controlled study has established the optimum selection or dosage.[113]

Pericarditis — Subacute Bacterial Endocarditis

Autopsy protocols have confirmed the fact that pericarditis may supervene in the course of subacute bacterial endocarditis.[114-116] This sequence of events has been explained by several mechanisms: mycotic aneurysm of the ascending aorta, rheumatic fever, myocardial infarction, and uremia.[117] Although very unusual, massive effusion as well as tamponade have occurred.[118, 119] These cases of pericarditis, which develop from subacute bacterial endocarditis, are usually due to streptococci, particularly *Streptococcus viridans*.

A recent report from the New York Hospital has established the fact that a regimen consisting of crystalline penicillin G, administered as 2 million units intravenously every four hours, plus streptomycin, 1 gm. intramuscularly for two weeks, followed by penicillin alone for an additional two weeks resulted in extraordinary success.[120] In patients who have renal insufficiency or evidence of eighth nerve damage the streptomycin should be omitted. When patients are sensitive to penicillin, therapy should consist of vancomycin in a dose of 0.5 gm. intravenously every six hours for four weeks. The therapeutic dosage is adjusted to produce serum dilution bactericidal levels of $\frac{1}{16}$ or greater.[121] Vancomycin does penetrate pericardial fluid in therapeutic concentra-

tions,[102] and has been employed successfully in the treatment of life threatening streptococcal and staphylococcal endocarditis. Adjunctive treatment would consist of the
management of congestive heart failure and cardiac tamponade.

Tuberculous Pericarditis

Tuberculous pericarditis has been studied and described by some of the world's most
eminent cardiologists.[122-124] In spite of this, no characteristic pattern of signs or symptoms has emerged that would be of definitive value for today's clinician. There are
many reasons for this situation: this disorder is rare, limiting detailed evaluations; a
large number of the reported cases were based on assumptions that were not absolutely
confirmed; the majority of medical publications antedates the present chemotherapeutic era; to some extent, the diagnosis has been established according to the principle of "guilt by association" (the patient had a positive family history of tuberculosis;
the patient had prior tuberculosis; the presence of a positive skin test; the presence of a
concomitant pulmonary infiltrate having the appearance of tuberculosis; the presence
of tuberculosis in other organs; the response of the process to antituberculous therapy
and the demonstration of granuloma in excised pericardial tissue or at necropsy); and
the ability of the organism to elicit an acute, subacute, or chronic pericarditis, with or
without effusion.[125]

Absolute proof of a tuberculous etiology demands growth of the organism from the
pericardial fluid or pericardial tissue. Stains and microscopic appearance of host tissue
are not specific. Other organisms have the ability to demonstrate the acid-fast property
and granuloma formation, with or without caseation necrosis, which has been described
in many disorders.[126] Unfortunately, however, there are documented cases of tuberculous pericarditis in which the pericardial fluid, although intensely studied both by culture medium and guinea pig inoculation, failed to grow the organism.[127] If that were not
enough of a problem for the clinician, there are situations in which pericardial tissue has
demonstrated only nonspecific fibrosis, where convincing evidence supported the diagnosis of tuberculous pericarditis.[54, 128]

Tuberculous pericarditis develops most frequently from direct extension of mediastinal or hilar nodes.[129, 130] Less frequently it results from direct contact from tuberculous lungs or as a manifestation of miliary disease.

Clinical Presentation

A recent review of the subject has described the symptoms and signs of tuberculous
pericarditis, as well as their relative frequencies.[65] What must be emphasized, however,
is the fact that there are no absolutes. Various authors and students of this disease have
stressed certain clinical aspects: constitutional symptoms are relatively insignificant;[128]
the disease usually has an insidious onset;[131, 132] tachycardia is almost invariably present;[65, 122, 124] the most prominent symptom at the onset of the disorder is shortness of
breath;[122] significant murmurs are absent;[130, 133, 134] the heart is normal in size and the
pericardium, as evaluated by x-ray following air injection, is thickened;[130, 133] the pericardial fluid is most commonly bloody;[134] the pericardial fluid tends to recur after aspiration;[127, 133, 135] and the majority of the white blood cells of the pericardium are lymphocytes.[122, 131, 132] There are, however, reports that negate the value of all of these "diagnostic clues." Symptoms can develop acutely,[131, 136] and the disease can simulate viral
pericarditis because of the presence of severe recurrent chest pain.[136] The hallmark of
this disease is its variable nature.[135] Tuberculosis pericarditis must always be considered in the differential diagnosis of a pericarditis or a fever of unknown origin.[137]

Prognosis and Treatment

Tuberculosis is regarded as the most common identifiable organism that produces chronic constrictive pericarditis.[124] Although tuberculous pericarditis can spontaneously undergo complete resolution,[128, 130, 138, 139] the untreated disease usually results in death from disseminated disease or myocardial failure.[122, 134, 138, 140] A review of 37 cases of tuberculous pericarditis found in the literature by Stepman and Owyang[133] disclosed that 63 per cent died within six months, and at least 84 per cent ultimately had fatal outcomes. A followup study at Johns Hopkins on 71 patients with untreated clinically significant tuberculous pericarditis showed that 39 died within two years of the onset of the disease, usually with disseminated disease, less commonly from cardiac compression.[141]

It is apparent from the natural history of the disease that therapy must be directed at the control of the tuberculous activity (role of chemotherapy) and relief of the cardiac embarrassment (pericardiocentesis for acute cardiac tamponade and percardiectomy for constrictive pericarditis). Effective antituberculous agents have been available for 25 years, and a modest number of reviews of the drug treatment of tuberculous pericarditis have appeared in the medical literature.[65, 142-144] The optimum chemotherapeutic approach to this disorder has not been resolved, however. Published articles have established important therapeutic guidelines: drugs have unequivocally improved the prognosis of tuberculous pericarditis; ambulatory treatment, following the initial period of disease activity, is not deleterious; multiple drugs must be administered simultaneously; treatment should be started as soon as initial studies have been completed; inadequate drug dosage and delay in treatment are important factors contributing to constrictive pericarditis and dissemination of the disease; clinical response to therapy is usually slow; chemotherapy should be continued for 18 months after all signs of active disease have subsided; and a poor prognosis following the exclusive medical therapy of this disease has resulted when hepatomegaly, ankle edema, paradoxical pulse, and ascites were detected.[145]

Isoniazid remains the keystone of therapy of tuberculosis and should be included in the initial treatment regimen, pending antimicrobial susceptibility testing. The usual oral adult dose of isoniazid is 300 mg. or 5 to 8 mg./kg. daily. To minimize the risk of polyneuritis from isoniazid, pyridoxine in doses of 100 mg. daily should be given. Additional untoward reactions attributed to isoniazid include the following: nervous system (seizures, psychoses, memory loss, interference with autonomic function), hematologic system (Coombs positive hemolytic anemia, hypochromic microcytic anemia with megaloblastoid features), and musculoskeletal system (simulate rheumatoid arthritis or lupus-like syndrome). Of greatest importance, however, is the isoniazid hepatitis hypersensitivity syndrome, as this has resulted in deaths.

Because aminosalicyclic acid (PAS) causes frequent adverse gastrointestinal effects and hypersensitivity reactions, most experts now use ethambutal in preference to PAS in antituberculous combinations. Although optic neuritis has been associated with the use of ethambutal, it is likely to occur only with doses higher than the 15 mg./kg. daily now recommended for initial treatment. Unfortunately, however, there are no data available concerning the ability of this drug to penetrate the tuberculous pericardium.

The other major antituberculous drugs are streptomycin and rifampin. Streptomycin, which must be given by injection, can damage the vestibular and the auditory divisions of the eighth cranial nerve, sometimes irreversibly. This drug is given in daily doses of 1 gm. for adults with normal renal function. In patients with preexisting renal impairment, nephrotoxicity and ototoxicity are augmented so that the dose of the drug must be regulated carefully. Limited data suggest that streptomycin penetrates pericardial fluid.[62]

Rifampin has proven to be a highly effective and safe drug, when used in combination with other agents, for the therapy of tuberculosis. The adult dose of rifampin is 600 mg. (2 capsules) once a day, administered one hour before breakfast. Rifampin can be used, in combination with INH, for onset treatment of tuberculosis and certainly should be employed in the combination of drugs for the retreatment of patients who have relapsed or who have failed to respond to the initial drug regimen.[146] No data are available regarding the ability of rifampin to penetrate the infected pericardium, but it distributes well into body tissue and fluids.[147]

Accordingly, some investigators of this disease treat patients with triple drug therapy consisting of INH plus ethambutal and streptomycin,[65] and others administer INH plus PAS and streptomycin.[144] Another area of dispute is the use of corticosteroid in conjunction with specific antituberculous agents. Some publications support their use,[144, 148, 149] but no well designed prospective controlled studies have documented their true value.

Surgery has continued to be of vital importance for the management of tuberculous pericarditis. It has been shown conclusively that surgical resection can be performed in the presence of active disease without danger of dissemination.[150] The contribution that surgery makes to the treatment of constrictive pericarditis is unquestioned.[150, 151] The unresolved issue is the proper time to offer surgery for the patient with tuberculous pericarditis, with or without effusion. Some surgeons have recently advocated a more aggressive approach. The indications would be the relief of pain; the prevention of the sequence of effusion progressing to organization, which in turn progresses to obliteration of the pericardial cavity; and the obtaining of tissue for biopsy and relief of chronic tamponade.[152]Cardiologists recommend pericardiectomy for "persistent enlarged heart size, progressive congestive heart failure and increasing venous pressure when heart size is decreasing,"[144] and surgeons suggest that "all reasonable-risk patients with tuberculous pericarditis would benefit from prompt surgical intervention following institution of chemotherapy."[153] The surgeons build their case on the following facts: progression to constriction, which makes surgery technically hazardous, can occur insidiously and thus not be well recognized, and it can occur despite adequate chemotherapy. Only well designed future studies will resolve these divergent points of view.

Histoplasmosis Pericarditis

The pericarditis caused by *Histoplasma capsulatum* can be a manifestation of an acute self-limited primary infection,[154-161] of chronic pulmonary disease,[162, 163] or of progressive disseminated disease.[164] Pericarditis is not a common feature of progressive disseminated histoplasmosis, however.[165] The pericarditis can have an acute onset or develop insidiously. It shares many similar characteristics with tuberculous pericarditis: the pericarditis can represent direct extension from hilar nodes or be an expression of hematogenous dissemination; effusions can develop; concomitant hilar lymph nodes, mediastinal lymph nodes, and pulmonary infiltrates can exist; constriction with or without calcification of the pericardium can develop;[157, 162] and the tissue response can be fibrosis and/or caseating or non-caseating granuloma.[157]

The pericardial effusion has invariably had a predominance of lymphocytes, and a protein content that exceeds 3 g%[159, 160, 166] Smears of the pericardial fluid[162] and pericardial tissue,[157, 164, 166] as well as cultures of the pericardial fluid,[166] have demonstrated the organism, but not consistently.

The latex agglutination test is a valuable serologic test in acute histoplasmosis, that form of the disease in which most cases of pericarditis have been described.[167] A single titer of 1:32 or greater is strong evidence for active or recent histoplasmosis. Latex agglutination titers become positive at about two to three weeks. This test is particularly appropriate because of the following reasons: positive sputum cultures in the acute form of the disease are rare; the complement fixation test detects only 50 per cent of the cases of the acute pulmonary form of the disease;[168] the skin test has significant defects.[169] The diagnosis can be supported by isolation of the organism from the peripheral blood or bone marrow, or the presence of a complement-fixation titer of $1:8$ or greater.

Skin and serologic testing are of considerably less value than cultural studies to establish the diagnosis of progressive disseminated histoplasmosis.[165] Cultures of bone marrow, peripheral blood, urine, liver, and oral lesions are particularly rewarding. The organism has even been seen in a Wright-stained peripheral blood smear.[170]

The drug treatment of pericarditis caused by *Histoplasma capsulatum* is determined by the clinical stage of the disease. Acute pulmonary histoplasmosis is usually a benign, self-limited infection requiring no specific therapy, in spite of the fact that hematogenous dissemination occurs in a sizable portion of the cases.[171] Careful observation of patients is necessary to detect progressive dissemination of disease or the development of chronic respiratory disease. Evidence of progressive dissemination include persistent fever and debility, hepatosplenomegaly, mucosal ulcerations, renal function abnormalities, anemia, thrombocytopenia, and leukopenia.

A fatal outcome is to be expected without drug treatment of progressive disseminated disease. The treatment of choice for this form of histoplasmosis is the intravenous administration of amphotericin B. The details regarding administration of this polyene macrolide have recently been published.[172] For the progressive disseminated stage of the disease a total dose of between 35 and 40 mg./kg. of body weight has been suggested.[173] Amphotericin B administration is attended by immediate unpleasant and occasionally serious side effects. The most common untoward events attributed to this compound include chills, fever, headache, nausea, vomiting, thrombophlebitis, anemia, hypokalemia, and nephrotoxicity.[174] Because of its appreciable toxicity, amphotericin B should be given under close clinical supervision, with frequent determination of the serum potassium and creatinine, as well as hematocrit.[172]

It is important to stress that tuberculosis[175] is frequently found in association with histoplasmosis, and adrenal function must be evaluated in every patient with disseminated histoplasmosis, as adrenal insufficiency represents a common cause of death.[173]

SUMMARY

Infections of the pericardium can occur as incidental findings in patients with systemic disease or dominate the clinical situation, representing a major threat to life. These infections appear to arise from the contiguous spread of infected tissue or from hematogenous dissemination. The clinical manifestations can resemble the "textbook description," but more often are subtle, nonspecific, or altered by the patient's basic disease. The diagnosis should never be discarded because dyspnea or chest pain are not elicited, friction rub and pulsus paradoxus are not detected, and chest x-rays and electrocardiograms are not "confirmatory."

It is generally conceded that there has been a recent shift in the etiology of infectious pericarditis. This change has been attributed to the increased average age of hospitalized patients, modern diagnostic and therapeutic advances, and the impact of antibiotics. However, three concepts have stood the test of time: accurate diagnosis is the cornerstone of treatment; the availability of antibiotics must not relegate the role of surgery to a secondary position; and therapy must be directed against the pericarditis and the additional sources of infected tissue.

ACKNOWLEDGMENT

I wish to express my thanks and appreciation to Paul Vaiginas of the Lemuel Shattuck Hospital's Medical Library and Barbara Paxton of the Faulkner Hospital's Medical library for their extensive library research and to Phyllis Rotman and Geraldine Weinberg of the Lemuel Shattuck Hospital for their secretarial assistance.

REFERENCES

1. VIETZKE, W. M.: *Gonococcal arthritis with pericarditis.* Arch. Intern. Med. 117:270, 1966.

2. CROSSLEY, K., BIGOS, T., AND JOFFE, C. D.: *Hemophilus influenzae pericarditis.* Am. Heart J. 85: 246, 1973.

3. DUKE, M., AND DONOVAN, T. J.: *Hemophilus influenzae pericarditis with cardiac tamponade.* Am. J. Cardiol. 31:778, 1973.

4. ALSEVER, R. N., STIVER, G., DINERMAN, N., ET AL.: *Hemophilus influenzae pericarditis and empyema with thyroiditis in an adult.* J.A.M.A. 230:1426, 1974.

5. KILLAM, H. A. W., CROWDER, J. G., WHITE, A. C., ET AL.: *Pericarditis due to vibrio fetus.* Am. J. Cardiol. 17:723, 1966.

6. KHAN, A., ROSEN, K. M., RAHIMTOOLA, S. H., ET AL.: *Listeria bacteremia with acute pericarditis.* Chest 60:496, 1971.

7. BRAUNSTEIN, H., TUCKER, E., AND GIBSON, B. C.: *Infections caused by unusual beta hemolytic streptococci.* Am. J. Clin. Pathol. 55:424, 1971.

8. SUSENS, G. P., AL-SHAMMA, A., AND ROWE, J. C.: *Purulent constrictive pericarditis caused by nocardia asteroides.* Ann. Intern. Med. 67:1021, 1967.

9. KNODELLE, R. G., AND MANDERS, S. J.: *Staphylococcal pericarditis in a patient with systemic lupus erythematosus.* Chest 65:103, 1974.

10. HARRIS, C. L., BENCHIMOL, A., AND DESSER, K. B.: *Bacteroides pericardial effusion and cardiac tamponade in a patient with chronic renal failure.* Am. Heart J. 89:629, 1975.

11. BOYLE, J. D., PEARCE, M. L., AND GUZE, L. B.: *Purulent pericarditis: review of literature and report of eleven cases.* Medicine 40:119, 1961.

12. HANCOCK, E. W.: *Constrictive pericarditis.* J.A.M.A. 232:176, 1975.

13. BARTLETT, R. C.: *Contemporary blood culture practices,* in SONNENWIRTH, A. L. (ED.): *Bacteremia: Laboratory and Clinical Aspects.* Charles C Thomas, Springfield, Ill., 1973.

14. SUTTER, V. L., ATTEBERY, H. R., ROSENBLATT, J. E., ET AL.: *Anaerobic bacteriology manual.* UCLA School of Medicine, Los Angeles, 1972.

15. ROBERTS, G. D., AND WASHINGTON, J. A., II: *Detection of fungi in blood cultures (abstract).* 14th Interscience conference on antimicrobial agents and chemotherapy, San Francisco, Sept. 11–13, 1974.

16. CARLETON, J., AND HAMBURGER, M.: *Unmasking of false-negative blood cultures in patients receiving new penicillins.* J.A.M.A. 186:157, 1963.

17. MURRAY, M., AND MOOSNICK, F.: *Simultaneous arterial and venous blood cultures.* J. Lab. Clin. Med. 26:382, 1940.

18. BEESON, P. B., BRANNON, E. S., AND WARREN, J. V.: *Observations on the sites of removal of bacteria from the blood in patients with bacterial endocarditis.* J. Exp. Med. 81:9, 1945.

19. LOURIA, D. B.: *L-forms, spheroplasts and aberrant forms in chronic sepsis.* Adv. Intern. Med. 17:125, 1971.

20. PORTNOY, J., WOLF, P. L., WEBB, M., ET AL.: *Candida blastospores and pseudohyphae in blood smears.* N. Engl. J. Med. 285:1010, 1971.

21. BENNETT, I. L., JR., AND BEESON, P. B.: *Bacteremia: a consideration of some experimental and clinical aspects.* Yale J. Biol. Med. 26:241, 1954.

22. SMITH, J. W., AND UTZ, J. P.: *Progressive disseminated histoplasmosis.* Ann. Intern. Med. 76:557, 1972.

23. HEINLE, E. W., JENSEN, W. N., AND WESTERMAN, M. P.: *Diagnostic usefulness of marrow biopsy in disseminated tuberculosis.* Am. Rev. Resp. Dis. 91:701, 1965.

24. CUCIN, R. L., COLEMAN, M., ECKARDT, J. J., ET AL.: *The diagnosis of miliary tuberculosis: Utility of peripheral blood abnormalities, bone marrow and liver needle biopsy.* J. Chronic Dis. 26: 355, 1973.

25. SASLOW, S., AND PERKINS, R.: *The gastric smear for acid-fast bacilli in the presumptive diagnosis of tuberculosis.* Am. J. Med. Sci. 243:470, 1962.

26. JONES, F. L., JR.: *The relative efficacy of spontaneous sputa, aerosol-induced sputa, and gastric aspirates in the bacteriologic diagnosis of pulmonary tuberculosis.* Dis. Chest 50:403, 1966.

27. GILKERSON, S. W., AND KANNER, O.: *Improved technique for the detection of acid-fast bacilli by fluorescence.* J. Bacteriol. 86:890, 1963.

28. WEED, L. A., AND MACY, N. E.: *Tuberculosis – problems in diagnosis and eradication.* Am. J. Clin. Pathol. 53:136, 1970.

29. LEVINE, H., SZARTO, P. B., AND CUGELL, S. W.: *Tuberculous pleurisy.* Arch. Intern. Med. 122:329, 1968.

30. LEVINE, H., METZGER, W., LACERA, D., ET AL.: *Diagnosis of tuberculous pleurisy by culture of pleural biopsy specimen.* Arch. Intern. Med. 126:269, 1970.

31. BERGQUIST, S., AND NORDENSTOM, H.: *Thoracoscopy and pleural biopsy in the diagnosis of pleurisy.* Scand. J. Respir. Dis. 47:64, 1966.

32. DE CAMP, P. T., MOSELEY, P. W., SCOTT, M. L., ET AL.: *Diagnostic thoracoscopy.* Ann. Thorac. Surg. 14:79, 1973.

33. WIJSMULLER, G.: *The negative tuberculin test.* J. Med. Assoc. State Alabama 41:353, 1971.

34. HOLDEN, M., DUBIN, M. R., AND DIAMOND, P. H.: *Frequency of negative intermediate-strength tuberculin sensitivity in patients with active tuberculosis.* N. Engl. J. Med. 285:1506, 1971.

35. STEAD, W.: *Tuberculosis. An old disease returns to main stream of medicine.* J. Chronic Dis. 25:249, 1972.

36. SMITH, J. A., AND REICHMAN, L. B.: *Lymphocyte transformation.* Am. Rev. Resp. Dis. 106:194, 1972.

37. PARK, B. H., FIKRIG, S. M., AND SMITHWICK, E. M.: *Infection and nitroblue-tetrazolium reduction by neutrophils.* Lancet 2:532, 1968.

38. MATULA, G., AND PATERSON, P. Y.: *Spontaneous in vitro reduction of nitroblue tetrazolium by neutrophils of adult patients with bacterial infection.* N. Engl. J. Med. 285:311, 1971.

39. MANDELL, G. L., AND FULLER, L. F.: *Nitroblue tetrazolium dye test: A diagnostic aid in tuberculosis.* Am. Rev. Resp. Dis. 105:123, 1972.

40. Segal, A. W.: *Nitroblue-tetrazolium tests.* Lancet 2:1248, 1974.

41. DORFF, G. H., COONROD, J. D., AND RYTEL, M. W.: *Detection by immunoelectrophoresis of antigen in sera of patients with pneumococcal bacteremia.* Lancet 2:519, 1971.

42. WEINSTEIN, L., AND TSAO, C. L.: *Effect of types of treatment on development of antistreptolysin in patients with scarlet fever.* Proc. Soc. Exp. Biol. Med. 63:449, 1946.

43. DILLON, H. C., JR., AND REEVES, M.S.A.: *Streptococcal immune responses in nephritis after skin infection.* Am. J. Med. 56:333, 1974.

44. KAPLAN, E. L., ANTHONY, B. F., CHAPMAN, S. S., ET AL.: *The influence of the site of infection on the immune response to group A streptococci.* J. Clin. Invest. 49:1405, 1970.

45. HAKKILA, J., FRICK, H. M., AND HALONEN, P. I.: *Pericarditis and myocarditis caused by toxoplasma: report of a case and review of the literature.* Am. Heart J. 55:758, 1958.

46. JONES, T. C., KEAN, B. H., AND KIMBALL, A. L.: *Pericarditis associated with toxoplasmosis.* Ann. Intern. Med. 62:786, 1965.

47. SABIN, A. B., AND FELDMAN, H. A.: *Dyes as microchemical indicators of a new immunity phenomenon affecting a protozoan parasite (toxoplasma).* Science 108;660, 1948.

48. FELDMAN, H.: *Toxoplasmosis.* N. Engl. J. Med. 279:1431, 1968.

49. LUNDE, M. N., GELDERMAN, A. H., HAYES, S. L., ET AL.: *Serologic diagnosis of active toxoplasmosis complicating malignant diseases.* Cancer 25:637, 1970.

50. KAGAN, I. G.: *Serologic diagnosis of parasitic diseases.* N. Engl. J. Med. 282:685, 1970.

51. HUNDER, G. G., MULLEN, B. J., AND MCDUFFIE, F. C.: *Complement in pericardial fluid of lupus erythematosus.* Ann. Intern. Med. 80:453, 1974.

52. LIGHT, R. W., MACGREGOR, M. I., LUCHSINGER, P. C., ET AL.: *Pleural effusions: The diagnostic separation of transudates and exudates.* Ann. Intern. Med. 77:507, 1972.

53. NACHUM, R., LIPSEY, A., AND SIEGEL, S. E.: *Rapid detection of gram-negative bacterial meningitis by the limilus lysate test.* N. Engl. J. Med. 289:931, 1973.

54. CHEITLIN, M. D., SERFAS, L. J., SEBAR, S. S., ET AL.: *Tuberculous pericarditis: Is limited pericardial biopsy sufficient for diagnosis?* Am. Rev. Resp. Dis. 98:287, 1968.

55. BRANCH, C. F.: *A brief review of the essential pathology of pericarditis.* N. Engl. J. Med. 208:771, 1933.

56. BISGARD, J. D.: *Pyopericarditis: an analysis of cases treated by pericardiotomy.* Am. J. Surg. 17:1, 1932.

57. KAUFFMAN, C. A., WATANAKUNAKOIN, C., AND PHAIR, J. P.: *Purulent pneumococcal pericarditis.* Am. J. Med. 54:743, 1973.

58. GOULD, K., BARNETT, J. A., AND SANFORD, J. P.: *Purulent pericarditis in the antibiotic era.* Arch. Intern. Med. 134:923, 1974.

59. CHATARD, J. A.: *Acute pericarditis complicating acute lobar pneumonia.* Johns Hopkins Hosp. Rep. 15:155, 1910.

60. HAHN, R. S., HOLMAN, E., AND FRENICKS, J. B.: *The role of the bronchial artery circulation in the etiology of pulmonary and pericardial suppuration.* J. Thorac. Surg. 27:121, 1954.

61. ORY, E. M., MEADS, M., BROWN, B., ET AL.: *Penicillin levels in serum and in some body fluids during systemic and local therapy.* J. Lab. Clin. Med. 30:809, 1945.

62. TAN, J. S., HOLMES, J. C., FOWLER, N. O., ET AL.: *Antibiotic levels in pericardial fluid.* J. Clin. Invest. 53:7, 1974.

63. NIEMAN, E. A.: *Penicillin-resistant staphylococcal pericarditis.* Lancet 1:1330, 1957.

64. TETZNER, K. H.: *Zur antibiotischen behandlung mit erycinum.* Medizinische 831, 1956.

65. FOWLER, N. O., AND MANITSAS, G. T.: *Infectious pericarditis.* Progr. Cardiovasc. Dis. 16:323, 1973.

66. ADAMS, R., AND POLDERMAN, H.: *Suppurative pericarditis.* N. Engl. J. Med. 225:897, 1941.

67. ROBERTS, K. B., AND NEFF, J. M.: *Meningococcal pericarditis without meningitis in a child.* Am. J. Dis. Child. 124:440, 1972.

68. MILLER, H. I.: *Acute pericarditis as a presenting feature of meningococcal septicemia.* Isr. J. Med. Sci. 9:1570, 1973.

69. NARAGI, S., AND KABINS, S. A.: *Acute meningococcal pericarditis without meningitis.* Arch. Intern. Med. 135:314, 1975.

70. PIERCE, H. I., AND COOPER, E. B.: *Meningococcal pericarditis.* Arch. Intern. Med. 129:918, 1972.

71. SASLOW, S., AND DISERENS, R. V.: *Purulent pericardial effusion complicating meningococcal meningitis.* N. Engl. J. Med. 263:1074, 1960.

72. LUKASH, W. M.: *Massive pericardial effusion due to meningococcic pericarditis.* J.A.M.A. 185:598, 1963.

73. BEAL, L. R., USTAH, T. J., AND FORKER, A. D.: *Meningococcemia without meningitis presenting as cardiac tamponade.* Am. J. Med. 51:659, 1971.

74. HERRICK, W. W.: *Meningococcic pericarditis, with report of 12 cases. Medical service of the base hospital, Camp Jackson, S. C.* Med. Clin. North Am. 2:411, 1918.

75. WANSBROUGH-JONES, M. H., AND WONG, O. P.: *Meningococcal pericarditis without meningitis.* Br. Med. J. 2:344, 1973.

76. MARON, B. J., MACONE, K. L., AND BENARON, P.: *Unusual complications of meningococcal meningitis.* Johns Hopkins Med. J. 131:64, 1972.

77. ORGAIN, E. S., AND POSTON, M. A.: *Pericarditis with effusion due to the meningococcus.* Am. Heart J. 18:368, 1932.

78. MORSE, J. R., ORETSKY, M. I., AND HUDSON, J. A.: *Pericarditis as a complication of meningococcal meningitis.* Ann. Intern. Med. 74:212, 1971.

79. PENNY, J. L., GRACE, W. J., AND KENNEDY, R. J.: *Meningococcic pericarditis.* Am. J. Cardiol. 18:281, 1966.

80. WOODWARD, T. E., AND WISSEMAN, C. L., JR.: *Chloromycetin (chloramphenicol).* Medical Encyclopedia, Inc., New York, 1958.

81. SCOTT, L. P., KNOX, D., PERURY, L. W., ET AL.: *Meningococcal pericarditis.* Am. J. Cardiol. 29:104, 1972.

82. WEISS, E. J., AND SILBER, E. N.: *Acute constrictive pericarditis.* J. Pediatr. 58:548, 1961.

83. GERSONY, W. M., AND McCRACKEN, G. H.: *Purulent pericarditis in infancy.* Pediatrics 40:224, 1967.

84. VAN REKER, D., STRAUSS, A., HERNANDEZ, A., ET AL.: *Infectious pericarditis in children.* J. Pediatr. 85:165, 1974.

85. RUBIN, R. H., AND MOELLERING, R. C., JR.: *Clinical, microbiologic and therapeutic aspects of purulent pericarditis,* Am. J. Med. (in press).

86. ABU-NASSAR, H. J., YOW, E. M., ALEXANDER, J. K., ET AL.: *Primary staphylococcal pericarditis complicating cardiotomy.* Ann. Intern. Med. 60:135, 1964.

87. THOMAS, G. I., GREGORES, B. J., PERRY, D. M., ET AL.: *Pericardiectomy for acute constrictive staphylococcal pericarditis.* N. Engl. J. Med. 267:440, 1962.

172

88. MORGAN, J.: *Pericardial tamponade: A complication of staphylococcal pericarditis.* Can. Med. Assoc. J. 90:1082, 1964.

89. SANYAL, S. K., KAUR, I., HOOJA, V., ET AL.: *Staphylococcal pericarditis with cardiac tamponade in children.* Arch. Dis. Child. 45:198, 1970.

90. SLIM, M. S., RIZK, G., UWAYDAH, M., ET AL.: *Mediastinal complications of staphylococcal infection in childhood: experience with six consecutive cases.* Surgery 69:755, 1971.

91. WATANAKUNAKOIN, C., TAN, J. S., AND PHAIR, J. P.: *Some salient features of staphylococcal aureus endocarditis.* Am. J. Med. 54:473, 1973.

92. FITZGERALD, J. D., AND McNICOL, M. W.: *Acute suppurative pericarditis with death from ruptured mycotic aneurysm of the aorta.* Postgrad. Med. J. 40:36, 1964.

93. CAIRD, R., CONWAY, N., AND McMILLAN, I. K. R.: *Purulent pericarditis followed by early constriction in young children.* Br. Heart J. 35:201, 1973.

94. UTLEY, J. R., AND MILLS, J.: *Annular erosion and pericarditis.* J. Thorac. Cardiovasc. Surg. 64:76, 1971.

95. CLUFF, L., REYNOLDS, R. C., PAGE, D. L., ET AL.: *Staphylococcal bacteremia and altered host resistance.* Ann. Intern. Med. 69:859, 1968.

96. ZINNER, S. H., DENNY-BROWN, B. C., BRAUN, P., ET AL.: *Risk of infection with intravenous indwelling catheter: effect of application of antibiotic ointment.* J. Infect. Dis. 120:616, 1969.

97. BENTLEY, D. W., AND LEPPER, M. H.: *Septicemia related to indwelling venous catheter.* J.A.M.A. 206: 1749, 1968.

98. GILBERT, D. N., AND SANFORD, J. P.: *Methicillin: critical appraisal after a decade of experience.* Med. Clin. North Am. 54:1113, 1970.

99. GUMP, D. W., AND LIPSON, R. L.: *The penetration of cephalothin into synovial and other body fluids.* Curr. Ther. Res. 10:583, 1968.

100. WISE, R. I.: *Modern management of severe staphylococcal disease.* Medicine 52:295, 1973.

101. GERACI, J. E., NICHOLS, D. R., AND WELLMAN, W. E.: *Vancomycin in serious staphylococcal infections.* Arch. Intern. Med. 109:53, 1962.

102. GERACI, J. E., HEILMAN, F. R., NICHOLS, D. R., ET AL.: *Some laboratory and clinical experiences with a new antibiotic, vancomycin.* Antibiotics Ann. 90, 1956–1957.

103. BERGMAN, M., AND CHARNAS, R. M.: *Acute staphylococcal pericarditis.* Arch. Surg. 81:93, 1960.

104. SYMBAR, P. N., WARE, R. E., AND DI ORIO, D. A.: *Purulent pericarditis: a review of diagnostic and surgical principles.* South. Med. J. 67:46, 1974.

105. RIFF, L. J., AND JACKSON, G. G.: *Pharmacology of gentamicin in man.* J. Infect. Dis. 124 (Suppl.):98, 1971.

106. CHAN, R. A., BENNER, E. J., AND HOEPRICH, P. D.: *Gentamicin therapy in renal failure: a nomogram for dosage.* Ann. Intern. Med. 76:773, 1972.

107. SABATH, L. D., CASEY, J. I., RUSH, P. A., ET AL.: *Rapid microassay of gentamicin, kanamycin, neomycin, streptomycin, and vancomycin in serum or plasma.* J. Lab. Clin. Med. 78:457, 1971.

108. NOONE, P., PARSONS, T. M. C., PATTISON, J. R., ET AL.: *Experience in monitoring gentamicin therapy during treatment of serious gram-negative sepsis.* Br. Med. J. 1:477, 1974.

109. FELNER, J. M., AND DOWELL, V. R., JR.: *Anaerobic bacterial endocarditis.* N. Engl. J. Med. 283:1188, 1970.

110. CASTLEMAN, B., AND McNEELY, B. U. (EDS.): *Case records of the Massachusetts General Hospital Weekly Clinicopathological Exercises Case 27-1970.* N. Engl. J. Med. 282:1477, 1970.

111. ALTEMEIER, W. A., SCHOWENGERDT, C. G., AND WHITELEY, D. H.: *Abscesses of the liver.* Arch. Surg. 101:258, 1970.

112. BENNER, E. J.: *Benzylpenicillin therapy of bacteroides infections (abstract).* 14th Interscience Conference on Antimicrobial Agents and Chemotherapy, San Francisco, Sept. 11–13, 1974.

113. GLECKMAN, R. A.: *Warning–chloramphenicol may be good for your health.* Arch. Intern. Med. (in press).

114. ROBINSON, M. J., AND RUEDY, J.: *Sequelae of bacterial endocarditis.* Am. J. Med. 32:922, 1962.

115. BUCHBINDER, N. A., AND ROBERTS, W. C.: *Left-sided valvular active infective endocarditis.* Am. J. Med. 53:20, 1972.

116. BECK, D.: *Pericarditis and subacute bacterial endocarditis.* J. Mt. Sinai Hosp. N. Y. 8:364, 1942.

117. McCALL, I.: *Pericarditis due to a mycotic aneurysm in subacute bacterial endocarditis.* Guys Hosp. Rep. 107:34, 1958.

118. TYKOT, H. B., AND RELKIN, R.: *Massive pericardial effusion in subacute bacterial endocarditis.*

J.A.M.A. 184:898, 1963.

119. ROSE, R. L., HIGGINS, L. S., AND HELGASON, A. H.: *Bacterial endocarditis, pericarditis and cardiac tamponade.* Am. J. Cardiol. 19:447, 1967.

120. WOLFE, J. C., AND JOHNSON, W. D.: *Penicillin sensitive streptococcal endocarditis.* Ann. Intern. Med. 81:178, 1974.

121. JAWETZ, E.: *Assay of antibacterial activity in serum: useful guide for complex antimicrobial therapy.* Am. J. Dis. Child. 103:81, 1962.

122. HARVEY, A. M., AND WHITEHILL, M. R.: *Tuberculous pericarditis.* Medicine 16:45, 1937.

123. WHITE, P. D.: *Chronic constrictive pericarditis.* Circulation 4:288, 1951.

124. ANDREWS, G. W. S., PICKERING, G. W., AND SELLORS, T. H.: *The aetiology of constrictive pericarditis, with special reference to tuberculous pericarditis, together with a note on polyserositis.* Q. J. Med. 17:291, 1948.

125. SCHEPERS, G. W. H.: *Tuberculous pericarditis.* Am. J. Cardiol. 9:248, 1962.

126. SIMON, H. B., AND WOLFF, S. M.: *Granulomatous hepatitis and prolonged fever of unknown origin: a study of 13 patients.* Medicine 52:1, 1973.

127. SUZMAN, S.: *Tuberculous pericardial effusion.* Br. Heart J. 5:19, 1943.

128. PEEL, A. A. F.: *Tuberculous pericarditis.* Br. Heart J. 10:195, 1948.

129. BELLET, S., McMILLAN, T. M., AND GONLEY, B. A.: *Tuberculous pericarditis: a clinical and pathologic study based upon a series of seventeen cases.* Med. Clin. North Am. 18:201, 1934.

130. ELLMAN, P.: *Tuberculous pericarditis with effusion.* Br. Heart J. 7:147, 1945.

131. WOOD, J. A.: *Tuberculous pericarditis.* Am. Heart J. 42:737, 1951.

132. McGUIRE, J., KOTTE, J. H., AND HELM, R. A.: *Acute pericarditis.* Circulation 9:425, 1954.

133. STEPMAN, T. R., AND OWYANG, E.: *Clinically primary tuberculous pericarditis.* Ann. Intern. Med. 27: 914, 1947.

134. HEIMANN, H. L., AND BINDER, S.: *Tuberculous pericarditis.* Br. Heart J. 2:165, 1947.

135. SPODICK, D.: *Tuberculous pericarditis.* Arch. Intern. Med. 98:737, 1956.

136. JANOVSKY, R. C., BOETTNER, J. F., AND VAN-ORDSTRAND, H. S.: *Recurrent tuberculous pericarditis.* Ann. Intern. Med. 37:1268, 1952.

137. PETERSDORF, R. G., AND BEESON, P. B.: *Fever of unexplained origin: report of 100 cases.* Medicine 40: 1, 1961.

138. MYERS, T. M., AND HAMBURGER, M.: *Tuberculous pericarditis.* Am. J. Med. 12:302, 1952.

139. GERACI, J.: *Some present-day problems in infectious heart disease.* J. Lancet 85:385, 1965.

140. BARRETT, A. M., AND COLE, L.: *A case of tuberculous pericarditis.* Br. Heart J. 6:185, 1944.

141. CARROLL, D.: *Streptomycin in the treatment of tuberculous pericarditis.* Bull. Johns Hopkins Hosp. 88: 425, 1951.

142. GOYETTE, E. M.: *The treatment of tuberculous pericarditis.* Prog. Cardiovasc. Dis. 3:141, 1960.

143. FRANKL, W. S., AND CORTES, F. M.: *Treatment of infectious pericarditis.* Mod. Treat. 4:135, 1967.

144. ROONEY, J. J., CROCCO, J. A., AND LYONS, H. A.: *Tuberculous pericarditis.* Ann. Intern. Med. 72:73, 1970.

145. HOGEMAN, J. H., D'ESPO, N. D., AND GLENN, W. W. L.: *Tuberculosis of the pericardium.* N. Engl. J. Med. 270:327, 1964.

146. LOUDON, R. G.: *The place of rifampin.* Chest 61:524, 1972.

147. FURESZ, S., SCOTTI, R., PALLANZA, R., ET AL.: *Rifampicin: a new rifamycin: absorption distribution and elimination in man.* Arzheim. Forsch. 17:534, 1967.

148. MINET, J., LINQUETTE, M., GOULDEMAIN, M., ET AL.: *Effects symptomatiques remarkquables de la cortisone dans un cas de pericardite tuberculeuse.* Soc. Med. Nord. 57:1137, 1951.

149. VARMA, B. N., AND SMITH, J. M.: *Tuberculous pericarditis—a review of 17 cases.* Tubercle 48:160, 1967.

150. HOLMAN, E., AND WILLETT, F.: *Treatment of active tuberculosis pericarditis by pericardiectomy.* J.A.M.A. 146:1, 1951.

151. SCHRIRE, V.: *Pericarditis (with particular reference to tuberculous pericarditis).* Aust. Ann. Med. 16: 41, 1967.

152. FINNEY, J. O., JR., YARBROUGH, R., AND SCOTT, C. W.: *Tuberculous pericarditis.* South. Med. J. 64: 49, 1971.

153. CARSON, T. J., MURRAY, G. F., WILCOX, B. R., ET AL.: *The role of surgery in tuberculous pericarditis.* Ann. Thorac. Surg. 17:163, 1974.

174

154. FRIEDMAN, J. L., BAUM, G. L., AND SCHWARZ, J.: *Primary pulmonary histoplasmosis.* Am. J. Dis. Child. 109:298, 1965.

155. KAPLAN, M. M., AND SHERWOOD, L. M.: *Acute pericarditis due to histoplasma capsulatum.* Ann. Intern. Med. 58:862, 1963.

156. BABBITT, D. P., AND WAISBREN, B. A.: *Epidemic pulmonary histoplasmosis.* Am. J. Roentgenol. Radium Ther. Nucl. Med. 83:236, 1960.

157. WOOLEY, C. F., AND HOSIER, D. M.: *Constrictive pericarditis due to histoplasma capsulatum.* N. Engl. J. Med. 264:1230, 1961.

158. CRAWFORD, S. E., CROOK, W. G., HARRISON, W. W., ET AL.: *Histoplasmosis as a cause of acute myocarditis and pericarditis.* Pediatrics 28:92, 1961.

159. LEEDOM, J. M., PRITCHARD, J. C., AND KEER, L. M.: *Probable histoplasma pericarditis with effusion.* Arch. Intern. Med. 112:652, 1963.

160. OWEN, G. E., SCHERR, S. N., AND SEGRE, E. J.: *Histoplasmosis involving the heart and great vessels.* Am. J. Med. 32:552, 1962.

161. VANEK, J., AND SCHWARZ, J.: *The gamut of histoplasmosis.* Am. J. Med. 50:89, 1971.

162. WEBB, W. R., AND HERRING, J. L.: *Pericarditis due to histoplasmosis.* Am. Heart J. 64:679, 1962.

163. RIEGEL, N., AND SCHRIEVER, H. G.: *Fatal pericarditis due to histoplasmosis.* Am. Rev. Resp. Dis. 95:99, 1967.

164. DIX, J. H., AND GURKAYNAK, N.: *Histoplasmosis with massive pericardial effusion and systemic involvement.* J.A.M.A. 182:687, 1962.

165. SMITH, J. W., AND UTZ, J.P.: *Progressive disseminated histoplasmosis.* Ann. Intern. Med. 76:557, 1972.

166. GREGORIADES, D. G., LANGELUTTIG, H. V., AND POLK, J. W.: *Pericarditis with massive effusion due to histoplasmosis.* J.A.M.A. 178:331, 1961.

167. BENNETT, D. E.: *The histoplasmin latex agglutination test: clinical evaluation and a review of the literature.* Am. J. Med. Sci. 251:175, 1966.

168. HILL, G. B., AND CAMPBELL, C. C.: *Commercially available histoplasmin sensitized latex particles in an agglutination test for histoplasmosis.* Mycopathologia 18:169, 1962.

169. BENNETT, D. E.: *Laboratory diagnosis of histoplasmosis: a review.* South. Med. J. 59:922, 1966.

170. JACOBS, H. S.: *Histoplasma in circulating blood.* J.A.M.A. 207:1916, 1969.

171. LOOSLI, C. G.: *Histoplasmosis.* J. Chronic Dis. 5:473, 1957.

172. BENNETT, J. E.: *Chemotherapy of systemic mycoses.* N. Engl. J. Med. 290:30, 1974.

173. SAROSI, G. A., VOTH, D. W., DAHL, B. A., ET AL.: *Disseminated histoplasmosis: results of long-term followup.* Ann. Intern. Med. 75:511, 1971.

174. UTZ, J. P.: *Amphotericin B toxicity.* Ann. Intern. Med. 61:334, 1964.

175. GOODWIN, R. A., JR., SNELL, J. D., JR., HUBBARD, W. W., ET AL.: *Relationship in combined pulmonary infections with histoplasma capsulatum and mycobacterium tuberculosis.* Am. Rev. Resp. Dis. 96:990, 1967.

Acute and Chronic Cardiac Tamponade

Leslie A. Kuhn, M.D.

Of the variety of clinical syndromes produced by diseases of the pericardium, the most dramatic is that of cardiac tamponade. There are few similar instances in medicine where accurate recognition of the disease and prompt therapy can be considered life saving.

PATHOPHYSIOLOGY

A full discussion of the pathophysiology of cardiac tamponade is provided elsewhere in this volume, but certain salient features warrant repetition as they are basic to rational therapy and prophylaxis.

The normal pericardium may contain 20 to 50 ml. of fluid. A number of studies have suggested that at least 80 to 100 ml. of fluid may accumulate within the pericardium without producing cardiac compression.[1] This is greater than the usual stroke volume of 60 to 80 ml. Elastic fibers within the pericardium allow some stretching to occur if effusions accumulate slowly. Analysis of pressure volume curves of the pericardial sac (Fig. 1) indicates initial slight rises of intracardiac pressure with substantial increases in volume. The pressure rise then becomes increasingly large with further small volume increments. Pericardial "stretching" has been demonstrated experimentally by the observation that increments of intrapericardial fluid must be added progressively to maintain elevation of venous pressure.[2]

Both clinical and experimental observations have provided information as to the hemodynamic alterations which occur during pericardial effusion. The hemodynamic effects of effusion are related to the speed of accumulation of the fluid. The rapid accumulation of 150 to 200 ml. may produce acute cardiac tamponade whereas the slow accumulation of a liter or more may be well tolerated, and in some cases as much as 4 liters has not interfered too greatly with cardiac function. Fluid generally accumulates inferiorly, anteriorly, and laterally, particularly on the left. Little fluid generally accumulates directly behind the heart because of firm attachments here, but posterolateral protrusions of fluid do occur.

When intrapericardial pressure is increased, diastolic filling of the ventricles is impeded, resulting in a rise of ventricular pressure and diminution in cardiac output. At a critical level of intrapericardial pressure, there is a precipitous fall of arterial pressure, a rise of left and right intracardiac pressures, and eventually a flowless system. Additional factors interfering with cardiac function include premature closing of the A–V valves because of abrupt rise of intraventricular pressure and reduction of coronary

177

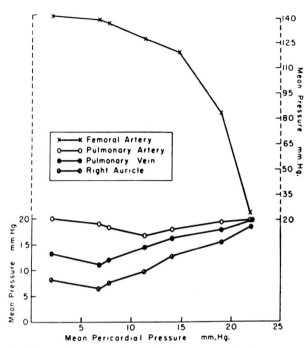

Figure 1. Hemodynamic effects of intrapericardial saline injection in a dog. Note the precipitous fall of arterial pressure and the rise in atrial and pulmonary arterial pressures as intrapericardial pressure is increased. Eventually, a "flowless" system is obtained. (From Metcalf, J. P., et al.: Circulation 5:518, 1952. Reprinted by permission of American Heart Assn., Inc.)

flow. The latter may result from diminution of coronary perfusion (aortic) pressure and perhaps compression of the coronary arteries. Both right and left ventricular functions are impaired, as measured by stroke work-filling pressure curves. A clinical correlate is that at a certain stage ventricular functional impairment may be rectified in pericardial tamponade by vasopressor agents which act to increase the inadequate coronary perfusion.[3]

Indirect effects accompany tamponade. As venous pressure is increased, fluid and sodium retention occur, leading to peripheral edema.[4] Subsequently, renal arteriolar constriction may accentuate this tendency. Tachycardia usually occurs relatively early along with reactive vasoconstriction, the latter acting to maintain arterial pressure until the final stages of the disorder. Recent experimenal investigations have indicated progressive deterioration of cardiac performance with increments of intrapericardial fluid, with significant changes noted when the pericardial sac contained one-half to three-fourths of the volume needed to produce terminal electromechanical dissociation. With abrupt rises of intrapericardial and intracardiac pressures, heart rate slowed abruptly and myocardial performance deteriorated, a "late" clinical sign. The administration of atropine produced improvement in myocardial performance and an increase in the amount of fluid the pericardial sac would accommodate, suggesting that a cardiac depressor reflex (vagally mediated) contributes to the deterioration of cardiac function late in the course of cardiac tamponade.[5] The important clinical point to be emphasized is that during the compensated phase, cardiovascular adjustments are quite delicately balanced and sudden increases in cardiac load, such as with exercise or a small further accumulation of intrapericardial fluid, may cause rapid and disastrous decompensation.

ETIOLOGY

There are many etiologies of acute and chronic cardiac tamponade. Tamponade results from inadequate compensatory responses to the previously delineated factors. It is associated with a rising ventricular diastolic pressure and a falling cardiac output. Generally, peripheral venous pressure at this point is about 150 mm. H_2O but right heart filling cannot be maintained because of the increasing intracardiac pressure. The major causes of acute tamponade are indicated in Table 1. Each of the "main" causes in turn may have a variety of etiologies. Preexisting pericardial thickening, as in tuberculous pericarditis, may be important in the production of tamponade when a relatively small effusion is added.

Table 1. Causes of acute cardiac tamponade

Acute pericarditis
Hemopericardium
  Following myocardial infarction
  Aortic rupture
  Luetic or dissecting aneurysm
    Coarctation with rupture above aortic valve
    Marfan's syndrome
  Trauma
Neoplasm
Chylopericardium (trauma, neoplasm)

Chronic tamponade may result from chronic, massive pericardial effusion. This may be caused by a variety of conditions as indicated in Table 2. These syndromes may last for many years and they may or may not present with signs and symptoms of tamponade or they may do so intermittently. Generally, when the signs and symptoms produced are those of chronic cardiac compression they are of a lower order of magnitude than those of acute tamponade, but at other times the clinical picture may be more acute mimicking that of acute pericardial tamponade. Because of the different pace of development, chronic cardiac compression may be associated with extensive changes in many organs of the body, particularly the development of extracellular fluid expansion characterized by ascites and edema. These latter findings are unusual in the rapidly developing acute cardiac tamponade. Impairment of renal function is greater in the chronic condition.

Many of the patients with chronic pericardial effusion do not have a known etiology. It is felt that some of these cases may result from initial acute idiopathic pericarditis.

Table 2. Causes of chronic massive pericardial effusion

Unknown etiology
Cardiac and pericardial neoplasms
Tuberculosis, mycotic diseases
Myxedema
"Cholesterol" pericarditis
Thoracic trauma
"Collagen" disease
Chylopericardium
Postirradiation
Post-myocardial-infarction syndrome
Postcardiotomy syndrome

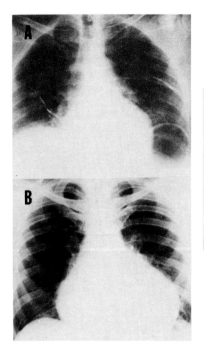
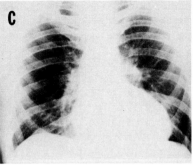

Figure 2. Chest films of patient with acute myocardial infarction who developed massive pericardial effusion of more than 2 liters within a few weeks following acute myocardial infarction. He required open pericardial "window" procedure for relief of recurrent pericardial effusion. A, 10/18/74, Shortly after admission for acute anterior myocardial infarction (portable film). B, 12/20/74, Readmission to hospital because of dyspnea. No evidence of new infarction. C, 5/16/75, Following removal of 2 liters of serosanguineous pericardial fluid by pericardiotomy after fluid reaccumulated following pericardiocentesis.

Cholesterol pericarditis is of interest. Cholesterol-containing pericardial fluid may be associated with myxedema, but more often the patients are euthyroid. Experimentally, chronic pericarditis with effusion has been produced by inserting suspensions of cholesterol into the pericardium of dogs.[6] Such deposits can be seen with a wide variety of illnesses causing pericarditis. It is probable, however, that the cholesterol noted clinically is related to inflammatory changes interfering with absorption of cholesterol deposits. Uremic patients may have recurrent pericarditis with effusion or chronic pericardial effusion, particularly those receiving intermittent hemodialysis. In my own experience, this is an increasingly frequent cause of "chronic" tamponade as dialysis becomes more widely applied. Occasionally, chronic massive pericardial effusion may occur in the post-myocardial-infarction syndrome (Dressler's syndrome). Figure 2 illustrates such an instance in a 46-year-old man with anterior myocardial infarction who had a large chronic pericardial effusion of at least 2 liters for many months after the initial infarction. He presented with signs of chronic, relatively moderate cardiac compression and required pericardiocentesis and open pericardiotomy for relief.

CLINICAL MANIFESTATIONS

Most of the clinical manifestations of acute or chronic pericardial tamponade are related directly to the hemodynamic alterations produced by the effusion. In very rapidly accumulating effusion, the only symptoms are apt to be those associated with profound circulatory failure and the shock state. In more slowly accumulating effusion, initial symptoms include precordial oppressive pain which may be due to pericardial stretching. Various positions of relief are commonly, but not invariably, adopted; and their absence certainly should not eliminate pericardial tamponade from diagnostic consideration. These positions include sitting up and leaning forward. The patient may "spread out" on hands and knees, the "signe de la prière Mahométane." Dyspnea and orthopnea occur because of compression and displacement of the lung parenchyma or atelectasis. There may be tracheobronchial encroachment producing cough and, at times, airway obstruction. In very large effusions, esophageal pressure produces dysphagia. Hoarseness occurs because of pressure on the recurrent laryngeal nerve. There may be impingement on the phrenic nerve with hiccoughs and nausea and abdominal pain due to liver congestion.

Clinical signs of pericardial effusion include neck vein engorgement; generally this is of a greater degree than that seen in the great majority of instances of congestive heart failure. Occasionally, in advanced compression, precordial venous distention and a precordial bulge may be noted. There may be edema and ascites but the latter is usually a manifestation of chronic constrictive pericarditis. Characteristically, in acute tamponade the pulse pressure is diminished and the pulse rapid. Two other characteristic signs include pulsus paradoxus and inspiratory distention of the neck veins. Normally, inspiration produces a more negative intrapleural pressure and a more positive intra-abdominal pressure, both of which result in increase of right atrial filling. Inspiratory distention of the neck veins occurs because right atrial filling is impeded and the right atrium (and ventricle) cannot accommodate the increased volume. As is well known, but may bear some repetition here, pulsus paradoxus is a misnomer because it is in fact an exaggeration of a normal response. However, it is a useful clinical guide in certain instances of pericardial tamponade. Normally, despite the inspiratory increase in venous return and right ventricular output, the capacity of the pulmonary vascular bed increases to a greater extent and there is a resultant fall in left ventricular stroke output, and a fall of arterial systolic pressure of about 5 mm. Hg. With hemodynamically significant pericardial effusion, inspiratory right ventricular volume is increased less than normal because of impaired ventricular filling, but the increased capacity of the pulmonary vascular bed with inspiration is not impaired. In addition, the inspiratory increment in right ventricular filling which does occur results in some expansion of the intrapericardial contents, causing some degree of left ventricular compression. The result of both of these effects is depression of left ventricular stroke volume and hence greater than normal fall of systolic pressure on inspiration. Studies of simultaneous pulmonary venous and left atrial pressure during experimental cardiac tamponade have demonstrated a reversal of normal gradient during inspiration, permitting a reversal of the normal flow in the pulmonary veins.[7] In addition, there may be inspiratory traction of the diaphragm, altering the cardiac silhouette to cause diminution of left ventricular output and fall in aortic pressure during this phase.[8]

A sign sometimes evident is an increase of cardiac "dullness" on recumbency in the second and third left intercostal spaces, diminishing when a sitting position is assumed. This is difficult to elicit and is an inconstant finding.

Because of the effusion and possible early closure of the A–V valves, the first heart sound may be diminished in intensity as may the second sound. An early diastolic third heart sound may be evident due to interference with ventricular filling. In those instances where tamponade results from pericarditis, a pericardial friction rub may be heard. Its presence in no way excludes cardiac tamponade due to massive pericardial effusion.

The so-called Ewart sign (more correctly, the Bamberger-Pins-Ewart sign) consists of an area of dullness and bronchial breathing at the left lung base, below the ninth rib. This may be noted on the right as well. Angiographic studies have shown that the sign usually results from lung compression, initially by a retrodisplaced heart and subsequently by posterior bulging of the lateral portion of the pericardium.[9]

The electrocardiogram will usually show low voltage. A more specific finding in pericardial effusion is total electrical alternans involving P waves as well as QRS complexes. It is seen with large pericardial effusion and is most probably due to alteration of the anatomic position of the heart.

The clinical demeanor of the patient is related to the speed with which tamponade develops. In rapidly developing tamponade the patient may appear to be in shock with cyanosis, rapid respiration, and sometimes syncope. The neck veins are engorged. They may pulsate or show inspiratory distention on sitting up. The retinal veins may also be engorged. The classic Beck triad of a quiet heart, increased venous pressure, and diminished arterial pressure may be present but is nonspecific as it may occur with severe congestive heart failure and may be absent in pericardial tamponade. The cardiac silhouette is usually considerably enlarged but not invariably so, since a relatively small amount of pericardial fluid accumulating rapidly may cause tamponade.

Longstanding cardiac compression produces the same general hemodynamic disturbances as does acute tamponade. In both instances there is impaired ventricular filling, and both demonstrate similar intracardiac pressure curves. However, because of the slow pace of development of chronic tamponade, there is time for circulatory adjustments to develop and patient survival is usually not the immediate problem. There are, of course, instances in which a relatively indolent process may exacerbate.

With chronic cardiac compression, blood volume may increase and there is usually time for ascites and edema to develop. Commonly there is great elevation of venous pressure, to some of the highest levels seen clinically with the possible exception of vena caval obstructions; peripheral venous pressures to 30 or 40 cm. H_2O are not uncommon, whereas in acute tamponade, the venous pressure rarely exceeds 15 to 18 cm. H_2O, death generally intervening before the pressure becomes much higher. Deficits of renal sodium excretion are much more prominent in the patient with chronic cardiac compression. In chronic compression, the degree of myocardial functional impairment may also play a role in altering the clinical and hemodynamic findings obtained. In this regard, it should be appreciated that both right and left ventricles are commonly involved by the compression process and there are almost equal abnormalities of both ventricles. There is generally uniform elevation of right atrial, right ventricular end diastolic, left atrial, pulmonary artery diastolic, and pulmonary venous pressures. There is consistent elevation of left ventricular diastolic pressure. The jugular venous pressure therefore is a reasonable reflection of the status of both ventricles. Characteristically, ventricular pressures demonstrate an early diastolic "dip," a high, mid, and late diastolic plateau, and usually somewhat elevated systolic pressures. These indicate the limitation imposed on ventricular filling. These features give rise to the well known "square root" appearance of the ventricular pressure curves. With atrial contraction, there may be a short presystolic pressure rise, but there is usually little increment of cardiac output produced by atrial contraction when the ventricles are compressed.

Chronic and acute cardiac compression interfere with the transport function of both atria. Atrial pressure curves in the presence of sinus rhythm show an elevated mean pressure and characteristic high peaks and steep descents producing an M or W configuration. However, with advanced cardiac compression, the atrial pressure troughs tend to be elevated towards the level of the peaks so that the characteristic configuration may not be apparent.

Although pulmonary arterial and venous hypertension are commonly present because of compression of both ventricles, clinical pulmonary edema is a most unusual event, possibly because of interference with right ventricular filling. Analysis of pulmonary artery curves usually shows moderate hypertension, often with rapid early diastolic descent.

The markedly elevated systemic venous pressure is secondary to elevated caval pressures. However, other physiologic responses may contribute to the elevation. There is increased venous volume and there may be venoconstriction, possibly related to diminished cardiac output causing adrenal medullary secretion and sympathetic nervous system stimulation. The extremities may appear cyanotic because of venous stasis, even though the arterial blood is generally fully saturated. (Occasionally, however, because of venous shunting or abnormal ventilation-perfusion areas, the arterial oxygen saturation may be reduced.) Venous compression by ascites or edema may elevate further the measured venous pressure. There is usually a markedly abnormal hepatojugular reflux because of the effects of small increases of volume in the already distended venous system.

Tachycardia is a common accompaniment of cardiac compression because of the low stroke volume. Because the compressed heart cannot increase its stroke volume, it responds to the need for increased output by tachycardia. Therefore, small degrees of activity may result in disproportional tachycardia.

Systolic arterial pressure may be low to normal, although in response to low cardiac output and a "compensatory" rise in systemic resistance, diastolic pressure may be elevated, thereby lowering the pulse pressure. Occasionally hypertension has been reported. With extensive or sudden compression, arterial pressure will fall to critical levels. The normal arterial pressure response to the Valsalva maneuver (increased pressure, followed by a fall and then a rebound elevation above initial levels) cannot be elicited with significant cardiac compression. Usually there is no change in arterial pressure and no "overshoot." Similar responses are elicited with poor myocardial function due to other causes. Because of increased blood plasma volume, moderate anemia is not uncommon with chronic cardiac compression.

Although it is difficult to separate clinically the effects of cardiac compression from those of myocardial dysfunction, there is evidence that there may be considerable myocardial functional abnormality in patients with cardiac compression. Evidence for poor myocardial function includes anatomic studies showing subepicardial (and sometimes transmural) inflammation, fibrosis, and atrophy; ECG abnormalities of the ST segments, P waves, and cardiac rhythm; abnormal apexcardiogram; cardiomegaly; some improvement with digitalis administraton; and slow or inadequate clinical improvement following relief of cardiac compression. The cause of the myocardial dysfunction may be atrophy of myocardial cells, myocardial injury due to the underlying disease process causing the cardiac compression, possibly inadequate coronary perfusion secondary to low coronary perfusion pressure, and high transmural pressure interfering with coronary filling. These result in a variety of manifestations of myocardial dysfunction including prolonged ejection time, ventricular kymographic and apexcardiographic abnormalities and diminished myocardial compliance.

Phonocardiograms have shown inspiratory increase in splitting of the second heart sound due to early aortic valve closure. This is secondary to shortening of the ejection period of the left ventricle, whereas the pulmonic component of the second sound is unchanged or changed very slightly because of relatively little alteration of the right ventricular ejection period. A triple rhythm is often noted because of an abnormal early diastolic sound. This is not a constant finding and it may not be audible if there is a substantial volume of pericardial fluid. It may vary in intensity, ranging from barely audible to a loud "knock." The sound coincides with the rapid ventricular filling peak of the apexcardiogram. It is reasonably attributable to diminished ventricular expansion following its rapid filling. Occasionally, an abnormal presystolic sound is detected, most probably related to atrial contraction in the presence of a high pressure in the ventricles.

There are a variety of systemic manifestations of chronic cardiac compression.

Pleural effusion, usually left-sided or bilateral, may be prominent and contribute to dyspnea. Generally the fluid is a transudate due to high venous pressure and the renal effects of sodium and water retention. Possibly, azygos vein compression may play a role. In those instances of chronic tamponade associated with initial inflammatory pericarditis, the process may involve adjacent pleura, producing adhesive pleuritis. There may be pulmonary vascular plethora but, as indicated previously, clinical pulmonary edema is most uncommon. In chronic cases there is some degree of interstitial fibrosis. These effects result in pulmonary functional impairment with reduction of vital capacity and, in some instances, poor gaseous diffusion.

Because of the chronicity and extent of hepatic venous hypertension, chronic cardiac compression may produce liver lesions and dysfunction. Hepatic changes include venous congestion as well as parenchymal destruction and fibrosis, i.e., cardiac cirrhosis, or pericapsular fibrosis. Generally, the liver is enlarged and palpable but at other times it may be of normal size or small. Therefore, the absence of an enlarged liver does not exclude the diagnosis of chronic cardiac compression. There may or may not be associated ascites. Splenomegaly is a frequent but not invariable clinical finding; this is attributable to associated portal hypertension as well as general venous hypertension. At times, the hematologic manifestation of "hypersplenism" may be evident.

Because of renal venous hypertension, proteinuria is a common clinical finding and occasionally, a nephrotic syndrome is evident. The sodium and water retention secondary to renal dysfunction contribute importantly to the edema and expanded extracellular volume noted in chronic cardiac compression. Renal blood flow is diminished, glomerular filtration rate usually less so, leading to a high filtration fraction. Aldosterone secretion related to diminished cardiac output and venous hypertension contribute to edema formation.

Manifestations of a malabsorption syndrome may be noted with protein-losing enteropathy and steatorrhea due to gastrointestinal and pancreatic congestion as well as lymphatic congestion. Hypoalbuminemia is frequently noted in patients with chronic pericardial tamponade. All the aforementioned mechanisms may lead to edema. However, there may be considerable cardiac compression without detectable edema. It is well established that ascites may be present in the absence of edema, probably related to more selected and more marked hepatic venous obstruction.

DIAGNOSIS AND DIFFERENTIAL DIAGNOSIS

The most common problem in differentiating acute and chronic tamponade from other disorders generally is to decide whether or not the signs and symptoms produced are due to pericardial compression or to myocardial dysfunction. At times, there may be cardiac compression by scarring and calcification which can mimic the findings of compression by fluid. There may be combinations of fluid and scar compression and, frequently, an initial inflammatory effusion may progress to constrictive pericarditis. Because of the different therapeutic approaches to myocardial dysfunction as compared to pericardial compression, it is of considerable importance that an early and precise diagnosis be made.

Acute tamponade will usually be preceded by an obvious cause such as trauma, dissecting aneurysm, acute pericarditis, or tumor. Hypotension is generally more sudden and more marked and venous pressure somewhat less elevated than in the most advanced form of constrictive pericarditis. Low pulse pressure and pulsus paradoxus are nearly always evident but are not specific findings. A variety of cardiac silhouette configurations may be noted in acute tamponade, from relatively normal to quite large. Pulsations are usually but not invariably diminished to a considerable extent.

In chronic tamponade, the effusions are substantial with very large cardiac silhouettes and markedly diminished cardiac pulsations. Since advanced myocardial dysfunction can produce similar signs and symptoms, the differential diagnosis usually involves determining whether or not there has been preexisting significant cardiac disease and whether or not fluid is present. It is difficult to determine this from conventional chest x-rays alone. A variety of cardiac diseases may mimic chronic pericardial compression. These include idiopathic myocardial hypertrophy, restrictive syndromes in which ventricular filling is interfered with by endocardial fibroelastosis or endomyocardial fibrosis, chronic myocarditis, or amyloidosis. In some instances, intracardiac tumors have produced high venous pressure and intracardiac obstruction and have been confused with the syndrome of cardiac compression. With myocardial disorders, specific chamber hypertrophy may be noted in the electrocardiogram, chest x-ray, or angiogram and there may be intraventricular conduction disturbances or Q waves present. Cardiac murmurs are generally more prominent. Medical treatment with diuretics and digitalis may be quite effective, at least in the initial stages. Dyspnea and orthopnea, particularly paroxysmal nocturnal dyspnea, are usually absent in pericardial disease or, if present, are not as marked in chronic pericardial effusion as in myocardial dysfunction. Acute pulmonary edema is rarely seen in purely or predominantly pericardial disease. Venous pressures are generally higher in chronic compressive syndromes than in myocardial failure. End diastolic pressure is usually higher in cardiac compression than in heart failure. In many instances the ratio of right ventricular end diastolic pressure to systolic pressure is greater than 1:3 in compression disorders. However this is not a fully reliable differential diagnostic sign and cannot be used definitively for this purpose.

Since the symptoms and signs of chronic cardiac tamponade are not specific, demonstration of intrapericardial fluid is essential to establish the diagnosis and to differentiate this disorder from other conditions which mimic it. It should be appreciated, however, that substantial amounts of intrapericardial fluid may be present without production of cardiac compression, probably owing to the slow rate of accumulation. Moreover, the fluid may coexist with myocardial dysfunction or pericardial constriction which may be responsible for symptoms of cardiac compression. Therefore, relief of symptoms and signs of compression with removal of fluid is necessary to establish that these manifestations are, in fact, due to the pericardial effusion.

The differential diagnosis is aided considerably by roentgenographic, radioisotopic, and echocardiographic studies. Physical signs and hemodynamic findings are of lesser aid in the differential diagnosis although they may be of some assistance. Lange and associates[10] attempted to determine the specificity of physical signs among patients with constrictive pericarditis, "lax" (noncompressive) pericardial effusion, acute tamponade, obstructive airway disease, myocardial disease, and those with extreme obesity. A third heart sound occurred only in the groups with constrictive pericarditis and myocardial disease. In constrictive pericardial disease, the third heart sound tended to occur somewhat closer to the second heart sound than in myocardial failure but the quality of the sound did not permit differentiation. High venous or right atrial pressure (greater than 12 mm. Hg) was common in constrictive pericarditis, was noted in all cases of acute tamponade and was also present in myocardial disease and obesity. Kussmaul's sign, defined as a regular inspiratory increase in venous pressure with tranquil respiration, was seen in about one third of the patients with constrictive pericarditis but not in the other groups. Pulsus paradoxus (greater than a 20 mm. Hg decrease in systolic arterial pressure with quiet inspiration) was found in patients with lax effusion, acute tamponade, airway obstruction, and in extreme obesity. In this series, it was not seen with constrictive pericarditis (but it has been reported in this condition by other

185

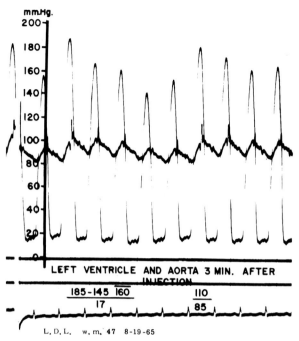

Figure 3. Note pulsus paradoxus in left ventricular pulse not reflected by equivalent changes in aortic pulse or pulse pressure in this patient with severe calcific aortic stenosis. (From Lange, et al.[10] with by permission of American Heart Assn., Inc.)

authors) or with myocardial disease. It was absent only in one (of 16) patients with acute tamponade, and in this individual there was severe aortic stenosis. There was a 50 mm. Hg variation of left ventricular systolic pressure with respiration in this latter patient but the aortic valvular obstruction prevented its transmission to the aortic pulse. Figure 3 demonstrates pulsus paradoxus of the left ventricle in this patient, not fully reflected by changes of aortic pressure. Figure 4 shows the pulsus paradoxus obtained

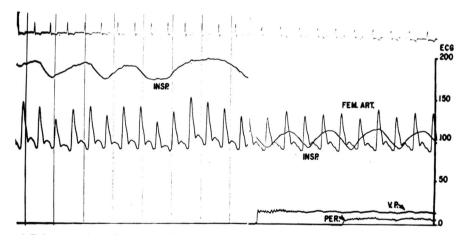

Figure 4. Pulsus paradoxus in acute cardiac tamponade secondary to aortic dissection. The femoral artery shows a paradoxical pulse prior to removal of 45 ml. of blood from pericardium. Following pericardiocentesis (right panel) pulsus paradoxus is no longer evident. (From Lange, et al.[10] with permission of American Heart Assn., Inc.)

186

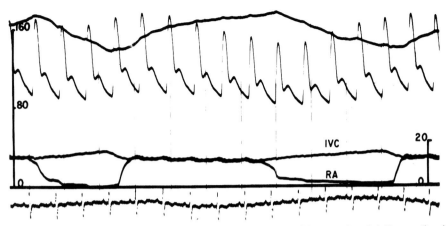

Figure 5. Spurious signs of cardiac compression in extreme obesity without pericardial disease (inspiration downward). Brachial artery, inferior vena caval, and right atrial pressures show pulsus paradoxus and inspiratory IVC-RA pressure gradient. (From Lange, et al.[10] with permission of American Heart Assn., Inc.)

in a patient with acute tamponade secondary to aortic dissection. Following removal of 45 ml. of intrapericardial blood, pulsus paradoxus was considerably lessened. Figure 5 indicates the pulsus paradoxus obtained in a patient with extreme obesity (weight 287 pounds, height 72½ inches). In this instance, there was evidence of thoracic inlet obstruction with rise of inferior vena caval pressure with inspiration.

An interesting physical sign in large chronic pericardial effusion has been described by Bonner and associates.[11] These authors recorded a sharp precordial pulsation in early diastole coinciding with the anterior excursion of the heart within the pericardial sac. Analysis of apexcardiograms and echocardiograms indicated that the pulsation and its accompanying early diastolic sound resulted from a "swinging heart" striking the anterior pericardium and chest wall. Pulsus alternans has also been described in effusive pericarditis, in this case in association with pneumococcal pericarditis.[12] However, significant underlying cardiac dysfunction due to myocarditis may have been a contributing factor.

Chest x-rays and echocardiography are the principal noninvasive techniques for diagnosing the presence of pericardial effusion. Radiologic studies of developing pericardial effusion have shown rapid increases in the size of the cardiac silhouette, reaching its maximum within a few days.[13] The shape of the heart changes suddenly with early obliteration of the left border and, to a somewhat lesser extent, the right border. Dilatation of the inferior vena caval shadow is also an early sign. The posterior border of the cardiac shadow is often indistinct in contrast to a more distinct posterior border in cardiac enlargment (Fig. 6). However, there is no consistent shape or size of the cardiac silhouette with pericardial effusion, and differentiation from that due to cardiac enlargement is difficult. It is generally thought that the cardiac silhouette will not change unless at least 250 ml. of fluid is present within the pericardial sac. Changes of the cardiac contours with tilt and recumbency are often seen with pericardial effusion, but this finding does not consistently differentiate the enlarged cardiac silhouette in pericardial effusion from that due solely to cardiac enlargement. Although the cardiac silhouette may increase in size progressively with cardiac failure, a rapid and substantial increase in size of the cardiac silhouette is more likely due to pericardial effusion. Epicardial fat lines deep within the cardiac silhouette have sometimes been noted in instances of pericardial effusion.

Fluoroscopy will not definitely distinguish between cardiac enlargement and peri-

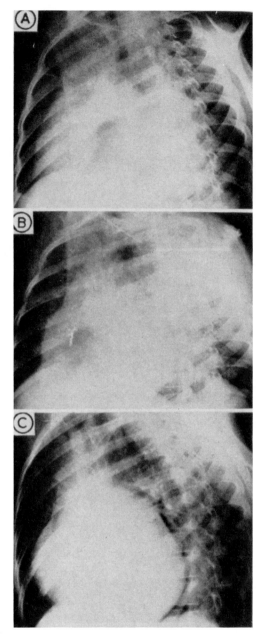

Figure 6. Oblique views of chest x-rays showing "hazy" posterior cardiac border at height of pericardial effusion (A) and during resolution of effusion (B). A film in a patient with cardiac enlargement but no pericardial effusion is seen in C. (From Besterman, et al.[13] with permission of British Medical Association.)

cardial effusion, but demonstration of a significant shadow (greater than 5 mm.) between the outer border of the cardiac silhouette and the right border of the heart by the use of dye, CO_2, or radioactive isotope is quite helpful (Fig. 7). In some instances of pericardial effusion, lateral positioning may show poor anterior pulsations and relatively normal posterior pulsations of the posteriorly displaced heart whereas in large

188

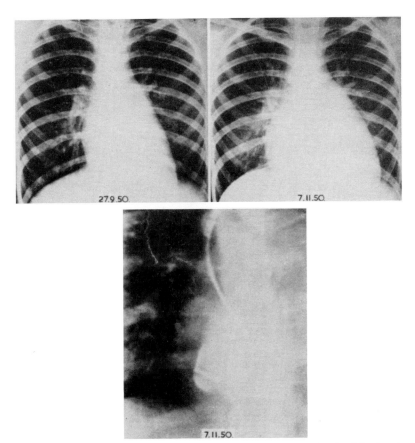

27.9.50. 7.11.50.

7.11.50.

Figure 7. Chest x-rays showing increase of size of cardiac silhouette. Intracardiac dye injection demonstrates that this is due to pericardial effusion. (From Besterman, et al.[13] with permission of British Medical Association.)

shadows due to cardiac decompensation, both borders will generally (but not invariably) show diminished pulsations.

Echocardiography has afforded a useful and generally highly accurate noninvasive technique for evaluating the presence and extent of pericardial effusion. The usefulness of echocardiography is based on the fact that the normal epicardium and parietal pericardium are close together. An echocardiogram shows the parietal pericardium and epicardium as one echo without an echo-free space between them. When there is accumulation of pericardial effusion an echo-free space appears, initially posteriorly in systole. With moderate sized effusion, there is posterior accumulation in systole and diastole. In more advanced effusion, there is an echo-free space both anteriorly and posteriorly. Small volumes of pericardial effusion have been detected (in some reports, as little as 20 ml.), and the technique may be used semiquantitatively with a reasonable degree of accuracy. Figure 8 demonstrates an echocardiogram in a patient without pericardial effusion. There is no echo-free space between the pericardium and epicardium. Figure 9 shows a large pericardial effusion with a large posterior and smaller anterior echo-free space. There is a "flat" (minimally moving) pericardium.

Additional echocardiographic findings have been reported in cardiac tamponade. D'Cruz and associates[14] have described cyclic respiratory changes affecting the diastolic motion of the mitral valve with a decrease of its anterior excursion during inspira-

189

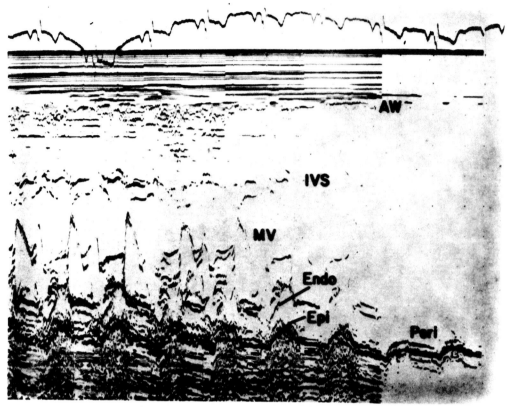

Figure 8. An echocardiogram indicating absence of pericardial effusion. There is no "echo-free" space between the epicardium and pericardium. (From Kerber, R. E., et al.: Circulation 52:823, 1975. Reprinted by permission of American Heart Assn., Inc.)

tion and a diminution of its E-F slope, the latter representing the rate of left ventricular filling. These authors indicated an increase in right ventricular dimension and a decrease in left ventricular dimension during inspiration in tamponade, these findings not being evident following pericardiocentesis. Figure 10 demonstrates the inspiratory diminution of diastolic excursion, an abnormally small E-F slope of the anterior mitral valve leaflet and the enlarged right ventricular dimensions and lessened left ventricular dimensions. Figure 11 shows the absence of these phasic changes following pericardiocentesis. These findings are consistent with the view that tamponade results in diminished left ventricular filling during inspiration. However, other authors have reported right ventricular compression, as determined by echocardiographic dimensions, with cardiac tamponade.[15]

The prognosis of acute tamponade is obviously very grave if unrelieved. However, the clinical spectrum ranges from the most severe in which the patient may survive for only a few minutes (generally due to major arterial bleeding into the pericardial sac) to a somewhat more indolent course in which there is ample time to make a prompt diagnosis and institute appropriate therapy.

In chronic tamponade, when the effusion is due to noninflammatory cause, the course and prognosis are generally those of the underlying disease. Inflammatory effusions have a varied and somewhat unpredictable course. Sometimes they clear spontaneously; at other times one or more pericardiocenteses may be required before resolution of the disorder. In some instances rapid reaccumulation of fluid occurs with resultant car-

190

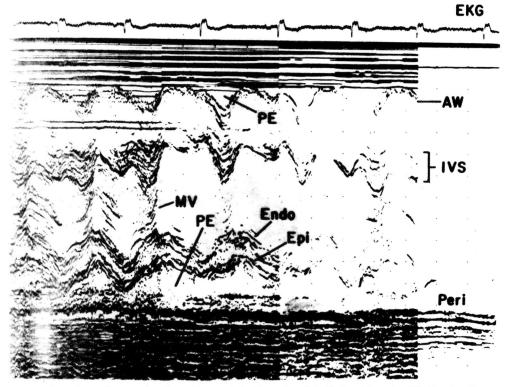

Figure 9. An echocardiogram showing evidence of sizable pericardial effusion. There is a "flat" pericardium, a large posterior echo-free space and a smaller anterior echo-free space. PE = pericardial effusion. (From Kerber, R. E., et al.: Circulation 52:823, 1975. Reprinted by permission of American Heart Assn., Inc.)

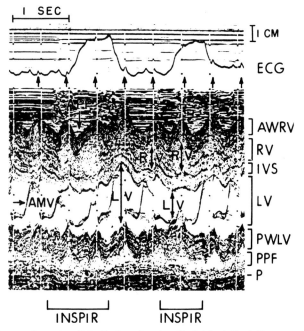

Figure 10. Echocardiogram in pericardial effusion showing diminished diastolic excursion of anterior mitral leaflet (AMV) during inspiration as well as enlarged right ventricular (RV) and diminished left ventricular (LV) dimensions. PPF = posterior pericardial fluid. (From D'Cruz, et al.[14] with permission of American Heart Assn., Inc.)

191

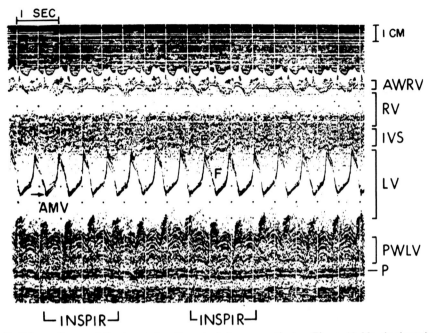

Figure 11. Echocardiogram following pericardiocentesis in same patient as Figure 10. No phasic variation in ventricular dimension or in anterior mitral leaflet motion can be seen. (From D'Cruz, et al.[14] with permission of American Heart Assn., Inc.)

diac compression and there may be associated constrictive pericarditis. Therefore the patients must be observed carefully and generally for a prolonged interval. Constriction may be suspected by increasing signs of cardiac compression with a stable (or "shrinking") cardiac silhouette.

TREATMENT

Treatment in acute tamponade can be life-saving but must be instituted promptly. The diagnosis must be suspected when there is a reasonable underlying cause for tamponade (trauma, dissecting aneurysm, previous pericarditis with or without effusion). It should be quickly confirmed by the presence of the characteristic physical findings outlined previously and by chest x-ray and/or echocardiography. It should be appreciated, however, that the size of the cardiac silhouette may vary considerably and there need not be a very large silhouette in acute tamponade if fluid or blood accumulates rapidly before appropriate cardiovascular adjustments occur. Pericardiocentesis should be performed promptly. A variety of sites have been used for this purpose. I believe the preferred site is the angle between the xiphoid process and the left costal arch. In this region there is no lung tissue over the heart. There will be no confusion with pleural effusion if fluid is obtained. Fluid often accumulates earliest in the inferior surface so that fluid may be obtained even when there is an effusion which is not very large. Alternative sites include the 5th left intercostal space, about 2 cm. inside the left border of dullness, the 5th or 6th left intercostal or right intercostal space at the sternal margin, the 7th or 8th left intercostal space at the midscapular line, or the right 4th intercostal space about 1 cm. medial to the right border of cardiac dullness. These sites can be used, depending on the x-ray of the cardiac silhouette, if fluid cannot be obtained via the subxiphoid approach. Occasionally, fluid can be aspirated from one of these sites and not via the subxiphoid route, but this is unusual.

Asepsis is essential and the usual procedure is to employ local anesthesia. An 18 or 16 gauge aspirating needle is generally used. The needle is introduced cautiously until the pericardial membrane is penetrated, gentle suction then being employed. Usually this membrane is noted at a depth of 2 to 4 cm. At times a wider bore trocar may be necessary for thick effusions. In the subxiphoid approach the needle is directed posteriorly and inward towards the right sternoclavicular joint. A helpful technique is to monitor the pericardiocentesis with continuous electrocardiography. A "V" lead is connected to the pericardial needle by alligator clamps and wire or by special electrodes. Elevation of the ST segments indicates a current of injury when the ventricular wall is contacted. There may also be premature ventricular beats. Atrial injury is manifested by elevated P-R segments and atrial premature beats. While this is a useful technique, it is not infallible. Instances have been established in which laceration of the myocardium occurred despite failure of an injury current to appear on a continuously monitored electrocardiogram. Electrically silent areas of the myocardium may be present,[16] or tumors may be penetrated which will not show expected changes of myocardial injury. Preexisting ECG abnormalities such as left ventricular hypertrophy pattern or bundle branch block may also mask injury currents. Fatal myocardial (right ventricle) laceration with resultant tamponade has been reported following attempts at subxiphoid pericardiocentesis in which continuous electrocardiographic monitoring did not show injury currents in an individual with left ventricular hypertrophy and additional ST segment changes attributed to digitalis.[17]

Often, depending on clinical circumstances, air is inserted, usually in a volume of about one half of the volume of fluid removed, and subsequent chest x-rays may be helpful in delineating tumors or chronic inflammation of the pericardium by outlining the walls of the pericardial sac. However, if blood is obtained on presumed pericardial aspiration, it must be definitely established that the needle has not entered the heart or a coronary artery before air is injected. It is best to avoid an injection if the aspirate is bloody.

Ancillary measures may be of some aid in treating acute tamponade. As previously indicated, the hypotension of acute tamponade may in part be related to poor myocardial function and perhaps restriction of coronary arterial inflow. Elevation of the depressed coronary perfusion pressure by expansion of plasma volume with fluids or blood or the use of vasopressor agents may offer temporary improvement and should be employed if there is significant hypotension. In addition, experimental evidence indicates that administration of atropine may improve cardiac performance in tamponade because of depressing vagal reflexes relatively late in its course.[5] There is experimental evidence that sympathetic blockade causes marked depression of cardiac performance with relatively small pericardial effusion, indicating the importance of adrenergic response in maintaining hemodynamic stability.[18]

The treatment of chronic tamponade usually resolves itself to treating its cause. The question often arises as to when to employ diagnostic (and therapeutic) pericardiocentesis and/or surgical procedures, such as pericardiotomy, pericardial "window," or pericardiectomy. Pericardiocentesis is indicated if the specific etiology is in doubt or if there are signs and symptoms of initial or recurrent cardiac compression not well tolerated by the patient. In general, the more conservative approach (pericardiocentesis) is elected initially, and only if that fails is an open method employed. There is considerable advantage of pericardiocentesis and/or short-term (24 to 48 hrs.) pericardial catheter drainage. It is simple to apply and there is less incidence of infection than noted with open techniques. With malignant effusion or those associated with uremia, the condition of the patient may make an open procedure more hazardous. A recent report describes good results in six consecutive patients with malignant effusion treated by pericardiocentesis with short-term catheter drainage in some instances.[19] A variety of antitumor agents has been injected into the pericardial sac after pericardiocentesis, particularly when malignant cells are found in the aspirate, but this is not uniformly necessary for relief of the effusion.

Local therapy with the nonabsorbable steroid, triamcinolone hexacetonide, combined with 24 to 48 hour pericardial catheter drainage has been successfully employed in instances of pericarditis with recurrent effusion not responding to systemic steroid therapy or to pericardiocentesis in uremic as well as in nonuremic patients.[20] Good results have been reported in these resistant patients with no recurrence in followup observation up to four years.

However, despite successes with conservative regimens, there should be no hesitation to use surgical methods when indicated. Surgery will generally be necessary in purulent pericardial effusion or when repeated pericardiocentesis or catheter drainage is insufficiently effective. In nonpurulent pericarditis, generally a left pleuropericardial window or a pericardial window through an anterior approach is the surgical technique first employed; but on some occasions this is ineffective and pericardiectomy may be necessary. The open techniques do afford the advantage of pericardial biopsy, should this be necessary to establish the diagnosis.

REFERENCES

1. FINEBERG, M. H.: *Functional capacity of the normal pericardium. An experimental study.* Am. Heart J. 11:784, 1936.
2. FOULGER, M., AND FOULGER, J. H.: *The blood pressure and electrocardiogram in experimental pericardial effusion.* Am. Heart J. 7:744, 1932.
3. BINION, J. T., MORGAN, W. J., JR., WELCH, G. H., ET AL.: *Effect of sympathomimetic drugs in acute experimental cardiac tamponade.* Circ. Res. 4:705, 1956.
4. FISHMAN, A. P., STAMLER, J., KATZ, L. N., ET AL.: *Mechanisms of edema formation in chronic experimental pericarditis with effusion.* J. Clin. Invest. 29:521, 1956.
5. FRIEDMAN, H. S., LAJAM, F., GOMES, J. A., ET AL.: *Experimental acute cardiac tamponade. II. Hemodynamic effects.* Clin. Res. 23:184A, 1975.
6. EHRENHAFT, J. G., AND TABER, R. E.: *Hemopericardium and constrictive pericarditis.* J. Thorac. Surg. 24:355, 1952.
7. GOLINKO, R. J., KAPLAN, N., AND RUDOLPH, A. M.: *The mechanism of pulsus paradoxus during acute pericardial tamponade.* J. Clin. Invest. 42:249, 1963.
8. DOCK, W.: *Inspiratory traction on the pericardium.* Arch. Intern. Med. 108:837, 1961.
9. STEINBERG, I.: *Pericarditis with effusion: New observations with a note on Ewart's sign.* Ann. Intern. Med. 49:428, 1958.
10. LANGE, R. L., BOTTICELLI, J. T., TSAGARIS, T. J., ET AL.: *Diagnostic signs in compressive cardiac disorders.* Circulation 33:763, 1966.
11. BONNER, A. J., JR., ESTEVEZ, C. M., DILLON, J. C., ET AL.: *An unusual precordial pulse and sound associated with large pericardial effusion.* Chest 67:829, 1975.
12. SCHWEITZER, S.: *Pulsus alternans in effusive pericarditis.* Chest 67:506, 1975.
13. BESTERMAN, E. M. M., AND THOMAS, E. G.: *Radiologic diagnosis of pericardial effusion.* Br. Heart J. 15:113, 1953.
14. D'CRUZ, I. A., COHEN, H. C., PRABHU, N., ET AL.: *Diagnosis of cardiac tamponade by echocardiography.* Circulation 52:460, 1975.
15. SCHILLER, N. B., AND BOTWINICK, E. H.: *Right ventricular compression: An echocardiographic sign of cardiac tamponade.* Clin. Res. 24:89A, 1976.
16. SOBOL, S. M., THOMAS, H. M., JR., AND EVANS, R. W.: *Myocardial laceration not demonstrated by continuous electrocardiographic monitoring occurring during pericardiocentesis.* N. Engl. J. Med. 292:1222, 1975.
17. GUERON, M., HIRSCH, M., AND WANDERMAN, K.: *Myocardial laceration not shown by ECG during pericardiocentesis.* N. Engl. J. Med. 293:938, 1975.
18. FRIEDMAN, H. S., LAJAM, F., GOMES, J. A., ET AL.: *Experimental acute tamponade. III. Effect of sympathetic blockade.* Clin. Res. 23:563A, 1975.

19. FLANNERY, E. S., GREGORATOS, G., AND CORDER, M. P.: *Pericardial effusion in patients with malignant diseases*. Arch. Intern. Med. 135:976, 1975.
20. BUSELMEIER, T. J., SIMMONS, R. L., NAJARIAN, J. S., ET AL.: *Local steroid therapy of chronic pericarditis*. Circulation 52 (Suppl. II):79, 1975.

Constrictive Pericarditis

Daniel E. Wise, M.D., and C. Richard Conti, M.D.

The first case of constrictive pericarditis was described by Chevers of Guy's Hospital in 1842.[1] Despite the earlier description, the disease has been referred to as Pick's Disease following his description of the clinical and pathologic features in 1896.[2] The modern clinical, pathologic, and physiologic concepts of constrictive pericarditis were described by Paul Dudley White in 1935 in his St. Cyres lecture at the National Heart Hospital in London.[3] Since that report, much has been written but the basic concepts of the disease remain the same. This communication reviews the recent literature on constrictive pericarditis and reports the findings of 22 additional patients personally seen by the authors.

CLINICAL PRESENTATION

Patients with constrictive pericarditis usually present in the second to the seventh decade of life with no predilection for any decade.[4] Of our 22 patients, the mean age was 35 years (14 to 71). Males predominate with a ratio of approximately 2:1. In our series, there were 14 males and 8 females.

The commonest presenting symptom is dyspnea. The other symptoms frequently encountered are presented in Table 1.[4] A clinical point worth noting is the observation that orthopnea is relatively uncommon and paroxysmal nocturnal dyspnea is rare, features that help differentiate chronic constrictive pericarditis from cardiomyopathies. Chest pain is also uncommon. However, Ikram points out that patients with nontuber-

Table 1. Symptoms

Dyspnea	78%
Edema	64%
Abdominal swelling	64%
Palpitations	22%
Fatigue	25%
Abdominal discomfort	32%
Cough	18%
Orthopnea	22%
Nausea	10%
Dizziness	6%
Vomiting	8%

Table 2. Physical examination

Physical findings	Number of patients	
	137*	22†
Elevated venous pressure	137	20
Hepatomegaly	134	22
Ascites	106	13
Peripheral edema	84	22
Pleural effusion	68	—
Cyanosis	19	—
Clubbing	3	—
Paradoxical pulse	40	10
Pericardial knock	20	13
Friction rub	7	—
Decreased precordial activity	—	9

*Wychulis, et al.
†Authors' experience

culous constrictive pericarditis developing over a short duration do experience chest pain typical of acute pericarditis.[5]

The hallmark of constrictive pericarditis on physical examination is the persistence of increased venous pressure after adequate diuresis.[6] Other commonly observed findings[7] which compare favorably with our findings are presented in Table 2. Of particular note is that hepatomegaly and ascites are observed more frequently than peripheral edema.

The clinical diagnosis of constrictive pericarditis should be suspected when a pericardial knock and a diminished precordial cardiac impulse are noted. The pericardial knock is an early diastolic sound which is heard approximately 0.09 to 0.12 second after the aortic component of the second heart sound. This sound occurs earlier, is higher pitched, and radiates wider than the usual third heart sound. It is sometimes mistaken for a mitral opening snap but is easily differentiated by the simultaneous recording of the phonocardiogram and the external jugular venous pulse tracing (the pericardial knock occurs at the trough of the Y descent of the venous pulse tracing) and the echocardiographic examination of the mitral valve.

Paradoxical pulsation, defined as a greater than 10 mm. Hg drop in systolic pressure during normal inspiration, is less commonly seen in constrictive pericarditis than in acute cardiac tamponade. The reason for this is unclear but may be related to elastic properties of the pericardium.

Kussmaul's sign (paradoxical distention of the neck veins during inspiration) is classically described in patients with chronic constrictive pericarditis but is not specific for constriction due to pericardial disease.

X-Ray Examination of the Chest

The cardiac silhouette of patients with constrictive pericarditis may be normal (45 percent), slightly enlarged (17 percent), moderately enlarged (32 percent), or greatly enlarged (6 percent).[4] In our patients, 11 of 22 had enlargement of their cardiac silhouette on chest x-ray.

Chest fluoroscopy may reveal decreased cardiac pulsation although this observation is not specific for constrictive pericarditis. The absence of this finding does not exclude pericardial constriction, as illustrated by 9 of our 22 patients having normal cardiac pulsation at fluoroscopic examination. Another radiographic clue to the diagnosis of constrictive pericarditis is the detection of calcium in the pericardium. Calcium has been

198

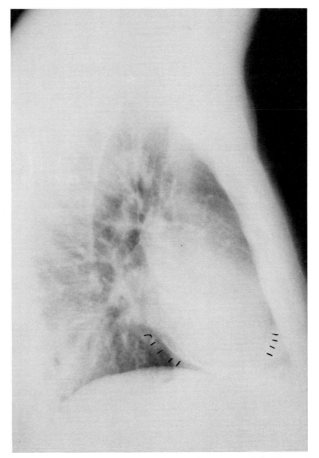

Figure 1. Lateral chest x-ray of a patient with proven constrictive pericarditis, illustrating pericardial calcification in the anterior and inferoposterior portion of the heart. (Outlined by black marks.)

detected in approximately 50 percent of patients with constriction[4] and was found in 11 of our 22 patients. Wood has suggested that in constrictive processes of greater than 2 years duration the incidence of pericardial calcium is as high as 70 percent.[8] A typical lateral x-ray showing calcium in the pericardium is seen in Figure 1.

Pleural effusions are nonspecific findings but are seen frequently. Paul reported effusions in 28 of 53 cases.[4]

Pulmonary vascular congestion has been reported in patients with constrictive pericarditis.[9] However, most series report this infrequently with only 12 of 137 patients from the Mayo Clinic demonstrating vascular congestion by chest x-ray.[7]

Electrocardiogram

Electrocardiographic abnormalities, while not specific, can be a helpful clue to the clinician. The most common abnormalities reported by Levine were nonspecific ST segment and T wave changes, that is, low, flat, biphasic, or inverted T waves in leads that normally have upright T waves.[10] In addition to the T wave changes, there were 12 of 57 patients with ST segment depression associated with the T wave changes. None of Levine's patients were reported to have ST segment elevation which is usually seen

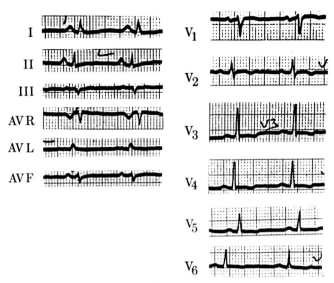

Figure 2. Electrocardiogram of a patient with proven constrictive pericarditis. Note low voltage in the standard limb leads and nonspecific T-wave abnormalities in the limb and precordial leads.

in acute pericarditis. Figure 2 is an illustrative example of a typical ECG. Low voltage was present on the ECG in 35 of the 57 patients. Changes compatible with right ventricular hypertrophy (12) or left ventricular hypertrophy (5), and notched P waves (28) were also observed. Rhythm disturbances were frequent, with atrial fibrillation being present in 19 of the 57 patients. Other atrial arrhythmias were also seen including atrial flutter (3) and paroxysmal atrial tachycardia (3). These findings were in close agreement with our own observations which are summarized in Table 3.

Abnormal Q waves in the electrocardiograms of patients with constrictive pericarditis are not uncommon.[10] Levine reported 7 patients with ECG patterns characteristic of myocardial infarction.[10] Five of these patients with suspected myocardial infarctions were studied at necropsy and found to have myocardial fibrosis thought to be related to the primary pericardial process rather than the usual etiology of ischemic heart disease. The absence of Q waves, however, did not predict the absence of myocardial fibrosis, since four of seven patients studied at necropsy showed myocardial fibrosis with only the nonspecific T wave changes.

LABORATORY INVESTIGATION

When the clinician suspects constrictive pericarditis, there are a number of laboratory tests both noninvasive and invasive to help confirm the diagnosis.

Table 3. Electrocardiograms (22 patients)

ST T-wave changes	20
Decreased voltage	9
Atrial fibrillation	10
RAD	4
RBBB	2

200

Jugular Venous Pulse and Phonocardiogram

One of the more useful techniques used to establish the diagnosis of constrictive pericarditis is simultaneous recording of the jugular venous pulse and the phonocardiogram. The analysis of the jugular venous pulse tracing alone often provides suggestive evidence of constrictive pericarditis. Characteristically the external jugular venous pulse resembles an M or W. The "a" wave usually is prominent and probably related to diminished compliance of the right ventricle secondary to the constricting process. The "x" descent of the venous pulse is variable. It may be shallow[8] or it may be sharper and deeper than the Y descent.[11] In patients with constrictive pericarditis and atrial fibrillation, the x descent is blunted. Because of the high venous pressure, the V wave is prominent in constrictive pericarditis. The V wave characteristically is followed by a steep Y descent with a prominent early Y trough. The Y trough occurs nearly coincident with the "diastolic dip" of the right ventricular pressure signal. The pattern is not specific for constrictive pericarditis since it occurs in any condition that restricts ventricular filling. It is particularly difficult to differentiate patients with constrictive physiology from those with restrictive physiology due to cardiomyopathy.

Lisa and colleagues[12] measured the duration from the aortic component of the second heart sound to the peak of the V wave of the simultaneously recorded jugular venous pulse and suggested that constrictive pericarditis usually could be differentiated from cardiomyopathies. If the A_2V time was less than 0.03 sec., constrictive pericarditis was favored, whereas an A_2V time greater than 0.03 sec. favored cardiomopathy. The physiologic explanation of these observations is as follows: Patients with cardiomyop-

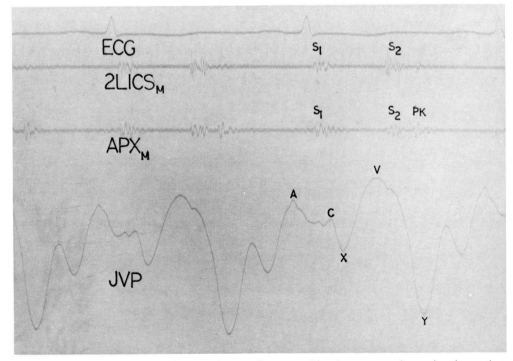

Figure 3. Simultaneous electrocardiogram, phonocardiogram, and jugular venous pulse tracings in a patient with proven constrictive pericarditis. S_1 = first heart sound. S_2 = second heart sound. PK = pericardial knock. The characteristic venous pulse waves are labeled A, C, and V with the corresponding venous troughs labeled X and Y. See text for full explanation.

athy usually have right ventricular systolic pressures that are higher than those found in patients with constrictive pericarditis. Right ventricular pressure must fall before the tricuspid valve opens. Thus, in patients with cardiomyopathy (high RV pressure) the isovolumetric relaxation period is relatively long and the measured A_2V time is prolonged. In patients with constrictive pericarditis (lower RV pressure), isovolumetric relaxation period is short and the measured A_2V time is short.

In many patients with constrictive pericarditis, a diastolic sound (pericardial knock) can be recorded. The pericardial knock occurs at the nadir of the Y descent of the jugular venous pulse. When these observations are made, the diagnosis of constrictive pericarditis is strongly suspected. A typical example of a characteristic jugular venous pulse and pericardial knock is seen in Figure 3.

Systolic Time Intervals

The use of systolic time intervals in detecting patients with constrictive pericarditis and differentiating them from cardiomyopathies has been evaluated recently by Armstrong, Lewis and Gotsman.[13] The usefulness of systolic time intervals is based on the observation that patients with severe cardiomyopathies have diminished left ventricular ejection fraction while patients with constrictive pericarditis usually have nearly normal ejection fractions. Assuming that systolic time intervals correlate well with ejection fractions, Garrard and associates demonstrated that patients with constrictive pericarditis have significantly shorter PEP, longer LVET and lower PEP/LVET ratios than did patients with cardiomyopathy.

Echocardiography

Echocardiography is the most sensitive method available to detect pericardial effusions. However, its use in the evaluation of constrictive pericarditis has not been as well established and reports are conflicting concerning its usefulness. Gibson and colleagues were unable to detect consistently pericardial thickening.[14] They reported that parodoxical septal motion was the only consistent echocardiographic abnormality in patients with constrictive pericarditis. On the other hand, Horowitz was able to detect two equally intense, parallel moving echos separated by 1 to 3 mm. in the region of the posterior parietal and visceral pleura in patients with effusive constrictive pericarditis.[15] The anatomic findings were confirmed at surgery, and Horowitz concluded that effusive constrictive cases could be differentiated by the echo free space between the two intense parallel moving echoes. He further concluded that differentiation from restrictive myocardiopathies could be made by measuring a smaller left ventricular end-diastolic dimension, greater systolic shortening of the diastolic diameter, and increased systolic septal thickening in patients with constrictive pericarditis as compared with cardiomyopathies. Figure 4 is an illustrative example of the echocardiographic findings of one of our patients with chronic constrictive pericarditis.

Fluoroscopy

Fluoroscopy may be of some value in evaluating patients with constrictive pericarditis. The detection of calcium in the pericardium is a useful sign when present but it is only found in approximately 50 percent of cases.[4] Lack of left ventricular movement has been advocated as a sign of constrictive pericarditis but it is not a sensitive method of detection since only 50 percent of patients with proven constrictive physiology demonstrate this finding.[4] Furthermore, many patients with cardiomyopathy with moderately or markedly enlarged silhouettes have diminished cardiac pulsations.

202

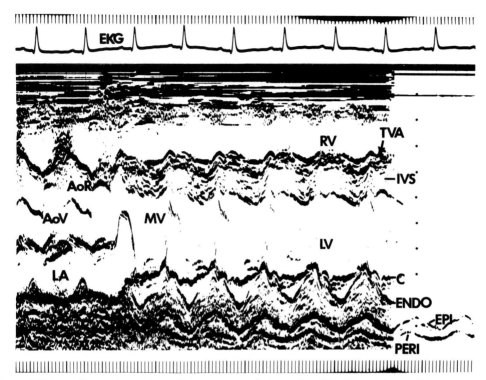

Figure 4. Echocardiogram in a patient with proven constrictive pericarditis. RV = right ventricle, TVA = tricuspid valve apparatus, IVS = interventricular septum, AOR = aortic root, AOV = aortic valve, MV = mitral valve, LA = left atrium, LV = left ventricle, C = chordae tendineae, ENDO = endocardium, EPI = epicardium, PERI = pericardium. The echocardiogram shows a small left ventricular cavity with good ejection fraction. In addition, note the two parallel moving lines labeled EPI and PERI with a 2 to 3 mm. clear space suggesting an effusive component to the constrictive process.

Hemodynamic Studies

The measurement of pressure and flow along with angiographic studies provide the most accurate methods to detect constrictive pericarditis in man. Because all diastolic expansion of the heart is restricted in patients with constrictive pericarditis, all diastolic pressures are elevated and in many instances, equal. There may be some difference between right and left sided diastolic pressures, but it is usually less than 6 mm. Hg. Our 22 patients showed this characteristic equalization of the diastolic pressures with less than 6 mm. Hg differences between the right and left atrial pressures. The right atrial pulse tracing has the same configuration that was described previously for the jugular venous pulse configuration. The ventricular pressure contour also has a characteristic appearance. The systolic portion of the tracing appears normal, but following return of the pressure to baseline, there is an abrupt elevation of the pressure in early diastole which is sustained throughout the diastolic filling period. This abrupt elevation of the pressure is due to the lack of compliance of the heart in diastole and gives the appearance of the mathematical symbol for "square root." Typical ventricular pressure contours of a patient with constrictive pericarditis are seen in Figure 5.

Moderate elevation of the right ventricular and pulmonary artery systolic pressures is commonly observed in patients with constrictive pericarditis. In the 22 patients studied, we observed an average pulmonary artery systolic pressure of 37 mm. Hg with a range of 23 to 65 mm. Hg.

Intracardiac Pressures - Constrictive Pericarditis

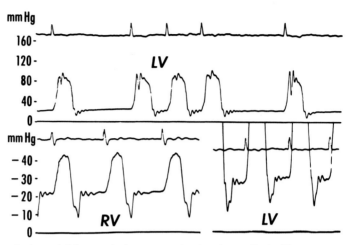

Figure 5. Left ventricular and right ventricular pressure tracings in a patient with proven constrictive pericarditis. LV = left ventricular pressure; RV = right ventricular pressure. Note the abrupt elevation of the pressure in early diastole which is sustained throughout the diastolic filling period.

Cardiac output in patients with constrictive pericarditis is usually normal or slightly below normal. The average cardiac index of our 22 patients was 2.4 L./min./m².

These hemodynamic findings are not specific for constrictive pericarditis because, once again, cardiomyopathies produce similar hemodynamic measurements. However, there are a number of helpful clues that usually allow differentiation of these two entities. These are listed in Table 4. Compared to patients with constrictive pericarditis, patients with cardiomyopathies tend to have lower cardiac outputs, higher pulmonary artery and wedge pressures, and more than a 6 mm. Hg difference between the right and left sided diastolic pressure.

We compared 22 patients with constrictive pericarditis to 31 patients with cardiomyopathy and plotted right atrial pressure versus pulmonary artery systolic pressure. This simple technique, which can be accomplished by using a Swan-Ganz catheter, produced a clean separation of the patients with constrictive pericarditis from the patients with cardiomyopathies (Figure 6). All patients with constrictive pericarditis had a ratio of PA systolic to RA mean pressures of less than 3.5 while all but three of the 31 patients with cardiomyopathy had a ratio greater than 3.5.

Table 4. Hemodynamic differences between cardiomyopathies and chronic constrictive pericarditis

	Cardiomyopathy	*Constrictive pericarditis*
Cardiac output	↓ ↓ ↓	normal to ↓
PCW	↑ ↑	↑
LA-RA	>6 mm. Hg	<6 mm. Hg
PA systolic/RA	>3.5	<3.5

PCW = Pulmonary capillary wedge pressure; LA-RA = Difference in mean left atrial and right atrial pressures; PA systolic/RA = Ratio of systolic pulmonary artery pressure to mean right atrial pressure

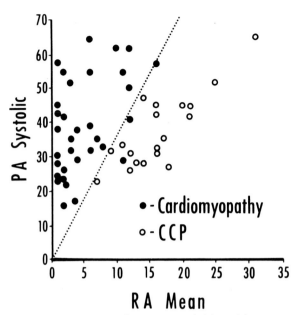

Figure 6. Comparison of pulmonary artery systolic pressure and right atrial mean pressure in patients with proven constrictive pericarditis and cardiomyopathy.

Angiography

Angiography provides supportive evidence for the diagnosis of constrictive pericarditis. The goal is to determine pericardial thickening. The thickness of the pericardium is most reliably determined and easiest to assess at the right atrial border. Thus, right atrial cineangiography in the AP projection will provide information about the contour, motion, and thickness of the atriopericardial border. In patients who have not had previous heart or lung surgery, thickening, straightening, and decreased motion of the right atrial border will be the result of constrictive pericarditis in most instances. Table 5 summarizes our own observations in 20 of the 22 patients; 17 had all three right atrial angiographic abnormalities and 19 had two of the three. Carbon dioxide injection into the right atrium can be substituted for radiopaque contrast material in situations where contrast injection is hazardous, for instance, proven allergic reaction. However, carbon dioxide injection does not allow assessment of the right atrial motion since cinefluorography is not used with this technique.

Ramsey and co-workers described another angiographic technique to assess pericardial thickening.[16] They reported observations during injection of the left anterior descending coronary artery. In normal man, the left anterior descending coronary artery is easily seen on the surface of the cardiac silhouette. In patients with thickened pericardium, the left anterior descending is positioned within the cardiac silhouette.

Obviously, all of these techniques have difficulty differentiating between pericardial

Table 5. Right
atrial angiography

RA border	
Thickened	19/20
Straight	17/20
Immobile	20/20

thickening, pericardial effusions with tamponade, and so-called effusive constrictive pericarditis. The use of echocardiography is of considerable help in determining the presence of pericardial effusions.[17] However, in the case of effusive constrictive pericarditis, as pointed out by Hancock, it is sometimes necessary to measure right and left sided pressures before and after a pericardiocentesis to determine whether it is the fluid or the visceral pericardium that is causing the hemodynamic changes.[18]

ETIOLOGY

The etiology of constrictive pericarditis is not much clearer today than it was when White gave his historic address at St. Cyres in 1935. In the past, most cases of constrictive pericarditis were felt to be tuberculous in origin. However, in more recent series of constrictive pericarditis, tuberculosis has become less and less common. Many other causes of pericardial constriction have been reported and are listed in Table 6. In recent years with the advent of chronic hemodialysis programs and the aggressive radiotherapy approach to many malignancies especially the lymphomas, uremia and radiation fibrosis have been associated with increased numbers of patients with constrictive pericarditis. Despite these iatrogenically produced cases of constrictive pericarditis, it is important to keep proper perspective and it must be pointed out that the overall incidence of constrictive pericarditis is low.

By the time the constrictive process manifests itself clinically, the acute process usually has subsided. Pathologic specimens of the pericardium thus reflect a chronic disease state. Pathologic examination of the pericardium of our 22 cases revealed only chronic inflammation and fibrosis. Two patients had proven but old pulmonary tuberculosis; 5 of 16 tested had a positive histoplasmin skin test. The remainder of the patients had no obvious etiology for the constrictive process.

The pathogenesis of constrictive pericarditis is poorly understood. The reason why one patient with acute pericarditis of whatever etiology later develops constriction and another patient with the same acute process remains free of sequelae is not clear. Hancock has made several observations which may be pertinent to the natural history of this disease.[18] He reported 13 patients with "subacute effusive constrictive pericarditis." All of these patients eventually came to surgery since medical treatment made no significant difference in their clinical courses. Of interest is the observation that four patients developed a noneffusive constriction in the later stages, suggesting that the natural history of this disease consists of progression through the subacute effusive constrictive state to the chronic constrictive noneffusive state.

PATHOPHYSIOLOGY

Isaacs and colleagues were able to produce experimental constrictive pericarditis in dogs by using plastic casts within the pericardial space.[19] They were able to produce all of the hemodynamic changes observed in patients with this disease. They observed

Table 6. Etiology of constrictive pericarditis

Post-viral pericarditis	Tuberculosis
Post-trauma	Post-bacterial pericarditis
Post-radiation	Post-Dressler syndrome
Uremia	Post-pericardiotomy syndrome
Metastatic malignancy	Rheumatoid arthritis
Fungus (histoplasmosis)	Systemic lupus erythematosus

that localized constriction of the right ventricle produced systemic venous hypertension and all of its consequences (hepatomegaly, ascites, and peripheral edema). When constriction was limited to the left ventricle, the animals developed rales, accentuated pulmonary closure sounds, and marked pulmonary hypertension. The animals with isolated left ventricular constriction were more prone to develop pulmonary edema than animals with left and right ventricular constriction. Constriction of both ventricles produced the combination of effects seen in the isolated right and left ventricular constriction, resembling those changes seen in patients with this disorder. They further showed that it was the constriction of the ventricles and not the atria which produced the hemodynamic changes. This experimental observation led them to postulate that the pathophysiology of the disease is related to the "mechanical defect" in ventricular diastolic filling on the basis of alteration of ventricular volume — elasticity characteristics of the pericardium.

THERAPY

The current therapy of chronic constrictive pericarditis is surgical, although it is possible to manage patients successfully with vigorous diuretic therapy. Patients with mild cases and few symptoms frequently can be managed for long periods of time with medical therapy alone. The exact time for surgery in these patients still remains an individual decision based on the general condition of the patient and the presence of incapacitating symptoms.

In recent years, the mortality associated with surgery of this condition has dropped steadily. Wychulis and associates[7] reported the mortality rate during 1936–1951 as 24 percent with a high of 50 percent in some series. From 1951–1960 the mortality rate decreased to 11 percent. From 1961–1969, it dropped to 6 percent. They found no significant difference between patients with calcific pericardial disease and those without a calcified pericardium. Not only has mortality decreased, but the overall clinical results from surgery have improved. During the years 1936–1950 14 of 35 operative survivors symptomatically improved, from 1951–1960 42 of 51 improved, and from 1961–1969 28 of 32 improved.

In our series, 1 of 22 patients died as a result of surgery and there was one late death. Eighteen of the survivors were either symptom free or minimally symptomatic and only two patients required continued drug therapy.

The improvement that patients experience following pericardiectomy is frequently apparent only after prolonged convalescent periods. The hemodynamic mechanism behind this has only recently been clarified by Viola.[20] He demonstrated that immediately following surgery there were no significant changes in the intraventricular pressure curves. For the first 24 to 48 hours all patients showed central venous pressures similar to the preoperative values. Between the second and fourth days, patients began to steadily drop their systemic venous pressures and by four weeks they were all back to normal. Subsequently, all patients were recatheterized and all were found to have marked hemodynamic improvement.

Many postulates have been made concerning the etiology for failure of surgical results. The two most prominent causes are (1) incomplete resection of the pericardium from the ventricles and atrioventricular groove and (2) the myocardial fibrosis which is frequently present. Whether the myocardial fibrosis is secondary to the primary process itself or secondary to partial ventricular immobilization is not clear.[21] The recent report by Viola suggests that the decreased compliance of the myocardium due to the immobilization of the ventricular muscle is at least partially reversible.[20] Whether the fibrosis is related to the duration of the constrictive process is difficult to determine, but if it is, then a stronger argument could be made for earlier surgical intervention prior to the onset of severe symptoms. As yet, however, this matter has not been satisfactorily resolved.

SUMMARY

Constrictive pericarditis, although still a relatively rare disease, continues to be a clinical problem that most practicing cardiologists may encounter. A major clinical clue to diagnosis is the continued elevation of the central venous pressure after adequate diuresis. The diagnosis is further supported by (1) prominent X and Y descents in the jugular venous pulse, (2) a relatively normal or only slightly enlarged cardiac silhouette in a patient with congestive heart failure, (3) pericardial calcification or significant congestive failure especially when the right sided signs predominate without obvious cause. When the disease is suspected, appropriate investigation should be undertaken using both the noninvasive and the catheterization studies. If the diagnosis is supported, then the choice of therapy at present is based primarily on severity of symptoms with surgical removal of the constricting pericardium being the therapy of choice in patients unable to be managed medically.

REFERENCES

1. CHEVERS, N.: *Observations on the disease of the orifice and valves of the aorta.* Guy's Hosp. Rep. 7: 387, 1842.

2. PICK, F.: *Uber chroniscke unter dem Bilde dem Ledercirrhose verlairpende Perikarditis (perikardische Pseudolebercirrhose) (Curschmann), Nebst Bemerkungen ube die Zuckergussleber.* Z. Klin. Med. 29: 385, 1896.

3. WHITE, P. D.: *Chronic constrictive pericarditis (Pick's disease) treated by pericardial resection.* Lancet 2:597, 1935.

4. PAUL, O., CASTLEMAN, B., AND WHITE, P. D.: *Chronic constrictive pericarditis, a study of 53 cases.* Am. J. Med. Sci. 216:361, 1948.

5. IKRAM, H., BANIM, S. O., AND MAKEY, A. R.: *Clinical features of non-tuberculous constrictive pericarditis.* Thorax 29:204, 1974.

6. CONTI, C. R., AND FRIESINGER, G. C.: *Chronic constrictive pericarditis, clinical and laboratory findings in 11 cases.* Johns Hopkins Med. J. 120:262, 1967.

7. WYCHULIS, A. R., CONNOLLY, D. C., AND MCGOON, D. C.: *Surgical treatment of pericarditis.* J. Thorac. Cardiovasc. Surg. 62:608, 1971.

8. WOOD, P.: *Chronic constrictive pericarditis.* Br. Heart J. 21:9, 1959.

9. GIMLETTE, T. M. D.: *Constrictive pericarditis.* Br. Heart J. 21:9, 1959.

10. LEVINE, H. D.: *Myocardial fibrosis in constrictive pericarditis — electrocardiographic and pathologic observations.* Circulation 48:1268, 1973.

11. GIBSON, R.: *Atypical constrictive pericarditis.* Br. Heart J. 21:583, 1959.

12. LISA, C. P., GOOD, G., AND TAVEL, M. E.: *The jugular pulse in pericardial constriction, its differentiation from that of cardiomyopathy.* Am. Heart J. 84:409, 1972.

13. ARMSTRONG, T. G., LEWIS, B. S., AND GOTSMAN, M. S.: *Systolic time intervals in constrictive pericarditis and severe primary myocardial disease.* Am. Heart J. 85:6, 1973.

14. GIBSON, T. C., GROSSMAN, W., MCLAURIN, L. P., ET AL.: *Echocardiography in patients with constrictive pericarditis.* Circulation 49 & 50 (Suppl. 3):86, 1974.

15. HOROWITZ, M. S., ROSSEN, R. M., AND HARRISON, D. C.: *Ultrasound evaluation of constrictive pericarditis.* Circulation 49 & 50 (Suppl.3):87, 1974.

16. RAMSEY, H. W., SBAR, S., ELLIOTT, L. P., ET AL.: *The differential diagnosis of restrictive myocardiopathy and chronic constrictive pericarditis without calcification.* Am. J. Cardiol. 25:635, 1970.

17. HOROWITZ, M. S., SHULTZ, C. S., STINSON, E. B., ET AL.: *Sensitivity and specificity of echocardiographic diagnosis of pericardial effusion.* Circulation 50:239, 1974.

18. HANCOCK, E. W.: *Subacute effusive constrictive pericarditis.* Circulation 43:183, 1971.

19. ISAACS, J. P., CARTER, B. N., AND HALLER, J. A.: *Experimental pericarditis: the pathologic physiology of constrictive pericarditis.* Bull. Hopkins Hosp. 90:259, 1957.
20. VIOLA, A. R.: *The influence of pericardiectomy on the hemodynamics of chronic constrictive pericarditis.* Circulation 48:1038, 1973.
21. SUMMERVILLE, W.: *Constrictive pericarditis with special reference to the change in the natural history brought about by surgical intervention.* Circulation 38 (Suppl. 5):102, 1968.

The Postpericardiotomy
and Similar Syndromes*

Mary Allen Engle, M.D., Arthur A. Klein, M.D., Seymour Hepner, M.D., and Kathryn H. Ehlers, M.D.

About 20 years ago, three clinically identical syndromes came to medical attention, each named for the setting in which it occurred: the postpericardiotomy syndrome, the postmyocardial infarction syndrome, and postpericardial trauma syndrome. Each is characterized by the appearance, a few days to a few weeks after the event, of fever and signs of pericarditis and pleuritis, often with sanguinous or serous effusions and sometimes with pulmonary parenchymal infiltrates. Nonspecific evidence of inflammation (elevated white cell blood count and sedimentation rate) accompany them, but signs of effusions or inflammation in other serous surfaces are conspicuously lacking; nor is there involvement of the reticuloendothelial system. The condition is self-limited after an average course of two to four weeks. When present, the manifestations range from so mild as to be detected only by a high index of suspicion and careful search, to a seriously debilitating illness with high fever, malaise, and such rapidly developing pericardial effusion or such a large effusion that cardiac tamponade occurs. Each may relapse in months and even over a period of two or three years, with no obvious antecedent event. Recurrence may mimic the original episode, even to recurrent pericardial effusions, but in general recurrences are mild. Late sequelae, such as constrictive pericarditis, apparently do not occur.

The advent of intracardiac surgery to relieve valvular stenosis created the "postvalvulotomy," "postcommissurotomy," or "postcardiotomy" syndrome, which was first reported in 1952.[1, 2] Because the operation was usually performed for severe mitral stenosis due to rheumatic heart disease, it was originally thought perhaps to represent reactivation of rheumatic fever. Then it was pointed out that this postoperative event followed surgery for nonrheumatic heart disease and that it could occur not just after valvulotomy or cardiotomy but after intrapericardial exploration alone. Since pericardiotomy was the common denominator in all these operations, the designation "postpericardiotomy syndrome" was given.[3, 4]

It was in 1956 that Dressler called attention to the syndrome that now bears his name and follows myocardial infarction in some patients.[5, 6] A similar condition was noted following penetrating injury to the heart or blunt precordial trauma: the postpericardial trauma syndrome.[7-10]

Reported incidence of the postoperative and post-traumatic syndromes has varied, but it is probably 20 to 30 percent.[1-4, 8, 11] That has been the occurrence rate of the postpericardiotomy syndrome over the years in our experience, which is chiefly in patients

*This work was supported in part by NIH Research Grant #5 ROI HL 16246.

with congenital heart disease.[3, 4, 12-17] Larson found that the syndrome occurred 78 times in 51 of 137 patients surviving mitral valvotomy, an incidence of 36 percent.[18] Segal and Tabatznik reported an incidence of 30 percent following traumatic hemopericardium.[8, 9] Recently Toole and Silverman studied 554 patients with myocardial infarction over a three-year period.[19] They encountered 40 patients (7.2 percent) with early pericarditis and in the survivors of that complication, an incidence of postmyocardial infarction syndrome of 15 percent. The incidence of the syndrome cited for all patients suffering a myocardial infarction is 1 to 4 percent.

Diagnosis of these syndromes is based on a high index of suspicion in patients recovering from one of the three events and on exclusion of other causes of pericardial involvement and fever, such as infection or endocarditis. To the radiologist the findings of "cardiomegaly" together with pleural effusion (usually on the left) and pulmonary parenchymal infiltrate suggest cardiac failure.[20] The physician at the bedside may also mistakenly diagnose congestive failure when the tachycardia, tachypnea, orthopnea, jugular venous distention, and hepatomegaly that accompany cardiac tamponade are observed. Echocardiography has been helpful in confirming the presence of pericardial effusion and in estimating its size.[21] Other causes of pulmonary infiltrate such as atelectasis, pneumonia, or infarction need to be excluded. We have found that the development of heart-reactive antibody in high titer is a confirmatory diagnostic test in the postpericardiotomy syndrome[15] (see later), and we have found the antibody to be similarly elevated in the few patients we have studied with postmyocardial infarction syndrome and in the one child with post-traumatic pericardial syndrome following a stab wound of the heart.

Etiology of these syndromes is still obscure. Similarity to "benign" viral pericarditis has been commented upon.[3-5, 14, 22, 23] It has also been suggested that the syndromes may represent an autoimmune phenomenon.[3, 4, 24-8] Features common to all three are trauma to pericardium and myocardium and the opportunity for intrapericardial bleeding.

Since etiology is unknown, therapy is empiric. Because the syndromes are self-limited, effects of any treatment are difficult to judge. Measures employed have included bed rest and use of diuretics, salicylates, and/or corticosteroids.[7, 13]

Our experience has been chiefly with the postpericardiotomy syndrome (PPS) in the pediatric age group. In order to better understand this condition, we began a prospective study of consecutive, long-term survivors of intrapericardial surgery. In an ongoing study we sought to determine whether there appeared in the serum postoperatively an antiheart antibody,[29] whether there was a significant rise in antiviral antibody, and if so, whether the rise in antibodies bore any relation to each other or to clinical signs of the syndrome. Immunologic, virologic, and clinical determinations were made on a triple-blind basis and periodically the results were compared.[15-17] Conditions of operative and postoperative management were standardized insofar as possible. Samples of blood were drawn preoperatively, postoperatively at 7 to 10 days, on the first two visits after discharge, and additionally as indicated. Antibiotics were administered for the first five days and not thereafter except on clear indication of bacterial infection. No other medications were given except for a diuretic, furosemide, when effusions were moderate.

Of 257 survivors of cardiac surgery in which the pericardium was entered, 66 had PPS, an incidence of 25.7 percent. In 22, the syndrome was mild; in 28, moderate; and in 16, severe. Antiheart antibody was not demonstrable preoperatively, and in 102 patients none was demonstrated postoperatively. However, in 62 patients heart-reactive antibody in high titer (greater than 2+ on a scale of 0 to 4+) appeared toward the end of the first week. It declined about a month postoperatively and disappeared by two to three months after surgery. In an intermediate group of 93 patients, the antiheart antibody appeared at the same time but did not exceed 2+ and disappeared earlier. None of

212

the patients with no detectable antibody had the syndrome, whereas all with heart-reactive antibody in high titer had clinical evidence of PPS, and three of the intermediate group had the syndrome in mild form. We concluded that appearance of a heart-reactive antibody in high titer correlated closely with clinical syndrome, and that its presence afforded a confirmatory diagnostic test of the condition. Figures 1 to 4 summarize the findings.

In 137 of these subjects we analyzed the same samples of serum for antibody to adenovirus, Coxsackie B1-B6, and cytomegalovirus. We found a fourfold or greater rise in titer to one or more viral agents in 5 percent of those with negative antiheart antibody and no syndrome, in 15 percent of those with intermediate level of antiheart antibody and no PPS, but in 68 percent of those with high antiheart antibody and the clinical syndrome (21 out of 31 patients). In 21 of these 31 with a significant rise there was no detectable antiviral antibody preoperatively, while in 10 others, antibody was present in low titer prior to surgery and became elevated afterward.[16] This suggests that

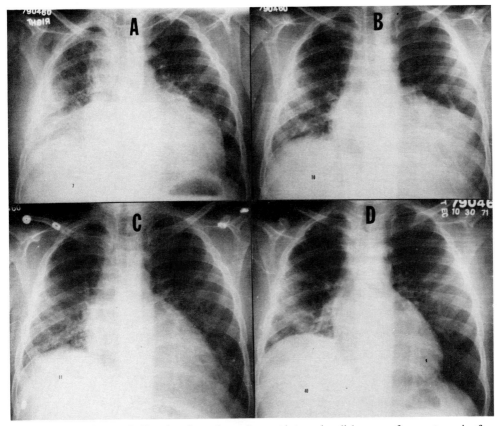

Figure 1. Serial radiologic findings in a boy who underwent intrapericardial surgery for anastomosis of ascending aorta to right pulmonary artery (Waterston procedure) because of the diagnosis of tricuspid atresia with inadequate pulmonary blood flow. A, Seven days postoperatively, showing "cardiomegaly" with right pleural effusion and high right diaphragm. Angiocardiogram obtained on this day is shown in Figure 2 and the electrocardiogram in Figure 3. Pericardiocentesis was performed on day 8. B, Ten days postoperatively showing return of pericardial effusion, prior to second pericardiocentesis for tamponade. C, Eleven days postoperatively with pericardial fluid again present. Steroids started at this time. D, the roentgenogram at discharge, comparable to that after institution of steroid therapy. Paralysis of right diaphragm persists, but there is no cardiomegaly, pericardial or pleural effusion.

213

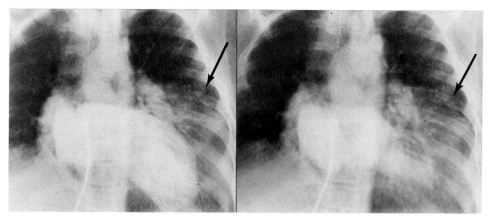

Figure 2. Angiocardiogram on 7th day after surgery as large pericardial effusion caused cardiac tamponade. Cardiac chambers (right and left atria, left ventricle) contain contrast medium, while large nonopacified shadow lateral to right and left heart borders represents the massive pericardial effusion. Diastole on left, systole on right side of photograph.

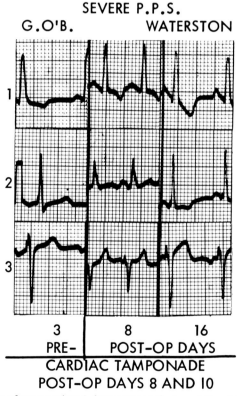

Figure 3. Electrocardiogram of same patient 3 days preoperatively and 8 and 16 days postoperatively. Because of his congenital anomaly, there is left axis deviation and TI is inverted. During tamponade on day 8, note sinus tachycardia, deeper inversion of TI, and decrease in voltage. Improvement in voltage on day 16 after pericardial effusion had disappeared.

214

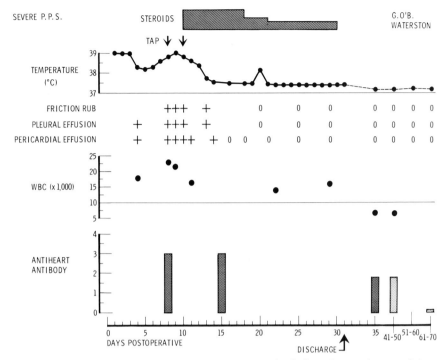

Figure 4. Course of patient in Figures 1 to 3 with days postoperative indicated across bottom of chart and the parameters observed shown on left side. Note disappearance of fever, friction rub, pericardial and pleural effusions, and leukocytosis with administration of corticosteroids from day 9 for three weeks. Elevation of antiheart antibody greater than 2+ was present at height of syndrome, was less in second month, and gone by third month postoperatively. (From Engle et al.[15] with permission.)

recent viral illness or reactivation of a latent illness may trigger the immunologic response that constitutes the PPS.

In this study[16, 17] we found a low incidence of only 1.6 percent of the condition in the 63 infants under the age of two years, whereas the incidence was around 30 percent in the older age groups (2 to 5, 6 to 10, 11 to 15, and 16+ years). Since the same kinds of operations were performed in the babies as in those over age two years, and because there was no indication of impaired immunologic competence in any of the patients, the difference in occurrence rates of the syndrome may be explained by the relatively short experience of the infants in exposure to and reaction to viral illness.

We noted a higher incidence of the syndrome in patients whose cardiac surgery involved greater myocardial trauma than in those with only an atriotomy for atrial septal defect or simple Mustard procedure or with pulmonary arteriotomy and valvotomy for valvular pulmonic stenosis. The risk of the syndrome was highest in those undergoing infundibular resection and patch-closure of the ventricular septal defect through a right ventriculotomy for repair of tetralogy of Fallott.[16]

In order to evaluate effects of therapy, other than those of rest, fluid restriction, and duiretics, we studied the clinical response and the behavior of the antiheart antibody in 12 patients with severe syndrome.[16] After the illness was well established, we treated six patients with salicylates for several weeks and six others with steroids (prednisolone) for three weeks. After the first week the dose of prednisolone of 2 mg./kg./day was cut by half, and again by half for the third week. Salicylates had the expected antipyretic effect but did not appreciably shorten the course nor cause a lowering of antiheart antibody titer. In contrast, steroids had a prompt effect on all clinical parameters, and the improvement was maintained after corticosteroids were discontinued at the end of three weeks. In addition, the level of antiheart antibody dropped more quickly and disappeared sooner than in other patients with severe manifestations who were treated nonspecifically or with salicylates. We believe that patients with the syndrome in severe form may benefit from a course of steroids such as that described.

Prevention of the syndrome is not accomplished by enforced bed rest early in the course. We found no difference in incidence between the first 100 patients who did not ambulate until they had been afebrile for 48 hours and the subsequent 100 who were permitted early ambulation. We do restrict ambulation, though, for those with large pericardial effusion. Prevention has been accomplished for some patients, however: the recent trend to open heart surgery early in infancy for symptomatic babies has meant their repair has been accomplished at an age when risk of the syndrome is minimal. The overall incidence of the syndrome in pediatric patients undergoing surgery that involves entry into the pericardium is now decreasing for the first time as a result.

We interpret the postpericardiotomy syndrome as an immunologically determined reaction in association with a recent or latent viral illness. The trauma consequent to the intrapericardial manipulations and perhaps the bleeding into the pericardial sac set the stage for the syndrome. The epicardial layer of myocardium responds by an inflammatory reaction, often accompanied by the outpouring of fluid. The pleural effusions, usually on the left, are viewed as a "neighborhood" response to the pericardial reaction. The postmyocardial infarction and the postpericardial trauma syndromes may have a similar mechanism. Recurrences may be triggered by a new, though at times clinically inapparent, viral illness.

SUMMARY

A syndrome of pericardial and often pleural reaction with effusions and with fever occurs in three different settings. It bears the descriptive term of the condition which it follows: the postpericardiotomy syndrome, the postmyocardial infarction syndrome, and the postpericardial trauma syndrome. The manifestations, incidence, theories of etiology, treatment, and possibility of prevention were discussed. The syndrome is probably due to an immunologic response with an associated viral illness, since in a prospective study of children undergoing cardiac surgery in which the pericardium was entered, we found that the development of heart-reactive antibody in high titer and a significant rise in antiviral antibody occurred in patients with clinically evident syndrome.

REFERENCES

1. JANTON, O. H., GLOVER, R. P., O'NEILL, T. J. E., ET AL.: *Results of the surgical treatment for mitral stenosis*. Circulation 6:321, 1952.

2. SOLOFF, L. A., ZATUCHNI, J., JANTON, O. H., ET AL.: *Reactivation of rheumatic fever following mitral commissurotomy*. Circulation 8:481, 1953.

3. ITO, T., ENGLE, M. A., AND GOLDBERG, H. P.: *Postpericardiotomy syndrome following surgery for non-rheumatic heart disease*. Circulation 17:549, 1958.

4. ENGLE, M. A., AND ITO, T.: *The post-pericardiotomy syndrome*. Am. J. Cardiol. 7:73, 1961.

5. DRESSLER, W.: *A post-myocardial-infarction syndrome. Preliminary report of a complication resembling idiopathic, recurrent, benign pericarditis*. J.A.M.A. 160:1379, 1956.

6. DRESSLER, W.: *The post-myocardial-infarction syndrome: A report on forty-four cases*. AMA Arch. Intern. Med. 103:28, 1959.

7. GOODKIND, M. J., BLOOMER, W. E., AND GOODYER, A. V. N.: *Recurrent pericardial effusion after non-penetrating chest trauma: Report of two cases treated with adrenocortical steroids.* N. Engl. J. Med. 263:874, 1960.

8. SEGAL, F., AND TABATZNIK, B.: *Postpericardiotomy syndrome following penetrating stab wounds of the chest: Comparison with the post-commissurotomy syndrome.* Am. Heart J. 59:175, 1960.

9. TABATZNIK, B., AND ISAACS, J. P.: *Postpericardiotomy syndrome following traumatic hemopericardium.* Am. J. Cardiol. 7:83, 1961.

10. PETER, R. H., WHALEN, R. E., ORGAIN, E.S., ET AL.: *Postpericardiotomy syndrome as a complication of percutaneous left ventricular puncture.* Am. J. Cardiol. 17:778, 1966.

11. SWAN, H., KORTZ, A. B., DAVIES, D. H., ET AL.: *Atrial septal defect, secundum: An analysis of one hundred patients undergoing open surgical repair.* J. Thorac. Surg. 37:52, 1959.

12. ENGLE, M. A., AND MARX, N. R.: *The postpericardiotomy and postperfusion syndromes.* Heart Bull. 14: 33, 1965.

13. ENGLE, M. A.: *Postoperative syndromes,* in MOSS, A. J., AND ADAMS, F. H. (EDS.): *Heart Disease in Infants and Children.* The Williams and Wilkins Co., Baltimore, 1968, pp. 1087–1101.

14. DRUSIN, L. M., ENGLE, M. A., HAGSTROM, J. W. C., ET AL.: *The postpericardiotomy syndrome. A six-year epidemiologic study.* N. Engl. J. Med. 272:597, 1965.

15. ENGLE, M. A., McCABE, J. C., EBERT, P. A., ET AL.: *The postpericardiotomy syndrome and antiheart antibodies.* Circulation 49:401, 1974.

16. ENGLE, M. A., ZABRISKIE, J. B., SENTERFIT, L. B., ET AL.: *Immunologic and virologic studies in the postpericardiotomy syndrome.* J. Pediatrics 87:1103, 1975.

17. ENGLE, M. A., ZABRISKIE, J. B., SENTERFIT, L. B., ET AL.: *Postpericardiotomy syndrome: A new look at an old condition.* Mod. Concepts Cardiovasc. Dis. 44:59, 1975.

18. LARSON, D. L.: *Relation of the postcommissurotomy syndrome to the rheumatic state.* Circulation 15: 203, 1957.

19. TOOLE, J. C., AND SILVERMAN, M. E.: *Pericarditis of acute myocardial infarction.* Chest 67:647, 1975.

20. ELLIS, K., MALM, J. R., BOWMAN, F. O., JR., ET AL.: *Roentgenographic findings after pericardial surgery.* Radiol. Clin. N. Am. 9:327, 1971.

21. FEIGENBAUM, H., WALDHAUSEN, J. S., AND HYDE, L. P.: *Ultrasound diagnosis of pericardial effusion.* J.A.M.A. 191:711, 1965.

22. KAHN, D. R., ERTEL, P. Y., MURPHY, W. H., ET AL.: *Pathogenesis of the postpericardiotomy syndrome.* J. Thorac. Cardiovasc. Surg. 54:682, 1967.

23. BURCH, G. E., AND COLCOLOUGH, H. L.: *Postcardiotomy and postinfarction syndrome-A theory.* Am. Heart J. 80:290, 1970.

24. DAVIES, A. M., AND GERY, I.: *The role of autoantibodies in heart disease.* Am. Heart J. 60:669, 1960.

25. GERY, I., DAVIES, A. M., AND EHRENFELD, E. N.: *Heart-specific autoantibodies.* Lancet 1:471, 1960.

26. ROBINSON, J., AND BRIGDEN, W.: *Immunological studies in the post-cardiotomy syndrome.* Br. Med. J. 2:706, 1963.

27. VAN DER GELD, H.: *Anti-heart antibodies in the postpericardiotomy and the postmyocardial-infarction syndromes.* Lancet 2:617, 1964.

28. FOWLER, N.: *Autoimmune heart disease (editorial).* Circulation 44:159, 1971.

29. McCABE, J. C., EBERT, P. A., ENGLE, M. A., ET AL.: *Circulating heart-reactive antibodies in the postpericardiotomy syndrome.* J. Surg. Research 14:158, 1973.

Uremic Pericarditis

Christina M. Comty, M.D., Ronald L. Wathen, Ph.D., M.D., and Fred L. Shapiro, M.D.

Pericarditis has been recognized as a serious complication of uremia since its first description by Richard Bright in 1836, and for many years was regarded as an indication that the disease was reaching a terminal phase, in both acute and chronic renal failure. With improved management of acute renal failure by prophylactic dialysis, pericarditis is an infrequent complication unless the patient is intensely catabolic as a result of sepsis or trauma.[1] With the widespread availability of chronic hemodialysis, uremic pericarditis has become one of several uremic complications which can be treated, usually with rapid resolution. Nevertheless, despite control of "uremia" by hemodialysis, pericarditis has remained a common problem. Patients already stabilized on dialysis are developing pericarditis after prolonged periods of treatment, with a high mortality.[2, 3]

INCIDENCE AND MORTALITY

The incidence of pericarditis in patients with chronic renal failure has fallen progressively since the introduction of chronic hemodialysis in 1960. Wacker and Merrill in 1954[4] reported pericarditis in 50 percent of their patients with chronic renal failure (Table 1). Between 1960 and 1968 other investigators reported an incidence of 41 percent.[5] More recent studies indicate a much lower incidence varying between 1.7 and 8.9 percent,[2, 3] reflecting improved conservative management by diet therapy, and elective initiation of chronic hemodialysis or transplantation before the patient becomes terminally ill. The incidence of pericarditis in the dialyzed patient is now higher than that of the untreated patient, most centers reporting an incidence of between 14 and 18 per-

Table 1. Incidence and mortality of uremic pericarditis

	1954[4]	1960–1967[5]	1966–1974[3]	1966–1970[2]	1971–1975[6]
Pericarditis before commencing chronic hemodialysis	50%	41%	1.7%	13.1%	8.9%
Pericarditis in patients receiving chronic hemodialysis	—	14%	17%	16.4%	18.0%
Mortality from pericarditis (% of cases)	—	—	20%	12.0%	8.0%

cent.[2, 3, 5] This figure has not changed significantly during the past five years despite improvements in dialysis technique.

The mortality from uremic pericarditis in the dialyzed patient has been considerable, varying from 8 to 20 percent. A comparison of mortality rates for the years 1966–1970 and 1971–1975, however, does show a decline in mortality (see Table 1). The causes of death have been cardiac tamponade, cardiac arrhythmias, myocarditis, and heart failure.

PATHOGENESIS

The etiology of uremic pericarditis is unknown despite repeated attempts to find a specific causative factor. Although it seldom occurs as a manifestation of untreated uremia until the blood urea nitrogen level is high, there is no direct correlation between the development of pericarditis and blood urea nitrogen levels. In uncontrolled uremia, generalized involvement of the serous membranes is common and a hemorrhagic tendency due to abnormal platelet function is frequently present. Most observers believe that the initiating factor in uremic pericarditis is a serositis, which is exacerbated and perpetuated by the hemorrhagic problems of the uremic patient and continued trauma to the inflamed pericardial surfaces by myocardial action. With the improvement of uremia by regular hemodialysis or successful transplantation,[2, 5] the platelet defect is rapidly reversed and pericarditis resolves in 70 percent of cases without complication.

The failure of pericarditis to resolve in some patients following control of uremia and the development of pericarditis in stable patients treated by chronic hemodialysis for months or years are not easily explained on a biochemical basis. Furthermore, pericarditis in the chronically dialyzed patient appears to differ from that occurring in the patient with uncontrolled uremia, since it is associated with more severe constitutional symptoms, is frequently unresponsive to medical management, and both acute and chronic complications are more frequent. Involvement of the underlying myocardium by the inflammatory process also tends to be more common in the dialyzed patient, and contributes significantly to the high mortality. In the dialyzed patient several factors have been implicated in the development of pericarditis (Table 2).

INADEQUATE DIALYSIS. The adequacy of dialysis therapy cannot be defined by any simple clinical parameter or laboratory measurement. Blood levels of creatinine and urea do not reflect the adequacy of uremic control in dialyzed patients since these parameters depend on such factors as dietary intake, body build, metabolic rate, and other factors. Measurements of peripheral nerve conduction velocity have been considered a better indicator of adequacy of dialysis.[7] Nevertheless, most observers have been unable to detect a significant difference in predialysis creatinine and urea levels of patients who develop pericarditis and those who do not, and serial measurements of nerve conduction velocity do not appear to reflect the individual patient's susceptibility to develop pericarditis.[2] There is, however, considerable evidence to support the "inadequate dialysis" hypothesis. Some investigators report a sharp decline in the incidence of pericarditis by increasing dialysis frequency from two to three times weekly, although pericarditis was observed under conditions of severe stress such as infection or surgery.[5] Other evidence to support inadequate dialysis as a cause of pericarditis is the experience in many centers that intensification of dialysis therapy causes a dramatic resolution of pericarditis in approximately 30 percent of cases without anti-inflammatory drugs or surgical interventions.[2, 5] Many of the "failures" to respond to intensive hemodialysis have been due to cardiac tamponade and myocarditis. The failure of myocardial involvement to regress with dialysis, or even successful transplantation, does not rule out inadequate control of uremia as the inciting factor.

Factors which tend to weaken the "inadequate dialysis" theory are those of many investigators indicating that the incidence of pericarditis in the dialysis patient has

Table 2. Factors implicated in the development of pericarditis in the dialyzed patient

Inadequate dialysis	Duration of dialysis
Infection	Hypercalcemia
Surgical procedures	Heparin
Age and sex	Multiple causes

changed very little over the years despite the widespread practice of performing hemodialysis three times a week. Repeated episodes of pericarditis have also been observed in stable patients while being dialyzed on a three times a week basis.[8] Furthermore, pericarditis has been found at autopsy despite intensive dialysis, many months after clinical manifestations have disappeared.[2, 5]

INFECTION. Many workers have investigated a possible bacteriologic or viral etiology of uremic pericarditis. Evidence for direct bacterial invasion in the majority of cases has been unconvincing. Some investigators have been unable to exclude contamination or secondary invasion after pericardiocentesis.[9] Isolated cases of bacterial pericarditis have been reported after severe transplant rejection[10] and in severely debilitated patients with generalized sepsis.[11, 12] In one study there was good evidence to suggest that cytomegalic virus (CMV) was a direct causative agent.[13] The majority of investigators have reported finding sterile pericardial fluid either at pericardiocentesis or at surgery. However, documented infection, either viral or bacterial, immediately preceded the onset of clinical pericarditis in 53 percent of patients in one study.[2]

SURGICAL PROCEDURES. Surgical procedures have been implicated as a factor predisposing to the development of pericarditis by some investigators,[5] although others have not observed a close correlation unless the postoperative course was complicated by sepsis.[2] Even uncomplicated surgical procedures cause a catabolic state and will tend to increase dialysis requirements.

AGE AND SEX. Age and sex appear to be related to the development of pericarditis in the dialyzed patient and previous reports showed a statistically higher incidence of pericarditis in patients on chronic hemodialysis under 30 years of age, especially young females.[2] These findings may reflect a tendency to prescribe similar dialysis requirements for the smaller young patients compared to older patients, despite the higher metabolic rate of the younger person, and thus indirectly reflect inadequate dialysis.

DURATION OF DIALYSIS. Duration of hemodialysis does not appear to be related to the development of pericarditis. Statistical analysis shows that the patient may develop pericarditis at anytime during the course of his dialysis, although the risk is slightly higher during the first year.[2]

HYPERCALCEMIA. Severe secondary hyperparathyroidism has been a frequent problem in patients developing acute pericarditis.[2] Pericarditis has also been observed in one patient with hypercalcemia from a "hard water syndrome,"[6, 14] suggesting the hypercalcemia per se is responsible. However, neither hypercalcemia nor secondary hyperparathyroidism can be regarded as direct causative factors since many patients with severe hyperparathyroidism requiring parathyroidectomy have not developed pericarditis. However, anorexia, nausea, vomiting, and malnutrition associated with hypercalcemia may cause the patient to become catabolic and indirectly increase dialysis requirements.

HEPARIN. The role of heparin in the development of pericarditis in dialyzed patients is controversial, although precipitation of hemopericardium by inadvertent anticoagulation in idiopathic pericarditis is well documented. Most observers agree that heparin is not the initiating factor, but that it probably perpetuates the inflammatory process by causing repeated bleeding from the inflamed pericardial surfaces. Although Alfrey and his associates were unable to obtain evidence of blood loss into the pericardial sac during dialysis in two patients with acute pericarditis, regional heparinization was used on these patients.[15] Their studies did not exclude the possibility of active blood loss into the pericardial sac if total heparinization is used as during a routine hemodialysis. However, Skov and coworkers claim no ill effects from total heparinization in their patients.[11] Heparin may be a major factor causing the high incidence of cardiac tamponade in dialyzed patients, and chronic complications such as constrictive pericarditis. Many investigators have reported acute often fatal tamponade in patients during or immediately after hemodialysis, which they have attributed to heparinization.[2, 16] The fact that pericardial tamponade has occurred even during peritoneal dialysis suggests that heparin alone is not the sole factor involved.[9]

An alternative explanation for the high incidence of tamponade during and after dialysis may be the mechanical effects of the ultrafiltration of hemodialysis which causes a reduction in blood volume and venous return, thereby abolishing compensation of cardiac compression.

MULTIPLE FACTORS. The possibility that uremic pericarditis does not represent a single disease entity has not been excluded. Many cases closely resemble acute idiopathic pericarditis. Other cases are undoubtedly related to inadequate dialysis, and a very small percentage are due to direct invasion by bacteria and viruses. The high incidence of pericarditis may be a reflection of increased susceptibility to pericarditis in the uremic individual. While cholesterol content of the fluid in hemorrhagic uremic pericarditis is high[15] as in cholesterol pericarditis, this may reflect the combination of pericarditis and blood in the pericardial cavity rather than cholesterol being the inciting agent.[17]

PATHOLOGY

The initial lesion in uremic pericarditis is an aseptic inflammatory process with fibrin formation. The so-called "bread and butter appearance" of the pericardium (Fig. 1) is a

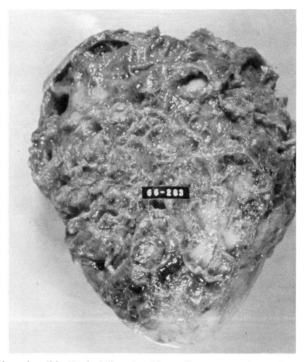

Figure 1. Acute uremic pericarditis. Typical "bread and butter" appearance in terminal uremia.

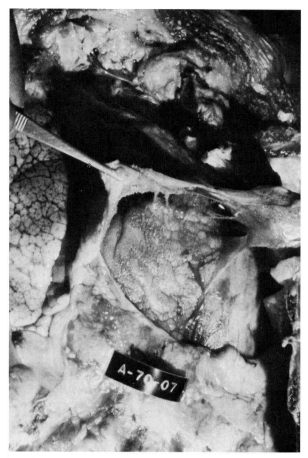

Figure 2. Acute uremic pericarditis showing extensive inflammation and hemorrhage and loculated blood clots.

typical finding in the untreated patient dying of chronic renal failure. In other cases the inflammatory process may be more severe with extensive thickening of both layers of the pericardium, with areas of hemorrhage. Fibrinous adhesions between the parietal and visceral pericardium are frequently extensive and adhesions between the visceral pericardium and epicardium are common. A pericardial effusion is usually present and may be serous, serosanguineous, or frankly hemorrhagic. The effusion is frequently loculated (Fig. 2). Histologically (Fig. 3) the pericardium is thickened by fibrin deposition with extensive formation of highly vascular granulation tissue.

Subacute constrictive pericarditis appears to result from failure of the acute lesion to heal. There may be active pericarditis and with fibrin formation, hemorrhage, vascularization of the pericardium, and pericardial fibrosis may be marked.[8]

Chronic constrictive pericarditis is a rare complication of uremic pericarditis.[2, 17, 18, 19, 20] Both layers of the pericardium are markedly thickened by fibrosis and adherent to each other and to the underlying epicardium. Calcification has not been reported in constrictive uremic pericarditis.

Myocarditis or myocardiopathy may occur in association with uremic pericarditis, as with pericarditis from other causes.[2, 21, 22] There may be extension of the inflammatory process to the underlying myocardium, with round cell infiltration of the epicardial and subepicardial regions, and occasionally frank myocardial necrosis.[23]

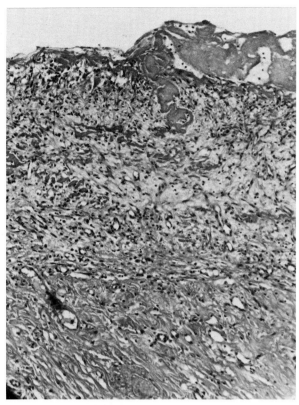

Figure 3. Histologic appearance of pericardium in uremic pericarditis showing the inflamed pericardium covered with vascular granulation tissue and fibrinous exudate.

CLINICAL FEATURES

Pericarditis is suggested when chest pain is a presenting complaint (Table 3). Chest pain is identical to that described in other types of pericarditis, and is frequently very severe, closely resembling the pain of myocardial infarction. Fever, leucocytosis, and cardiomegaly are frequently present at the time of presentation. A friction rub is present in 92 to 95 percent of cases of uremic pericarditis and a gallop rhythm is frequent.

Table 3. Clinical features of uremic pericarditis

	Comty, et al.[2] % of attacks	Ribot, et al.[3] % of attacks
Pain	64	71
Fever	96	76
Friction rub	92	95
Hypotension	56	—
Cardiac arrhythmia	28	19
Hepatomegaly	60	—
Elevated venous pressure	71	—
Cardiomegaly	92	100
Polymorphonuclear leucocytosis	71	62
Abnormal ECG	88	—

A friction rub may be transitory or absent in 5 to 8 percent of cases causing diagnostic problems. Signs of a pericardial effusion and even cardiac tamponade may be present at the time of developing chest pain.

The high mortality associated with uremic pericarditis as a result of cardiac tamponade, especially in dialyzed patients, emphasizes the importance of establishing a diagnosis early in the course of the disease. Although chest pain occurs in 70 percent of cases of uremic pericarditis, it may not be the initial manifestation. Furthermore there is a problem of diagnosing pericarditis in patients who do not manifest chest pain at any time. Some of the clinical manifestations which may alert the physician to the presence of uremic pericarditis are listed in Table 4.

All patients with chronic renal failure and a creatinine clearance of less than 10 ml./min. should be observed very closely since a slowly accumulating pericardial effusion may become very large without causing cardiac tamponade.[24] Hypertension requiring drug therapy, fluid overload, and heart failure from primary myocardial disease are common problems in patients with chronic renal failure and may make the diagnosis of pericarditis difficult. Nevertheless, pericarditis should be considered in the differential diagnosis in any patient with advanced chronic renal failure who demonstrates signs of increasing right heart failure associated with cardiomegaly or increasing heart size. Unexplained deterioration in renal function in previously stable patients may occur as a result of pericardial effusion with tamponade leading to decreased cardiac output, and should be investigated.

Pericarditis should always be included in the differential diagnosis when hypotension occurs. A fall in blood pressure may be more significant than hypotension per se since severe hypertension is common in chronic renal failure. Thus, either normalization of previously poorly controlled hypertension or a reduction in the required dosage of antihypertensive drug therapy may indicate the presence of a pericardial effusion with tamponade. Mental confusion has also been reported as a feature of pericarditis with effusion, and may cause a diagnostic problem in the patient with end-stage renal failure.

In the dialyzed patient, an early diagnosis of pericarditis can frequently be made from a careful scrutiny of the patient's dialysis flow sheets with respect to weight, temperature, and blood pressure. Fever which is frequently low grade may precede the onset of clinical pericarditis by several days in up to 50 percent of patients.[2] In many cases the patient may be afebrile before dialysis, and fever develops during treatment. Although there are many causes of fever in the dialyzed patient, pericarditis should always be considered in the differential diagnosis.

The significance of hypotension in the dialyzed patient is always difficult to evaluate,

Table 4. Unusual manifestations of uremic pericarditis

Undialyzed patient
 Cardiomegaly or increasing heart size
 Unexplained deterioration in renal function
 Alteration in blood pressure control
 Mental confusion
Dialyzed patient
 Fever
 Hypotension
 Weight gain
 Intolerance of ultrafiltration during dialysis
 Cardiac arrhythmia
 Cardiomegaly
 Mental confusion
 Access clotting
 Pleural effusion

especially when it occurs during hemodialysis, since hypotension may occur as a result of a pyrogen reaction, bacteremia, extracellular volume depletion, arrhythmia, and increasing congestive heart failure in addition to a pericardial effusion. However, hypotension may occur as an early manifestation of pericarditis in 50 percent of patients, even before a large pericardial effusion has developed.[2] Hypotension may be manifest in several different ways in the dialyzed patient, from frank shock unresponsive to volume expansion as occurs with cardiac tamponade, myocardial infarction, pyrogen reactions, and bacteremias. In other cases, the hypotension may be subtle. Some patients may be noted to have a low blood pressure prior to hemodialysis, even though there has been weight gain due to fluid retention between dialysis. Ultrafiltration may not be performed because of a low blood pressure, and the ensuing weight gain may be interpreted as a gain in tissue weight rather than fluid accumulation.

Cardiac arrhythmias, especially atrial flutter or fibrillation, have occasionally been a presenting feature of uremic pericarditis in some patients. The presence of a pericardial effusion should always be excluded in patients with cardiomegaly, or increasing heart size, despite the absence of other symptoms and signs of pericarditis. Mental confusion, lethargy, and occasionally disorientation as a result of a large pericardial effusion have been reported in several instances as a manifestation of pericarditis[9, 15] and require differentiation from other causes of mental confusion such as cerebrovascular disease, subdural hematoma, "disequilibrium syndrome," and other metabolic problems. Unexplained clotting of a blood access device may occasionally be a presenting problem. Pleural effusions may be unilateral or bilateral and are common in uremic pericarditis as well as in states of fluid overload, primary myocardial failure, and pulmonary disease. Such effusions do not assist in the differential diagnosis.

DIAGNOSIS

The electrocardiogram is of little value in diagnosis since the classic S-T segment elevation may not be present and most other findings are nonspecific.[8]

Attempts to document the presence of pericardial effusion should be made in all patients with clinical pericarditis or cardiomegaly, using currently available tests of which the echocardiogram is probably the most sensitive noninvasive procedure and can detect as little as 150 ml. of fluid in the pericardial sac.[25] Bacteriologic, fungal, and viral studies are negative in the typical case of uremic pericarditis. Occasionally, uremic pericarditis may complicate the course of patients with sepsis, in which case although blood cultures may be positive for the responsible organism, pericardial fluid cultures are negative. A diagnostic pericardiocentesis should not be performed routinely.

ACUTE COMPLICATIONS (Table 5)

Cardiac tamponade. The hemodynamic significance of a pericardial effusion requires critical evaluation. A very large pericardial effusion accumulating slowly may have less hemodynamic effect than the rapid accumulation of 150 ml. of fluid in the pericardial sac.[24] Cardiac tamponade is particularly liable to occur during or immediately after hemodialysis and may occur after peritoneal dialysis.[9] It is at this particular time that diagnostic and therapeutic problems arise in differentiating cardiac tamponade from hypovolemia, and increasing heart failure from fluid overload or primary myocardial disease. Clinical symptoms and signs are similar to those in tamponade occurring from other causes.[24] A loud friction rub with easily audible heart sounds is frequently present and does not exclude significant tamponade. A paradoxical pulse is usually present but its absence does not exclude tamponade if the patient is severely hypotensive. Radiologically the rapid increase in heart size, particularly with clear lung

226

Table 5. Complications of uremic pericarditis

Acute
 Cardiac tamponade
 Cardiac arrhythmia
 Myocarditis
 Heart failure
Chronic
 Subacute constrictive (restrictive) pericarditis
 Adhesive pericarditis
 Chronic constrictive pericarditis

fields, is suggestive. As in cardiac tamponade from other causes, the ECG is not diagnostic unless P, QRS, and T complexes all show alternans.

Central venous pressure may be high (in excess of 140 mm. of H_2O), but this elevation is not diagnostic since this may indicate fluid overload and myocardial failure. The differential diagnosis of hypotension due to cardiac tamponade, myocardial failure, or hypovolemia can be made in most cases by measurements of pulmonary artery, pulmonary capillary wedge, and right ventricular pressures using a Swan-Ganz catheter.[26]

CARDIAC ARRHYTHMIAS. Cardiac arrhythmias are a frequent complication of uremic pericarditis, and may be seen early in the course of the disease. They may be due to multiple causes in the uremic patient, including myocarditis, primary myocardial disease, and changes in serum potassium levels. Acute arrhythmias may also develop with the onset of cardiac tamponade. Cardiac arrest has been reported frequently during or after pericardiocentesis,[27] and may also occur with acute tamponade.

MYOCARDITIS. Myocarditis is a serious complication of uremic pericarditis and is manifest by intractable heart failure, hypotension, and serious arrhythmias. The condition is not always alleviated by drainage of the pericardial sac or pericardiectomy.[2] Steroids have been used with variable success, and in some instances the dramatic improvement may have been fortuitous. In other instances steroids have been ineffective, with death resulting from intractable myocardial failure or steroid complications.[2]

A reversible cardiomyopathy has been described by some investigators in patients with end-stage uremia maintained for prolonged periods of time on a low protein diet.[21, 22] The syndrome consists of massive cardiomegaly, gallop rhythm, fall in blood pressure, pericarditis, arrhythmias, and marked sensitivity to cardiac glycosides. In these patients, institution of dialysis resulted in a complete reversal of the abnormalities.

MOCARDIAL FAILURE. Heart failure may complicate the course of uremic pericarditis, as a manifestation of myocarditis,[21] and in other instances it may be a manifestation of primary myocardial disease. Acute left ventricular failure may occasionally occur during the treatment of uremic pericarditis, particularly after relief of the pericardial effusion by medical or surgical measures.[2] This phenomenon in the dialyzed patient closely resembles the "pericardial shock syndrome" reported by Spodik in nonuremic patients.[24] In uremic patients, it has been attributed to a sudden increase in venous return with relief of restriction in the presence of severe fluid overload used to maintain an adequate venous return and cardiac output.

CHRONIC COMPLICATIONS

Subacute uremic constrictive pericarditis may follow an acute episode immediately or appear several weeks or months later after apparent resolution. Hypotension particularly during hemodialysis becomes a problem and ultrafiltration may become difficult. Prominent complaints are weight gain, fatigue, and dyspnea and an increase in abdominal girth. Ascites, edema, hepatomegaly, and venous distention are prominent. A friction rub is frequently absent but may be heard intermittently. Chest pain occasionally occurs but is often absent. Serial chest x-rays may show a progressive reduction in size following the acute episode, although the heart size may remain enlarged or normal. The lung fields are characteristically clear without pulmonary vascular congestion. Heart scans may be positive or negative, depending whether or not a significant amount of pericardial fluid is present in addition to pericardial thickening. The major problem is in differentiating subacute constrictive pericarditis from congestive heart failure. This is important since cardiac tamponade is a hazard in cases of subacute uremic constrictive pericarditis although most cases have recovered spontaneously after a protracted period of time.[2] A precise diagnosis is important because of the danger of cardiac tamponade which is likely to occur when the patient is being treated in an outpatient dialysis facility or by home dialysis. This can be best made by angiocardiography and cardiac catheterization.

Adhesive pericarditis is an autopsy diagnosis. The pathologic process closely resembles that of acute and subacute or even chronic constrictive pericarditis but clinical manifestations usually are absent during life. Chronic constrictive pericarditis as a late complication of uremic pericarditis has been described with increasing frequency during the past few years as more patients have survived for longer periods of time on chronic hemodialysis after an episode of pericarditis.[2, 18, 19, 20] It is clinically indistinguishable from subacute constrictive pericarditis, chronic constrictive pericarditis from other causes, and congestive heart failure.

MANAGEMENT (Table 6)

Control of Uremia

In clinically significant acute renal failure the development of pericarditis can largely be avoided by the institution of regular and adequate dialysis on a prophylactic basis. Pericarditis may still occur, however, in patients who are intensely catabolic from sepsis or trauma, and their management is similar to that of patients treated by chronic hemodialysis.

Occasionally pericarditis may develop in patients with chronic renal failure which is not end-stage, who have not been following dietary protein restrictions, or in whom an acute temporary reduction in renal function has occurred as a result of infection or dehydration. In these cases appropriate dietary protein restriction, treatment of the acute insult, and occasionally a single peritoneal dialysis will result in clinical resolution of pericarditis.

If a patient with end-stage renal failure is acceptable for hemodialysis, the presence of pericarditis is an indication to institute dialysis therapy. The institution of dialysis therapy is highly effective in causing resolution of pericarditis in between 60 and 70

Table 6. Management of uremic pericarditis

1. Biochemical control: Dietary protein restriction; dialysis (initiate dialysis, augment dialysis)
2. Treat precipitating factors, e.g., infection
3. Maintain nutrition
4. Prevent bleeding: Discontinue oral anticoagulants; regional heparinization; peritoneal dialysis
5. Control hydration and heart failure
6. Use of anti-inflammatory drugs: indomethacin 25 mg. three or four times daily; prednisone 30 to 40 mg. daily orally
7. Pericardiocentesis: Simple aspiration; continuous drainage; ± intrapericardial steroids
8. Pericardiectomy: Simple window; subtotal pericardiectomy; total pericardiectomy

percent of cases, and many patients in this group do not develop a significant pericardial effusion.

In patients who have already been established on a dialysis program, the previous adequacy of dialysis should be reviewed, since in some instances inadequate dialysis may have resulted from a malfunctioning access or because of missed dialyses.[3] Measurements of peroneal nerve conduction velocity should be reviewed for evidence of progression of uremic neuropathy which would substantiate inadequate dialysis.

In most centers the initial step in the management of uremic pericarditis is to augment dialysis therapy by at least 30 percent of the previous requirements by either increasing the duration of dialysis or its frequency. Many centers are now performing dialysis on a daily basis in the treatment of uremic pericarditis. Frequently even large pericardial effusion with severe constitutional symptoms can be resolved by this method alone.[2, 5] However some controversy does exist as to the value of increased dialysis time in the resolution of uremic pericarditis. This therapeutic approach may be modified when a measurable parameter of the adequacy of dialysis is available. A possible precipitating factor such as infection should be vigorously irradicated and an adequate access provided.

Adequate Nutrition

Maintenance of an adequate nutritional status is essential since a diet lacking in calorific content will result in increased catabolism. With increased dialysis, losses of essential amino acids during dialysis may also be in excess of intake if the dietary content of high biologic value protein is inadequate, again resulting in a catabolic state. A daily dialysis schedule allows for a liberal intake of a wider variety of foods, and this will encourage the sick individual to eat. If necessary, the diet should be supplemented by amino acid mixtures in the severely debilitated patient.

Prevention of Bleeding

All anticoagulants should be discontinued until evidence of active pericarditis has resolved. The possible role of heparin in causing cardiac tamponade or continuation of the pericardial inflammatory process has been discussed in a previous section. The deleterious effects of heparin can be mitigated by performing hemodialysis using regional heparinization[28] or by using peritoneal dialysis.[16] The decision to use peritoneal dialysis to some extent depends upon the facilities available to the physician. It is, however, the treatment of choice for the initiation of dialysis therapy in patients with pericarditis since it avoids the dangers of heparinization in the presence of a hemorrhagic problem from uncontrolled uremia. If pain on recumbency is severe, peritoneal dialysis may be difficult, and is hazardous in patients with multiple adhesions from previous abdominal surgery. In other patients already being treated by hemodialysis, continuation depends entirely on whether or not a method of performing regional heparinization is available.[28]

Control of Hydration and Heart Failure

Achieving a balance between overhydration and heart failure on one hand, and maintaining an adequate blood volume to compensate for cardiac compression on the other can be both difficult and critical in uremic patients. In the dialyzed patient, problems with hydration and blood pressure stability are particularly related to the dialysis procedure itself where rapid changes of intravascular volume may precipitate cardiac tamponade.

229

In patients with stable, normal or high blood pressure, and either no effusion or a small effusion, control of hydration presents little problem. In the undialyzed patient daily weights provide a good guide to the presence of fluid retention. Regulation of sodium and fluid intake and the cautious use of potent diuretics serve to maintain a reasonably stable state of hydration. In the dialyzed patient, gradual ultrafiltration during dialysis with fluid restriction between dialyses can be used to maintain a body weight consistent with the patient's metabolic state.

Patients with unstable or low blood pressures, large effusions, cardiac arrhythmias, or evidence of severe fluid overload and myocardial failure require continuous monitoring especially during hemodialysis using either a central venous pressure monitor or Swan-Ganz catheter. When there is evidence of heart failure from fluid overload, some degree of fluid removal by ultrafiltration becomes essential. This may be better achieved by using a small volume dialyzer, gentle ultrafiltration performed during dialysis on a daily basis, and appropriate sodium and fluid restriction between dialyses. Surgical intervention should not be delayed where there are repeated problems with hypotension in the presence of a pericardial effusion, and an elective surgical procedure is the treatment of choice.

The use of digitalis and related drugs in the management of pericarditis is controversial, because of the theoretical possibility of a further reduction of venous return leading to decreased venous pressure.[28] Nevertheless, digitalis should not be withheld in patients with arrhythmias requiring its use, or patients where there is a possibility of myocardial failure as a result of myocarditis or primary myocardial disease. Its use in patients with renal failure requires modification, and careful attention must be given to serum potassium levels.

Use of Anti-Inflammatory Drugs

INDOMETHACIN. This drug is antipyretic, analgesic, and anti-inflammatory, and does not require dosage modification in renal failure. It has been used with success in the treatment of nonuremic recurrent pericarditis without effusion.[30] Although experience with its use in the treatment of uremic pericarditis is limited at the present time, some investigators have reported a good response with rapid amelioration of symptoms and reduction of pericardial effusion.[31] Although indomethacin has a significant number of side effects such as nausea, vomiting, abdominal pain, headaches, and occasional duodenal ulceration, it has a role in the treatment of uremic pericarditis. However, in the absence of more extensive experience the authors feel that its usage should not be continued in the face of progressive heart failure or increasing pericardial effusion with evidence of cardiac embarrassment.

STEROID THERAPY. Prednisone in oral doses of 40 mg. daily has been used with success for the treatment of pericarditis from other causes.[30] As with indomethacin there has been no large control study performed to determine its value in the management of the patient with uremic pericarditis. Nevertheless, based on the results of three groups of investigators,[2, 18, 31] prednisone is of value in the management of selected patients who develop uremic pericarditis. In dosages of 40 mg. daily, prednisone administration may be followed by a dramatic disappearance of pain, subsidence of fever, diminution of the friction rub, and reduction in heart size within a very short period of time (Fig 4). There appears to be no advantage to using doses of prednisone of greater than 40 mg. daily, or of increasing the dosage after the patient has failed to respond to 40 mg. daily. If the patient responds to steroids during the first week of therapy, steroids should be gradually tapered and withdrawn by the end of 4 to 6 weeks. On the other hand if the patient's condition deteriorates or hypotension and pericardial effusion persist, prednisone therapy should not be continued in lieu of appropriate surgical management. In

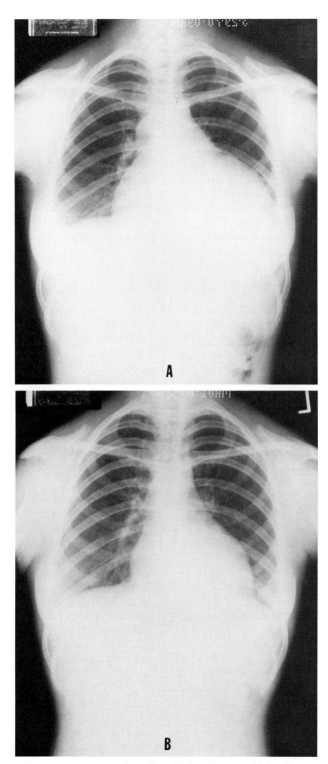

Figure 4. Effect of prednisone 40 mg. on uremic pericarditis in a 19-year-old girl. She was treated by intensive dialysis for 4 weeks (A), without improvement. After 1 week of prednisone therapy (B) she was afebrile and there was a marked reduction in heart size.

other cases where the patient has a recurrence of pericarditis after steroid therapy has been reduced or has been discontinued, our experience suggests that surgical intervention should be considered at this time.[6] Although early results suggest that prednisone may not be curative, with unsuspected adhesive pericarditis being present at autopsy in some instances,[2] there are too few autopsy studies available to make a definitive statement at this time.

INTRAPERICARDIAL STEROIDS. The administration of nonabsorbable steroids into the pericardial sac after pericardiocentesis has been used with success by some investigators.[19, 33] Nevertheless, from the limited experience available, its role in the treatment of uremic pericarditis is uncertain. In the limited studies reported it is not clear whether the pericardiocentesis per se was responsible for the improvement. Furthermore the dangers of pericardiocentesis are considerable, and will be discussed later. Although the healthy pericardium may be impervious to nonabsorbable steroids, it is possible that as with other serous membranes, significant absorption may occur across the inflamed pericardial surfaces and much of the effect of steroid administration is related to a systemic effect rather than local.

Surgical Management

Surgical management of uremic pericarditis is a highly controversial issue and may be related to the wide spectrum of pathology seen in uremic pericarditis, from the relatively benign "chemical" pericarditis with a serous effusion seen particularly in cases of untreated uremia, to the progressive hemorrhagic inflammatory process seen in many patients treated by chronic dialysis. The high mortality associated with uremic pericarditis, especially in dialyzed patients, is in sharp contrast to the mortality from other types of pericarditis, and testifies not only to the severity of the disease but also to the fact that treatment thus far may have been short of optimal, since the majority of deaths have been due to cardiac tamponade.

Pericardiocentesis

The role of pericardiocentesis in the management of uremic pericarditis and cardiac tamponade has aroused more controversy than any other treatment modality. The potential dangers of pericardiocentesis, which have been emphasized by many observers both in uremic and nonuremic pericarditis, include laceration of the heart or a coronary vessel, often with fatal consequences. If the effusion is loculated, relief of tamponade may be only temporary. Some investigators have either performed repeated pericardiocentesis[8] or pericardiocentesis with catheter drainage, and have reported a low mortality in uremic pericardial tamponade. Other workers have reported a mortality of as high as 75 percent, which they have attributed to pericardiocentesis.[27] However the pathology of uremic pericarditis is highly variable and suggests that those patients who have benefited from pericardiocentesis are those with either a serous effusion or a relatively benign form of hemorrhagic pericarditis without loculation and adhesions.

Unfortunately, uremic pericarditis which proceeds to tamponade is frequently grossly bloody and a very active inflammatory process is present, and further bleeding from the inflamed surfaces may be worsened by pericardiocentesis. Pericardiocentesis in severe cases of uremic pericarditis is not curative and potentially does not prevent the development of a subacute constrictive pericarditis with the risks of tamponade at a later date, or the eventual development of constrictive pericarditis.

The approach at many centers, including our own, regarding the role of pericardiocentesis in the management of uremic pericarditis can be summarized as follows. (1) Diagnostic pericardiocentesis may occasionally be necessary where there is a possibility that a purulent or tuberculous pericarditis may be present in a patient with chronic renal failure. In this situation the procedure should be undertaken using full precautions with a surgeon available to perform emergency thoracotomy if complications occur. (2) Without doubt, pericardiocentesis can be a life-saving procedure in the patient who develops cardiac tamponade from uremic pericarditis. If the effusion is serous or not loculated, a simple aspiration may be definitive care. If the fluid is frankly hemorrhagic, an open surgical procedure should be considered. Where clinical improvement fails to occur immediately or fluid reaccumulates, partial pericardectomy should be considered in preference to repeated pericardiocentesis. (3) Patients without tamponade who fail to respond to conservative management and anti-inflammatory drugs should be considered for elective pericardiectomy rather than simple pericardiocentesis.

Pericardiectomy

Pericardiectomy is now being used in many centers, and is claimed to be the most effective and definitive treatment of uremic pericarditis. The mortality has been low since the dialyzed patient tolerates surgical procedures very well.[34, 35] It must be emphasized, however, that a high percentage of patients will respond to conservative management and use of anti-inflammatory drugs with complete resolution of the inflammatory process. An open surgical approach should not be considered unless there is failure to respond to medical management, or tamponade supervenes.

A small pericardial window has been used with success by some investigators. However, window closure is frequent with recurrence of tamponade, incarceration, or strangulation of the heart. Subacute and chronic constrictive pericarditis continue to be possible complications. Creation of a small pericardial window should be considered in patients who are unfit for a more extensive procedure since this procedure can be performed quickly under local anesthesia.

The indications of partial pericardiectomy are shown in Table 7. Partial pericardiectomy is now considered as the treatment of choice for acute tamponade, unless initial pericardiocentesis is completely effective. Where window closure occurs, even in poor risk patients, partial pericardiectomy should be undertaken. Failure of a large pericardial effusion to respond to intensive hemodialysis and anti-inflammatory drugs is a further indication for an open surgical approach. In these cases partial pericardiectomy is curative, and the reduction in morbidity and mortality is significant. Where there has been a recurrence of pericardial effusion following withdrawal of steroids, the experience of some investigators[6] is that, as with nonuremic recurrent pericarditis, a partial pericardiectomy should be performed. Although resolution of subacute constrictive pericarditis may occur,[2] the patient may be incapacitated and miserable throughout the period of conservative management. In addition there has been a significant mortality from tamponade later. Because of this late mortality, which is unpredictable, a partial pericar-

Table 7. Indications for pericardiectomy

1. Acute tamponade
2. Large pericardial effusion unresponsive to intensive hemodialysis and prednisone 40 mg. daily
3. Recurrence of pericardial effusion following withdrawal of steroids
4. Subacute constrictive pericarditis with severe hypotension, hepatomegaly, ascites, and edema
5. Chronic constrictive pericarditis

diectomy should be an elective procedure if pericarditis persists longer than two months. Where there is evidence of a chronic constrictive pericarditis, the treatment of choice is a fairly extensive pericardiectomy.

REFERENCES

1. BULLOCK, M. L., AND SHAPIRO, F. L.: *Acute renal failure: Review of 375 cases.* In preparation.
2. COMTY, C. M., COHEN, S. L., AND SHAPIRO, F. L.: *Pericarditis in chronic uremia and its sequels.* Ann. Intern. Med. 75:173, 1971.
3. RIBOT, S., FRANKEL, H. J., GIELCHINSKY, I., ET AL.: *Treatment of uremic pericarditis.* Clin. Nephrol. 2: 127, 1974.
4. WACKER, W., AND MERRILL, J. P.: *Uremic pericarditis in acute and chronic renal failure.* J.A.M.A. 156: 764, 1954.
5. BAILEY, G. L., HAMPERS, C. L., HAGER, E. B., ET AL.: *Uremic pericarditis: Clinical features and management.* Circulation 38:582, 1968.
6. COMTY, C. M., SHAPIRO, F. L., AND WATHEN, R.: *Effect of varying therapeutic approaches on incidence and mortality in uremic pericarditis.* Presented to Am. Soc. of Nephrology, Nov. 1975. Manuscript in preparation.
7. JEBSEN, R. H., TENCKHOFF, H., AND HONET, H. C.: *Natural history of uremic polyneuropathy and effects of dialysis.* N. Engl. J. Med. 277:327, 1967.
8. BEAUDRY, G., NAKAMOTO, S., AND KOLFF, W. J.: *Uremic pericarditis and tamponade in chronic renal failure.* Ann. Intern. Med. 641:990, 1966.
9. HAGER, E. B.: *Clinical observations of five patients with uremic pericardial tamponade.* N. Engl. J. Med. 273:304, 1965.
10. LUFT, F. C., KLEIT, S. A., SMITH, R. N., ET AL.: *Management of uremic pericarditis with tamponade.* Arch. Intern. Med. 134:488, 1974.
11. SKOV, S. E., HANSEN, H. E., AND SPENCER, E. S.: *Uremic pericarditis.* Acta Med. Scand. 186:421, 1969.
12. HARRIS, C. L., BENCHIMOL, A., AND DESSER, K. B.: *Bacteroides pericardial effusion and cardiac tamponade in a patient with chronic renal failure.* Am. Heart J. 89:629, 1975.
13. PABICO, R. C., HANSHAW, J. B., AND TALLEY, T. E.: *Cytomegalovirus infection in chronic hemodialysis patients.* Abstract Western Dialysis and Transplantation Society, Oct. 9–10, 1971.
14. FREEMAN, R. M., LAWTON, R. L., AND CHAMBERLAIN, M. A.: *Hard water syndrome.* N. Engl. J. Med. 276:1113, 1967.
15. ALFREY, A. C., GOSS, J. E., OGDEN, D. A., ET AL.: *Uremic hemopericardium.* Am. J. Med. 45:391, 1968.
16. COHEN, G. F., BURGESS, J. H., AND KAYE, M.: *Peritoneal dialysis for the treatment of pericarditis in patients on chronic hemodialysis.* Canad. Med. Assoc. J. 102:1365, 1970.
17. BRAWLEY, R. L., VOSKO, J. S., AND MORROW, A. G.: *Cholesterol pericarditis: Consideration of its pathogenesis and treatment.* Am. J. Med. 41:235, 1966.
18. WOLFE, S. A., BAILEY, G. F., AND COLLINS, J. J., JR.: *Constrictive pericarditis following uremic effusion.* J. Thorac. Cardiovasc. Surg. 63:540, 1972.
19. LINDSAY, J., JR., CRAWLEY, I. S., AND CALLAWAY, G. M.: *Chronic constrictive pericarditis following uremic hemopericardium.* Am. Heart J. 79:390, 1970.
20. ESMOND, W. G., LEE, Y. C., AND HERNANDEZ, F.: *Successful pericardiectomy in chronic constrictive uremic pericarditis.* South. Med. J. 64:533, 1971.
21. BAILEY, G. L., HAMPERS, C. L., AND MERRILL, J. P.: *Reversible cardiomyopathy in uremia.* Trans. Am. Soc. Artif. Intern. Organs 13:263, 1967.
22. LANHEZ, L. E., LOWEN, J., AND SABBAGA, E.: *Uremic myocardiopathy.* Nephron 15:17, 1975.
23. LANGENDORF, R., AND PIRANI, C. L.: *The heart in uremia: An electrocardiographic and pathologic study.* Am. Heart J. 33:282, 1947.
24. SPODIK, D. H.: *Acute cardiac tamponade: Pathologic physiology, diagnosis and management.* Prog. Cardiovasc. Dis. 10:64, 1967.
25. ELLIS, K., AND KING, D. L.: *Pericarditis and pericardial effusion: Radiologic and echocardiographic diagnosis.* Radiol. Clin. North Am. 11:393, 1973.
26. BURTON, J. R., WANDS, J. R., VOIGT, G. C., ET AL.: *An approach to pericardial effusion in hemodialysis patients.* Johns Hopkins Med. J. 133:312, 1973.

27. SINGH, S., NEWMARK, K., ISHIKAWA, I., ET AL.: *Pericardiectomy in uremia.* J.A.M.A. 228:1132, 1974.

28. KJELLSTRAND, C. M.: *Simple method for regional heparinization during dialysis avoiding rebound phenomenon.* Am. Soc. Nephrology, Washington, D. C., 1969.

29. McMICHAEL, J., AND SHARPEY-SCHAFER, E. P.: *Action of intravenous digoxin in man.* Quart. J. Med. 37:123, 1945.

30. HATCHER, C. R., JR., LOGUE, R. B., LOGAN, W. D., JR., ET AL.: *Pericardiectomy for recurrent pericarditis.* J. Thorac. Cardiovasc. Surg. 62:371, 1971.

31. MINUTH, A. N. W., NOTTEBOHM, G. A., EKNOYAN, G., ET AL.: *Indomethacin treatment of pericarditis in chronic hemodialysis patients.* Arch. Intern. Med. 135:807, 1975.

32. ELIASSON, G., AND MURPHY, F. F.: *Steroid therapy in uremic pericarditis: A report of three cases.* J.A.M.A. 229:1634, 1974.

33. BUSELMEIER, T. J., SIMMONS, R. L., VON HARTITZSCH, B., ET AL.: *Persistent uremic pericardial effusion: Pericardial drainage and localized steroid instillation as definitive therapy.* Am. Soc. Nephrology, Washington D. C., 1973.

34. WRAY, T. M., HUMPHREYS, J., PERRY, J. M., ET AL.: *Pericardiectomy for treatment of uremic pericarditis.* Circulation 49 & 50 (Suppl. II): 268, 1974.

Pericarditis in the Rheumatologic Diseases*

Alan S. Cohen, M.D., and Juan J. Canoso, M.D.

Pericarditis is a well known accompaniment of many connective tissue diseases. It may be a presenting manifestation of systemic lupus erythematosus (SLE), an accompaniment of scleroderma, or simply an autopsy finding in rheumatoid arthritis. The variation in incidence and severity will be commented on further, but as we have analyzed the available literature and our own experience, it has become apparent that the connective tissue or rheumatologic diseases in which pericarditis is a major or frequent manifestation are limited in number. For this reason, rather than using the usual classification of all rheumatic diseases and their variants and reviewing pericarditis in each, we have devised a simplified scheme related to the frequency of pericarditis as a complication of the particular disorder (Table 1). Our arbitrary classification includes those connective tissue disorders in which pericarditis is frequent, i.e., rheumatoid arthritis,

Table 1

1. Rheumatologic disorders in which pericarditis is a major or frequent manifestation
    1. Rheumatoid arthritis
    2. Juvenile rheumatoid arthritis
    3. Systemic lupus erythematosus (SLE); Drug-induced SLE
    4. Scleroderma (progressive systemic sclerosis)
    5. Mixed connective tissue disease (MCTD)
    6. Sjögren's syndrome
    7. Whipple's disease
2. Rheumatologic disorders with occasional pericarditis
    1. Reiter's syndrome
    2. Ankylosing spondylitis
    3. Inflammatory bowel disease
    4. Serum sickness
    5. Wegener's granulomatosis
3. Rheumatologic disorders with rare pericarditis
    1. Vasculitis
    2. Polymyositis (dermatomyositis)
    3. Behçet's syndrome
    4. Familial Mediterranean fever
    5. Amyloidosis
    6. Gout

*Grants in support of these studies have been received from the USPHS, NIAMDD, NIH (AM-04599, TI-AM-5285 and RR-533), the Massachusetts Chapter of the Arthritis Foundation, and the Arthritis Foundation.

237

juvenile rheumatoid arthritis, systemic lupus erythematosus (including drug induced lupus), and scleroderma (progressive systemic sclerosis). Our detailed discussion centers about these diseases. The rheumatologic disorders with less frequent or occasional pericarditis were often difficult to separate from those in which pericarditis is rare, and in both instances re-evaluation will be appropriate when additional data are available. In the last group of essentially rare disorders, the clinically recognizable frequency was the major determining factor.

RHEUMATOLOGIC DISORDERS IN WHICH PERICARDITIS IS A MAJOR OR FREQUENT MANIFESTATION

Rheumatoid Arthritis (RA)

This chronic inflammatory articular disease affects approximately 1 percent of all adults, and is twice as common in females as it is in males. The etiology is unknown, and the pathogenetic mechanisms are just beginning to be elucidated.[1] Abnormalities in humoral and cellular immunity have been discussed in detail, though they have not been shown to be of primary etiologic significance. Antigammaglobulin antibodies (rheumatoid factors) which belong to the IgM immunoglobulin class can be easily identified by serologic techniques such as the latex fixation and the sheep cell agglutination tests. Rheumatoid factors belonging to other immunoglobulin classes can also be detected by special techniques.[2] The most severe cases of RA and certainly patients with systemic manifestations of the disease such as rheumatoid nodules, pneumonitis, pleuropericarditis, vasculitis, and others are usually seropositive, in high titer. On the other hand, persistent seronegativity carries a better prognosis, though this is not inevitable.

Of great interest has been the finding that synovial fluid complement is low in rheumatoid arthritis, and much more so in the seropositive patients.[3] This has been interpreted as the result of activation of the complement cascade by the gammaglobulin antigammaglobulin complexes. Similarly, very low levels of complement have been found in pleural[4] and pericardial[5] rheumatoid effusions as well as in serum in patients with rheumatoid vasculitis. In all, the hypothesis of complement activation by immune complexes has been put forward.

The diagnosis of RA is made on the basis of a cluster of clinical, radiologic, laboratory, and pathologic findings. Criteria for the classification of rheumatoid arthritis have also been established by the American Rheumatism Association.[6] In general, the early case will be identified by the appearance of protracted, usually symmetrical peripheral arthritis associated with morning stiffness which lasts hours, and easy fatigability. The sedimentation rate is high. Rheumatoid factor may or may not be present; if negative, a seroconversion will probably occur within 1 or 2 years, leaving a seronegative group which does not exceed 20 percent. The serum complement is normal or high except in patients with severe systemic disease, when it can be low. Low titer antinuclear antibodies can be present, but the LE phenomenon is usually negative.

The prognosis of patients with RA varies greatly depending upon local joint damage, systemic manifestations, and complications of therapy. In general, the life span of the uncomplicated patient with predominantly articular disease is not markedly diminished. Patients with systemic manifestations (other than nodules, which do not carry a prognostic implication) have a mortality rate twice as high as those without.[7]

The treatment of RA is a multidisciplinary endeavor with a goal-oriented strategy. Rest, graded exercises, and judicious use of heat decrease inflammation, maintain motion, and add comfort. Anti-inflammatory drugs are used to suppress and prevent tissue damage. Surgery is useful for specific joint deformities. Systemic manifestations, such as pericarditis, can be subtle or dramatic and often must be treated aggressively.

238

Rheumatoid pericarditis was first described in 1881 by Charcot,[8] who discussed a clinical case and reported 9 autopsies in which pericarditis was found in four. This original report presaged the dilemma of the incidence and significance of pericarditis in RA that baffled clinicians for almost a century, until newer methods of identifying occult disease in the asymptomatic patient yielded the answer.

Pathology

Sokoloff[9] in 1953 called attention to the frequency of pericarditis in an autopsy series of 101 cases of RA: 24.8 percent, as compared with 1.7 percent in 1154 controls. Subsequent studies confirmed this finding,[10, 11] with frequencies varying from 16 to 44 percent. Fibrous obliterative pericarditis predominated.[9-11] In operative specimens of patients with constrictive pericarditis, fibrous thickening of visceral and parietal layers was noted sometimes encasing a cavity lined by fibrin, or containing necrotic or fluid material.[12, 13, 14] Gross calcification has been exceptional[15] but focal calcium deposits have been common.[14] In patients with pericardial tamponade a variable amount of yellow to frankly hemorrhagic fluid under tension has been noted.[12, 14, 16] Histologically, the picture is nonspecific but consistent, i.e., fibrosis with focal perivascular aggregates of lymphocytes and plasmacytes.[5, 12, 13, 14] Rheumatoid granulomas were so infrequently found that they could not be relied upon for tissue diagnosis.[11, 14]

Acute Pericarditis

In contrast with its frequency at postmortem, *clinical* rheumatoid pericarditis is not common, although clinical awareness and thorough routine search have raised the yield of cases (see Subclinical Pericarditis). In large series of patients with severe disease, pericarditis was found in 1.6 to 2.4 percent of the patients.[7, 11] An example of the increased yield by routine methods (in a prospective study) is given by Kirk[17] who found pericarditis 10 times in 100 RA patients admitted consecutively, while only 1 case was diagnosed in a matched control series. However, 7 of the 10 with pericarditis were asymptomatic, 2 were identified due to symptoms of associated pleurisy, and 1 manifested fever alone. Although there are exceptions (in particular in young men with associated pleurisy), arthritis has usually been present for several years when pericarditis occurs.[17, 18] The pericarditis usually coincides with exacerbation of the articular disease.[5, 17, 18]

The clinical presentation usually includes chest pain, left-sided or substernal (55 to 100 percent of the cases), dyspnea (in 18 to 42 percent), and often fever. A pericardial rub was present in 65 to 81 percent of the cases, and manifestations of pleural effusion are often present.[5, 17, 18]

Chest films demonstrate cardiomegaly in over half of the cases, and associated pleural effusions (unilateral or bilateral) in 36 to 95 percent of the cases.[5, 17, 18] Visualization of nodules in the pericardium has been recorded once.[19] The electrocardiogram can show the classic concave elevation of the ST segment, but only in 12 to 33 percent of the cases;[5, 18] the ECG is sometimes normal, but most commonly nonspecific ST-T waves changes are seen.

The pericardial fluid has been analyzed in detail. The color varies from yellow to bloody and is almost always an exudate with a protein content of about 5.5 gm. %. White cell counts up to 88,100 per cu. mm. have been reported.[5, 14, 17, 20] The fluid may be frankly hemorrhagic.[21] As in rheumatoid pleural fluid,[22, 23] pericardial fluid glucose is low, usually below 20 mg.%[14, 17, 20] While the cause of the low sugar in pericardial fluid has not been established it is reasonable to postulate an inhibition of specific transport mechanism, as has been shown in rheumatoid pleural effusions.[24, 25] In two patients[14] with prolonged cardiac embarrassment, glucose was low in pericardial fluid and normal in pleural fluid, consistent with the congestive failure etiology of the latter. In one patient[26] who had acute rheumatoid pericarditis and pleuritis, glucose was low in both fluids. Another feature similar to rheumatoid pleural effusion[4] is the very low or undetectable complement level.[5, 20] Gamma globulin complexes similar to those found in synovial fluid were also identified and were probably responsible for the complement activation.[20] Another unusual feature of chronic rheumatoid pericardial effusions is a high cholesterol content, leading to the diagnosis of cholesterol pericarditis. This association is probably more than coincidental for rheumatoid synovial effusions[28] and pleural effusions[29] also show high cholesterol levels. Indeed, the appearance of a cholesterol pericarditis should make one search for clinical manifestations of rheumatoid arthritis.

The course of rheumatoid pericarditis is generally benign and self-limited. The pain and fever usually disappear within a month, as do the radiographic and electrocardiographic changes. A pericardial rub can persist, sometimes for several months. A few of the attacks recur within a few months.[17, 18] Corticosteroids have been advocated since most of the patients so treated in one series[5] improved, but there is no consensus about their effectiveness in suppressing the pericardial inflammation.[17] It is important that the patient's total disease process be treated.

Pericardial Tamponade

Tamponade in the course of rheumatoid pericarditis has been reported by a number of authors[5, 12, 14, 16, 17, 18, 30] and can be the initial, sometimes abrupt,[12, 17] presentation of the pericarditis. Its overall rate has varied in different series from 3 to 24 percent.[5, 17,, 18] Although sometimes relieved by pericardiocentesis,[5] this procedure may prove ineffective due to loculation or inspissated material. Under these circumstances, pericardiectomy should be immediately performed.[30] Corticosteroids, even intravenously and in massive dose, have only an ancillary role and one should not wait for steroid effectiveness when tamponade occurs.[16] It would seem logical, however, to use high dose corticosteroids as well when the tamponade is relieved by pericardiocentesis.

Constrictive Pericarditis

In the opinion of several authors, corticosteroids have not prevented the occurrence, or ameliorated the course, of rheumatoid constrictive pericarditis.[14, 17] Its frequency is similar to tamponade[5, 17] and good results have been obtained by pericardiectomy, except in patients who had associated disease such as rheumatoid aortic insufficiency[14] or coronary artery disease.[12] Clinically, it is often difficult in constrictive disease with RA to determine whether there is compression from accumulated fluid, thickened visceral pericardium and epicardium, or fibrous adherent pericardium. In any case, the surgical approach would often seem necessary.[27, 31, 32]

Subclinical Pericarditis

Goslings[33] explained the discrepancy between the common findings of pericarditis at autopsy, and its rarity in the living patient and negative electrocardiogram, by the brief duration of the physical signs, even in cases that showed pericarditis at autopsy. This may well be the case, for rheumatoid arthritis may last for decades during which only a brief hospital stay may occur where a random bout of pericarditis has a chance of being detected. The introduction of echocardiography, however, with its potential to detect small effusions, made it possible to reconcile these statistics. Bacon[34] showed that 50 percent of 22 patients with nodular disease had evidence of pericardial effusion by echocardiogram, as compared with 18 and 0 percent in non-nodular rheumatoid arthritis and osteoarthritis patients respectively. Similar work by other groups confirmed this finding and, in addition, demonstrated a possible dysfunction of the mitral valve in approximately one fourth of the patients,[35, 36] perhaps related to the rheumatoid granulomatous endocarditis described at postmortem by Cruickshank.[10]

Juvenile Rheumatoid Arthritis (JRA)

Pericarditis in JRA when looked for by modern techniques is a frequent finding. However, most writers have regarded it as clinically unusual and certainly not a serious manifestation of the disease.[37]

In 1881 Charcot[8] observed a 10-year-old child with chronic articular rheumatism who developed acute pericarditis concurrent with an exacerbation of the arthritis which subsequently became associated with nodules. In his original study, Still[38] emphasized the importance of pericarditis and found 3 definite and 5 possible instances in the 12 patients studied. According to Sury[39] in his review of the pre-1940 literature, adhesive pericarditis was found at autopsy but seldom described in vivo. Recent studies, however, reveal that pericarditis is associated most frequently with the acute systemic JRA, or Still's disease, rather than with the nodular, seropositive disease that is indistinguishable from the adult clinical form. A detailed study[40] has revealed that pericarditis occurred in 7 percent of 285 cases of JRA, a prevalence similar to the 8 percent[41] and 6 percent[42] noted earlier. Five of 11 autopsies cases, however, had definite evidence of pericarditis.[40] A striking clinical correlation was the association of pericarditis with systemic manifestations of the disease, i.e., rash, lymphadenopathy, splenomegaly, pulmonary and pleural disease, and amyloidosis. The mean duration of the pericarditis was 7.3 weeks with a range of 1 to 15 weeks. No circulatory embarrassment was found, nor was the development of constrictive lesions noted. Two patients autopsied in another series had fibrous pericarditis, although one had had only a short lived clinical pericarditis and no murmurs,[43] and at least two others in another large series[39] demonstrated fibrous pericarditis.

Two recent reports on Still's disease in the adult[44, 45] revealed the presence of clinical pericarditis in 25 percent of the patients. The high prevalence of pericarditis in Still's disease, and the observed high prevalence of pericarditis at autopsy have been corroborated in vivo as in adult RA by echocardiography.[46] In this latter series, 36 percent of 55 patients with JRA of various types had definite evidence of pericarditis. The clinical analysis of the cases showed that 81 percent of the patients with classic Still's disease had pericarditis, as compared with 21 percent and 10 percent in the polyarticular and oligoarticular forms, respectively.

Since it is clear that juvenile rheumatoid arthritis is a heterogeneous group of disorders with some individuals having juvenile ankylosing spondylitis, and so forth, it is likely that as better classification of cases occurs, clinically, serologically, and by histocompatability antigens (W-27), the relation of associated features such as pericarditis will be more clearly delineated.[47]

Finally, pericarditis does not seem to carry a serious prognostic implication in JRA.[40, 44, 48] It would appear that corticosteroid therapy should be reserved for the most severe cases and the rheumatoid disease as a whole should be the major object of treatment.

Systemic Lupus Erythematosus

General Manifestations

Systemic lupus erythematosus (SLE) is a diffuse connective tissue disease, characterized by remissions and exacerbations, involvement of skin, joints, kidney, nervous system, lungs, heart, and other organs to varying degrees. It is associated with a host of immunologic aberrations, particularly the presence of serum antinuclear antibodies. It affects females predominantly and peaks from the second through the fourth decades, but does not spare children and older people. Drug induced lupus is a syndrome associated with a number of pharmacologic agents, especially hydralazine, procainamide, and anticonvulsants, which produce an identical syndrome but far less renal, central nervous, and skin involvement. Drug induced SLE parallels the age distribution of the diseases for which the offending drug is used. Thus, procainamide induced lupus is seen predominantly in patients in their fifties and older.

While the etiology of SLE is presently unknown, its pathogenesis is better understood. Many of the manifestations are presumed to be due to the formation and deposition of immune complexes which lead to activation of the complement system and tissue damage, particularly in the kidney, central nervous system, articular, and serosal areas. Multiple types of antinuclear antibodies[49] are present and some may relate to disease activity (e.g., high titer of anti-DNA antibody correlates with active lupus nephritis), but their specific pathogenetic role, if any, has not been elucidated. Cellular immunity is also disturbed. Its role in the pathogenesis of the disease is unknown.

In addition to the disturbed immunity which underlies and is the hallmark of SLE, some forms of aggressive therapy, i.e., corticosteroids and immunosuppressive drugs, induce additional risk factors such as increased susceptibility to infection (a phenomenon relevant to pericarditis) and accelerate the atherosclerotic process,[50] also relevant to this discussion.

The American Rheumatism Association established classification criteria for SLE based on clinical and laboratory findings in order to differentiate this disease from others, especially rheumatoid arthritis.[51] They are useful for their intended purpose, i.e., comparison of series, drug trials, and epidemiology research. Their use as diagnostic criteria in individual patients, however, should be discouraged, since SLE may present fewer than the four required criteria in its milder forms. Systemic lupus will be diagnosed if a high index of clinical suspicion is followed by the appropriate laboratory tests. Virtually any type of system involvement can herald the disease, but classically patients have skin rash, articular involvement, renal, neurologic, and hematologic manifestations. Serosal involvement, including pericarditis, can be its earliest sign. A positive antinuclear antibody test in high titer in the presence of low serum complement is virtually confirmatory. It is important to note, however, that in drug induced lupus as well as in the mixed connective tissue disease syndrome[52] the serum complement is normal.

At times in a patient with seemingly viral or idiopathic pericarditis, careful anamnesis may elicit markers of connective tissue disease, i.e., arthralgia, Raynaud's phenomenon, "sicca" syndrome, a history of epilepsy, glomerulonephritis, false positive serology for syphilis, or a remote episode of purpura. Even in their absence, the physical examination may offer important clues: frontal or patchy alopecia, faint rash in malar distribution, oropharyngeal ulceration, adenopathy, splenomegaly, and soft retinal exudates. Common laboratory abnormalities that can be detected in the routine evaluation include leukopenia, urine sediment abnormalities or proteinuria, a prolonged partial thromboplastin test which may reflect a circulating anticoagulant, and a positive nontreponemal test for syphilis.

Prognosis in SLE depends on the presence of renal and neurologic involvement. In the absence of both, the 5 and 10 year survival are in the vicinity of 80 and 60 percent respectively.[53] The presence of either one or both of the above complications halves the 5 year survival, but there are exceptions since both central nervous system and renal involvement in SLE are heterogeneous manifestations. The treatment of SLE varies with the clinical and laboratory manifestations. While progressive renal disease and active nervous system involvement call for aggressive therapy including high dose corticosteroids with or without immunosuppressives such as cyclophosphamide or azathioprine, other manifestations can often be handled by salicylates, often in association with hydroxychloroquine or low dose corticosteroids.

Pathology

Pericarditis as a complication of SLE was first described by Keefer and Felty in 1924.[54] One of their three fatal cases had three bouts of pericarditis within a 4 month period, always in association with a flareup in the disease activity. The prevalence of pericarditis in autopsy series of patients with SLE varies from 47 to 75 percent.[49, 50, 55, 56, 57, 58] Recently, adhesive pericarditis has been found to predominate while exudative pericarditis (fibrinous or serofibrinous) was more common in the presteroid era, or in patients who died during active disease.[50, 58]

The inflammatory process is nonspecific except for the rare occurrence in the epicardium of *hematoxylin bodies,* the tissue equivalent of the LE phenomenon.[50, 59] Large effusions can occur and interfere with myocardial function. Rarely, the fibrotic process may enclose the heart leading to the constrictive pericarditis syndrome.[60] The proximity of the sinus node to the inflamed pericardium has been considered the cause of arrhythmias in a detailed clinicopathologic study.[61]

Pyogenic and tuberculous pericarditis have also been observed clinically[62] and at postmortem examination in patients with SLE, though frequently unsuspected during life.[50, 57, 63] Libman-Sacks endocarditis, myocarditis, and pericarditis frequently coexist.[50] The coronary vessels often show disease, mainly narrowing or occlusion of the extramural coronary arteries. At present, most of the occlusions are reported as atherosclerotic[50] although vasculitis has been observed.[64] Embolic occlusions have also been reported.[50] Most of the myocardial infarctions in patients with SLE seem to occur now on the basis of atherosclerotic disease and possibly are related to the prolonged corticosteroid therapy.[50] Another process related to the corticosteroids is an inordinate amount of subepicardial fat which seems to be clinically irrelevant except for the apparent increase in the cardiac size that can occur.[50]

Clinical Manifestations

Pericarditis is relatively rare as the initial manifestation of SLE, 1 to 4 percent in contrast with its frequency during the course of the disease, i.e., from 17 to 45 percent.[53, 57, 63, 65, 66, 67] In children, the overall rate of pericarditis seems to be lower.[68, 69, 70] In drug-induced lupus, pericarditis may also be less common than in spontaneous SLE[71] but all major agents capable of inducing lupus, i.e., procainamide, hydralazine, and isoniazid, have been associated with this complication, even leading to pericardial tamponade.[72]

In general, lupus pericarditis occurs during disease activity but it 'can occur during quiescent phases of the disease.[63] The clinical manifestations may be subtle or dramatic. The usual symptom is pain, either pleuritic or substernal. However, dyspnea and cardiac arrhythmias may predominate. On rare occasions the process is silent and the only abnormality is a pericardial friction rub. Sometimes, rapidly enlarging cardiac size or transient electrocardiographic changes, often atypical, are the only findings. An important clue to this possible presence of pericarditis is pleurisy, unilateral or bilateral, since pericarditis alone is relatively infrequent (i.e., in from 5 to 9 percent of cases). Pleuropericarditis, however, has been found in 15 to 27 percent.[53, 67] In turn, pericarditis has been considered a potential indicator of concurrent cardiac lesions, in particular Libman-Sacks endocarditis and, less frequently, myocarditis since the three types of lesions often coexist in autopsy specimens.[50] This view, however, may be very difficult to prove clinically unless echocardiography can detect valvular dysfunction associated with healed Libman-Sacks endocarditis.

Chest roentgenograms often reveal cardiomegaly, usually slight to moderate,[55] rarely massive. Unilateral or bilateral pleural effusions and areas of pneumonitis often coexist, and sometimes the pericardial sac seems sunken in the bilateral pleural effusions.[67]

The electrocardiographic changes are most often nonspecific, although in some series typical evolving patterns of pericarditis have been just as common. Large effusions are often associated with generalized loss of voltage. It has been said that the original voltage rarely recovers after a severe attack.[55]

The pericardial fluid is yellow to grossly bloody. The protein content is high and the glucose normal or moderately low. The complement level, usually measured as CH_{50} is low or undetectable.[73, 74] In general, the findings resemble those of pleural and synovial fluids.[4] Pericardial fluid was found able to activate the complement system when mixed in vitro with normal serum, probably due to the presence of immune complexes.[73] The white cell count is usually below 10,000/cu. mm., and consists mostly of polymorphonuclear leukocytes. LE cells have been repeatedly found on routine smears, both in spontaneous[19, 63, 75, 76, 77] and in drug induced lupus[78] pericardial effusions.

The usual course of lupus pericarditis is benign and responds to the same measures used for the treatment of other systemic manifestations. However, there are notable exceptions, and since the course is unpredictable and tamponade may occur, hospitalization and close observation are mandatory.

Tamponade

Tamponade is the most common complication and has been reported in spontaneous[53, 65, 74, 76, 79, 80, 81] and in drug induced lupus, the latter due to procainamide,[82, 83, 84] hydralazine,[78] and isoniazid.[72] In two of our cases as well as in others in the literature, tamponade has been the first manifestation or initial recognized feature of SLE both in spontaneous and in drug induced cases.[76, 78, 82, 83] Overall, tamponade occurs in about 7 percent of the clinically recognized cases of SLE pericarditis.[53, 65] Treatment is discussed below.

Constrictive Pericarditis

Constrictive pericarditis has been reported in three patients.[57, 60, 85] One of the patients was only briefly reported[57] and another had concurrent cardiovascular disease, i.e., atrial septal defect and rheumatic valvular disease.[85] It is interesting to note, however, that the three patients were male. Thus, it is an exceedingly rare complication of SLE.

Other Causes of Pericarditis in SLE

Uremia is a frequent event in late SLE as a complication of lupus nephritis and is the cause of death in 24 to 36 percent of the patients.[53, 63, 71] Thus uremic pericarditis is not an unexpected observation in SLE. In addition, opportunistic infections occur in SLE especially in patients treated with immunosuppressive agents. Bacterial pericarditis has been repeatedly found, usually as a clinically unrecognized autopsy finding.[50, 57, 62, 63] The diagnostic difficulty is compounded by the fact that renal failure, immunosuppressive agents, and infection often coexist, posing a dramatic clinical dilemma. Finally, episternocardiac pericarditis can occur as a result of atherosclerotic coronary disease, and rarely from coronary vasculitis, with infarction.

Management of Lupus Pericarditis

In the absence of tamponade, and if the SLE is clearcut and uncomplicated (i.e., no evidence of sepsis), the institution of full doses of salicylates or low dose corticosteroid agents will often suffice if only a rub is present. When an effusion is present and the etiology of the pericarditis is uncertain (namely when infection is suspected), careful paracentesis is indicated for the appropriate bacteriologic studies. Likewise, tamponade can often be treated by pericardial aspiration plus massive doses of intravenous corticosteroids. However, if the drainage is unsatisfactory or if cardiac embarrassment recurs, immediate thoractomy can be life-saving. Patients with lupus pericarditis should always be hospitalized and carefully followed.

Scleroderma

Scleroderma is a multisystem connective tissue disease which produces hardening and fibrosis of the skin, especially in distal upper extremities, and progressive visceral fibrosis especially in the lungs and gastrointestinal tract. Raynaud's phenomenon may precede (sometimes for several years) and most of the time accompany the skin changes. The visceral involvement may be subtle or clinically obvious. Dysphagia, reflux esophagitis, and aspiration relate to the motor dysfunction of the lower third of the esophagus. Dyspnea, hypoxemia, and pulmonary hypertension reflect fibrosis and vascular disease in the lung. Rapidly progressive renal insufficiency, marked protein-uria, and malignant hypertension — fortunately uncommon — herald the scleroderma kidney. Primary myocardial insufficiency and pericarditis are clinically uncommon events, but do occur and carry important prognostic significance. Scleroderma occurs predominantly in females; its incidence, which increases with age, is $1/50$ and $1/2.5$ of that of rheumatoid arthritis and systemic lupus erythematosus respectively. Scleroderma without pulmonary, heart, or kidney involvement carries an overall 5 year survival rate of 70 percent, pulmonary alone 48 percent, heart alone (including pericarditis) 25 percent, while patients affected by severe kidney disease as defined above die within a few months.[86]

The specific etiology and pathogenesis are unknown, but increased collagen production by scleroderma skin fibroblasts has been demonstrated and is one of a number of factors indicating collagen production (or degradation) abnormalities in this disorder. Vascular factors involving the capillary bed have also been implicated and some believe that vascular abnormalities leading to hypoxia can ultimately lead to the derangement in collagen metabolism.[87]

No definitive treatment for scleroderma is yet available. The inflammatory aspects can be treated with salicylates and occasionally low dose steroids while the vascular manifestations symptomatically improve with reserpine.

Scleroderma Pericarditis

Scleroderma heart disease, although described in the 19th century, was not firmly established as a clinicopathologic entity until the work of Weiss and colleagues[88] in 1943. Autopsy studies excluding patients who died of uremia have shown a prevalence of pericarditis or pericardial effusion of approximately 50 percent.[89, 90, 91] Histologically, the picture is nonspecific: thickened connective tissue and cellular infiltrates predominantly around vessels.[92, 93]

Clinically, pericarditis attributable to scleroderma occured in 5 to 7 percent of affected patients.[89, 91] In other series dealing only with patients who had cardiac involvement, pericarditis was found in 10 to 16 percent.[88, 94]

As in other connective tissue diseases, the scleroderma pericarditis may affect the sinus node. The depth depends upon the severity of the pericarditis. This in turn is at least a partial explanation for certain atrial arrhythmias and other types of sinus node malfunction.[95]

Recently McWhorter[91] distinguished two types of scleroderma pericardial disease. The first is an acute pericarditis which resembles viral or acute idiopathic pericarditis. Fever, chest pain, and pericardial friction rub were always present. The chest roentgenogram revealed cardiomegaly. The electrocardiograms showed nonspecific T wave changes. Two of the four reported patients died suddenly during the course of the pericarditis, presumably from cardiac arrhythmias. In one of our patients this type of pericarditis occurred preceded by severe weight loss, fever, anemia, polyneuropathy, and extreme elevation of the sedimentation rate.

The second type is the chronic pericardial effusion, previously reported by others.[92, 96] However, its prognostic significance was for the first time stressed. Chronic pericardial effusion was twice as frequent as in the acute type. The patients experienced no pain unless angina occurred. All patients had congestive heart failure, and early pericardial tamponade occurred in some. The chest roentgenogram uniformly showed cardiomegaly, plus pleural effusions in half of the patients. Electrocardiographic changes included low voltage in 64 percent of the patients, while 72 percent had nonspecific changes of the T wave. Chronic pericardial effusion was followed within 6 months by rapidly progressive renal insufficiency leading to death in 6 of 11 patients. Since rapidly progressive renal failure in scleroderma is accompanied by a drastic reduction in the cortical renal blood flow,[97] it was postulated that the cardiac failure, the pericarditis or its attendant diuretic therapy, or perhaps simultaneous microvascular changes in both organs could have been responsible for a critical reduction of the cortical renal blood flow.[91]

Pericardial effusions are rare, and in two cases angiocardiography disclosed their presence.[98] Pericardial aspiration in two patients[96] yielded a cloudy yellow fluid of high specific gravity and high protein content (5.9 and 6.8 gm.%) in association with a low cell count, i.e., 37 and 4 leukocytes/cu.mm.

Treatment of scleroderma pericardial disease includes mild anti-inflammatory agents and routine cardiac medications. Pericardial aspiration may be needed due to cardiac embarrassment in the chronic effusive type, while anti-inflammatory agents would seem a logical first choice in the acute type. This treatment is, however, empirical and the choice of agent would depend on the severity of the symptoms. In the sick patient, corticosteroids in moderately high dosage (rapidly decreased when improvement occurs), and with careful monitoring of renal function and blood pressure may be indicated. In the milder cases, analgesics or salicylates may suffice. In all cases, the patients should be hospitalized and followed carefully.

Mixed Connective Tissue Disease (MCTD)

This newly described syndrome combines features of scleroderma, dermatomyositis, and SLE.[52, 99] The age and sex distribution, although it is about 40 times less frequent, is similar to SLE. These patients often have tight skin, tapering digits, lower esophageal dysfunction, lid and digital erythemas, muscle weakness, high serum muscle enzymes, facial rash, photosensitivity, and arthralgias. Neurologic and renal involvement are quite uncommon. Serositis is present in about 25 percent of the patients and *acute pericarditis,* thought initially to be viral, was the initial presentation of several patients. The age and sex distribution are similar to SLE. It is characterized by a serum anti-RNP antibody.

Patients with MCTD respond well to low doses of corticosteroids and probably have a good prognosis. The diagnosis is made by the clinical symptom complex and a positive antinuclear antibody test with speckled pattern and normal complement. The ultimate identification depends on the demonstration of high titer of antibody to the RNase-sensitive component of an extractable nuclear antigen (i.e., anti-RNP antibody).

Sjögren's Syndrome

The sicca syndrome (dry eyes plus dry mouth as a result of the destructive lymphocytic infiltration of the tributary exocrine glands) can be seen as an isolated finding, or in association with a connective tissue disease such as rheumatoid arthritis, systemic lupus erythematosus, or scleroderma.[100, 101, 102] Thus, an association with pericarditis is to be expected on the basis of the associated disease alone. For example, in one series of 62 patients in which 39 patients presented associated connective tissue disease, two cases of clinical pericarditis occurred. Both had severe rheumatoid arthritis.[100] Such cases should be treated as described earlier.

Whipple's Disease

Whipple's disease is essentially a disorder of males, characterized by fever, abdominal pain, weight loss, arthralgias, diarrhea, ascites, and skin pigmentation. Clinical pericarditis can occur.[103] At autopsy the patient originally reported by Whipple[104] showed obliteration of pericardial and pleural cavities by gelatinous looking adhesions not dissimilar from the process involving the peritoneum. In a detailed review, evidence of pericarditis was found in 40 percent of autopsy cases.[105]

The diagnosis of this condition depends upon finding specific abnormalities, i.e., PAS positive inclusions or electron microscopic evidence of short rods,[106] in small bowel biopsy, lymph node, or other tissue biopsy. The disease can be suppressed, if not cured, by appropriate antibiotic therapy. The specific agent has not been isolated.

RHEUMATOLOGIC DISORDERS WITH OCCASIONAL PERICARDITIS

Reiter's Syndrome

A diagnosis of Reiter's syndrome is usually made when the triad of sterile urethritis, conjunctivitis, and arthritis is present, or when two of the above findings are associated with keratodermia blenorrhagica, uveitis, stomatitis, or balanitis circinata. Diarrhea may also be a prominent manifestation. While many patients seem to recover after the initial episode, perhaps more than 50 percent go on to develop a chronic form of arthritis which often includes ankylosing spondylitis.[107] Aortic insufficiency is a well known complication of Reiter's syndrome,[108] and many patients with ankylosing spondylitis who develop aortic insufficiency or A-V conduction disturbances or both after an earlier episode of myopericarditis were found to have features suggestive of Reiter's syndrome.[109]

Pericarditis was a reported abnormality in several reviews of the Reiter's syndrome literature. In the study of 344 patients by Paronen,[110] 23 patients had myopericarditis and 3 had pericarditis. Carditis occurred early in the disease, or up to 2 or 3 years after the onset. Other observers have reported[111] pericarditis in the setting of active disease.

The cause of Reiter's syndrome is unknown. While some cases have followed epidemic dysentery, such association is uncommon in this country. Most of the patients share an otherwise uncommon HLA antigen (W27), which also occurs in other types of spondylitis. The acute exacerbations respond at times to nonspecific anti-inflammatory drugs.

Ankylosing Spondylitis

Ankylosing spondylitis is easily diagnosed in the young male with a painful, stiff back who on x-ray shows bilateral sacroilitis. At other times only a careful search for the etiology of obscure aortic insufficiency or atrioventricular conduction disturbance will lead to the diagnosis.[112]

Pericarditis has been reported as an early complication of ankylosing spondylitis[109] or in association with exacerbations of the disease.[113] It is a rare event, however, since only 3 cases occurred among 519 patients.[108] Interestingly, however, aortic insufficiency and conduction disturbances were often late findings in the same patients who previously had myocarditis, with or without pericarditis. Since the patients with carditis often had peripheral polyarthritis and urethritis, one may speculate as to whether the underlying disease was Reiter's syndrome rather than "bona fide" ankylosing spondylitis.[110, 111] Detailed pathologic studies of patients with ankylosing spondylitis have not mentioned pericarditis as one of the complications of the disease.[114] Pericardial adhesions were seen only in patients who previously had thoracotomy.[111] This lends support to its extreme rarity.

Inflammatory Bowel Disease

Acute pericarditis, sometimes with tamponade,[115, 116] is an unusual extraintestinal complication of inflammatory bowel disease. Since erythema nodosum, arthritis, and uveitis can all be present, confusion with other rheumatologic conditions can occur. Little is known about the precise incidence of this manifestation, but clearly pericarditis is uncommon. Anti-inflammatory treatment, usually high dose steroids, will often be necessary to treat the primary disease and also the pericarditis with effusion.

Serum Sickness

Acute pericarditis of a benign type has been observed in severe serum sickness.[117, 118] This condition usually occurs 7 to 12 days after the administration of heterologous serum and is characterized by fever, urticaria, lymphadenopathy, myalgia, and arthritis. Neuritis, vasculitis, and glomerulonephritis can occur. The underlying mechanism is the deposition of soluble antigen-antibody complexes formed in antigen excess. Corticosteroid therapy is indicated in the severe form.

Wegener's Granulomatosis

Pericarditis has been found in Wegener's granulomatosis, a disease characterized by necrotizing granulomatous vasculitis of the upper and lower respiratory tracts in association with glomerulonephritis. In the classic series reported by Godman and Churg,[119] it was seen in 2 of 6 autopsied cases. In one, granulomatous inflammation with giant cells was present in the epicardium. The other showed focal pericarditis in association with patchy myocardial fibrosis. In a recent series, 3 of 18 patients had clinical pericarditis.[120] Two patients responded to therapy and one died of pulmonary hemorrhage. The recognition of Wegener's granulomatosis is of utmost importance since immunosuppressive agents such as cyclophosphamide are very effective therapy.

RHEUMATOLOGIC DISEASES WITH PERICARDITIS AS A RARE ASSOCIATION

Vasculitis

Pericarditis is not a feature of polyarteritis nodosa either in its primary form[121] or when it is associated with drug use,[122] Australia antigenemia,[123] or serous otitis media.[124] Rupture of a coronary artery aneurysm within the pericardial sac, leading to death, has been reported.[125] Also, epistenocardiac pericarditis secondary to arteritic myocardial infarction can be expected, as well as uremic pericarditis in patients who develop such renal arteritis leading to uremia.

Two observations of pericarditis in giant cell arteritis have been recorded. One was an autopsy finding[126] and the other, occurring during the course of temporal arteritis, responded to corticosteroid therapy.[127]

Acute pericarditis was observed in a case of Schönlein-Henoch purpura in the adult.[128] Finally, pericarditis with the characteristic histologic features was found at autopsy in a patient who died from allergic granulomatosis.[19]

Polymyositis

Pericarditis must be very rare if it does occur in association with polymyositis. Occasional cases have been mentioned.[129] However, systemic lupus erythematosus and scleroderma may occur with a predominantly myositic appearance which could conceivably lead to misclassification. In addition, pericarditis is frequently observed in the mixed connective tissue disease syndrome,[99] another possible source of confusion. No evidence of pericarditis was found in a detailed dermatomyositis necropsy series in children.[130]

Behçet's Disease

This interesting syndrome is diagnosed by the triad of iritis and painful ulcers of the mouth and the genitalia (scrotum and penis in the male, as opposed to the shallow painless ulcers of mouth and glans of Reiter's syndrome). A host of associated manifestations have been described and recent investigators have accepted looser criteria: two of the elements of the triad, plus one or more associations.

Pericarditis has been reported in Behçet's disease.[131, 132, 133] In one of the cases it was recurrent and posed a diagnostic dilemma. Other series have not included cases of pericarditis[134, 135] and its very existence has been questioned since the few reported cases could be coincidental. The etiology of the Behçet's syndrome is unknown and its therapy symptomatic.

Familial Mediterranean Fever (FMF)

Despite the fact that FMF is a clinical syndrome in which pericarditis might be expected (recurrent attacks of fever, in association with pleuritis, peritonitis, arthritis, and erysipelas-like erythema), pericarditis has been rarely reported.[136, 137] In fact, in a series of 470 patients studied in detail not a single instance of pericarditis was mentioned,[138] nor was it in a report from the same group 8 years later[139] or in a series of 100 cases.[140] Uremic pericarditis, however, is frequently observed when the associated renal amyloidosis leads to azotemia.

249

Amyloidosis

Amyloidosis, especially when primary or associated with multiple myeloma, frequently involves the heart.[141] In a series of 42 patients with the primary form, 67 percent had clinical heart disease at some time during the course of the illness,[142] but clinical pericarditis has not been reported.[141, 142, 143] It is interesting to note, however, that on postmortem examination the pericardium is often infiltrated.[144, 145] In one series, 7 of 15 patients with clinically significant cardiac amyloidosis examined at autopsy presented focal deposits of amyloid in the visceral pericardium, as well as in the epicardial nerve bundles of 4 patients.

On the other hand, several patients have been reported who underwent thoracotomy for suspected constrictive pericarditis only to have an infiltrated myocardium found.[142, 146]

Gout

Acute gouty pericarditis has been described;[147] however, the evidence presented for primary gouty pericarditis was slim and the patients most likely represented a coincidental association.

REFERENCES

1. WILLIAMS, R. C., JR.: *Rheumatoid Arthritis as a Systemic Disease.* W. B. Saunders Co., Philadelphia, 1974.

2. STAGE, D. E., AND MANNICK, M.: *Rheumatoid factors in rheumatoid arthritis.* Bull. Rheum. Dis. 23: 720, 1972.

3. RUDDY, S., AND AUSTEN, K. F.: *The complement system in rheumatoid synovitis. I. An analysis of complement component activities in rheumatoid synovial fluids.* Arthritis Rheum. 13:713, 1970.

4. HUNDER, G. G., McDUFFIE, F. C., AND HEPPER, N. G. G.: *Pleural fluid complement in systemic lupus erythematosus and rheumatoid arthritis.* Ann. Intern. Med. 76:357, 1972.

5. FRANCO, A. E., LEVINE, H. D., AND HALL, A. P.: *Rheumatoid pericarditis. Report of 17 cases diagnosed clinically.* Ann. Intern. Med. 77:837, 1972.

6. ROPES, M. W., BENNETT, G. A., COBB, S., ET AL.: *Revision of diagnostic criteria for rheumatoid arthritis.* Bull. Rheum. Dis. 9:175, 1958.

7. GORDON, D. A., STEIN, J. L., AND BRODER, I.: *The extra-articular features of rheumatoid arthritis. A systematic analysis of 127 cases.* Am. J. Med. 54:445, 1973.

8. CHARCOT, J. M.: *Clinical Lectures on Senile and Chronic Diseases,* translated by W. S. Tuke, pp. 172–175. The New Syndenham Society, Vol. 95, London, 1881.

9. SOKOLOFF, L.: *The heart in rheumatoid arthritis.* Am. Heart J. 45:635, 1953.

10. CRUICKSHANK, B.: *Heart lesions in rheumatoid disease.* J. Pathol. Bact. 76:223, 1958.

11. CATHCART, E. S., AND SPODICK, D. H.: *Rheumatoid heart disease. A study of the incidence and nature of cardiac lesions in rheumatoid arthritis.* N. Engl. J. Med. 266:959, 1962.

12. KENNEDY, W. P. U., PARTRIDGE, R. E. H., AND MATTHEWS, M. B.: *Rheumatoid pericarditis with cardiac failure treated by pericardiectomy.* Br. Heart J. 28:602, 1966.

13. BYWATERS, E. G. L.: *Constrictive pericarditis and other cardiovascular lesions in rheumatoid arthritis and the problem of post-inflammatory fibrosis.* Ned. Tijdschr. Geneeskd. 118:410, 1974.

14. THADANI, U., IVESON, J. M. I., AND WRIGHT, V.: *Cardiac tamponade, constrictive pericarditis and pericardial reaction in rheumatoid arthritis.* Medicine (Baltimore) 54:261, 1975.

15. ARTHUR, A., OSKVIG, R., AND BASTA, L. L.: *Calcific rheumatoid constrictive pericarditis with cardiac failure treated by pericardiectomy.* Chest 64:769, 1973.

16. THOMAS, P., AND HARSE, J.: *A case of rheumatoid arthritis and haemopericardium.* Rheumatol. Rehab. 13:32, 1974.

17. KIRK, J., AND COSH, J.: *The pericarditis of rheumatoid arthritis.* Q. J. Med. 38:397, 1969.

18. VRONINCKS, P., CATS, A., AND GOSLINGS, J.: *Les péricardites de la polyarthrite rhumatoïde. A propos d'une étude de 19 cas.* Rev. Rhum. Mal. Osteoartic. 39:351, 1972.

19. McKusick, V. A., and Harvey, A. M.: *Diseases of pericardium*. Adv. Intern. Med. 7:157, 1955.

20. Ball, G. V., Schrohenloher, R., and Hester, R.: *Gamma globulin complexes in rheumatoid pericardial fluid*. Am. J. Med. 58:123, 1975.

21. Stern, J. B., and Sobel, H. J.: *Hemorrhagic rheumatoid pericarditis*. Am. J. Cardiol. 8:670, 1961.

22. Carr, D. T., and Power, M. H.: *Pleural fluid glucose with special reference to its concentration in rheumatoid pleurisy with effusion*. Chest 37:324, 1960.

23. Lillington, G. A., Carr, D. T., and Mayne, J. G.: *Rheumatoid pleurisy with effusion*. Arch. Intern. Med. 128:764, 1971.

24. Dodson, W. H., and Hollingsworth, J. W.: *Pleural effusion in rheumatoid arthritis*. N. Engl. J. Med. 275:1337, 1966.

25. Carr, D. T., and McGuckin, W. F.: *Pleural fluid glucose. Serial observations of its concentration following administration of glucose to patients with rheumatoid pleural effusions and malignant effusions*. Am. Rev. Resp. Dis. 97:302, 1968.

26. Berger, H. W., and Seckler, S. G.: *Pleural and pericardial effusions in rheumatoid disease*. Ann. Intern. Med. 64:1291, 1966.

27. Liss, J. P., and Bachmann, W. T.: *Rheumatoid constrictive pericarditis treated by pericardiectomy*. Arthritis Rheum. 13:869, 1970.

28. Newcombe, D. S., and Cohen, A. S.: *Chylous synovial effusion in rheumatoid arthritis*. Am. J. Med. 38:156, 1965.

29. Stengel, B. F., Watson, R. R., and Darling, R. J.: *Pulmonary rheumatoid nodule with cavitation and chronic lipid effusion*. J.A.M.A. 198:1263, 1966.

30. Romanoff, H., Rozin, R., and Zlotnick, A.: *Cardiac tamponade in rheumatoid arthritis. A case report and review of the literature*. Arthritis Rheum. 13:426, 1970.

31. Burson, R. A., and Dennis, R. G.: *Rheumatoid constrictive pericarditis treated successfully by pericardiectomy*. South. Med. J. 66:1399, 1973.

32. Keith, T. A., III: *Chronic constrictive pericarditis in association with rheumatoid disease*. Circulation 25:477, 1962.

33. Goslings, J.: *Heberden round*. Ann. Rheum. Dis. 17:337, 1958.

34. Bacon, P. A., and Gibson, D. G.: *Cardiac involvement in rheumatoid arthritis*. Ann. Rheum. Dis. 33:20, 1974.

35. Nomeir, A., Turner, R., Watts, E., et al.: *Cardiac involvement in rheumatoid arthritis*. Ann. Intern. Med. 79:800, 1973.

36. Prakash, R., Atassi, A., Poske, R., et al.: *Prevalence of pericardial effusion and mitral valve involvement in patients with rheumatoid arthritis without cardiac symptoms*. N. Engl. J. Med. 289:597, 1973.

37. Calabro, J. J., Katz, R. M., and Maltz, B. A.: *A critical reappraisal of juvenile rheumatoid arthritis*. Clin. Orthop. 74:101, 1971.

38. Still, G. F.: *Form of chronic joint disease in children*. Med. Chir. Tr. (London) 80:47, 1897.

39. Sury, B.: *Rheumatoid arthritis in children*. Munksgaard, Denmark, 1952.

40. Lietman, P. S., and Bywaters, E. G. L.: *Pericarditis in juvenile rheumatoid arthritis*. Pediatrics 32:855, 1963.

41. Sairanen, E.: *On rheumatoid arthritis in children*. Acta Rheumatol. Scand. (Suppl.) 2:1, 1958.

42. Schlesinger, B. E., Forsyth, C. C., White, R. H. R., et al.: *Observations on the clinical course and treatment of 100 cases of Still's disease*. Arch. Dis. Child. 36:65, 1961.

43. Grokoest, A. W., Snyder, A. I., and Schlaeger, R.: *Juvenile Rheumatoid Arthritis*. Little Brown and Co., Boston, 1962.

44. Bywaters, E. G. L.: *Still's disease in the adult*. Ann. Rheum. Dis. 30:121, 1971.

45. Bujak, J. S., Aptekar, R. G., Decker, J. L., et al.: *Juvenile rheumatoid arthritis presenting in the adult as fever of unknown origin*. Medicine (Baltimore) 52:431, 1973.

46. Bernstein, B., Takahashi, M., and Hanson, V.: *Cardiac involvement in juvenile rheumatoid arthritis*. J. Pediatr. 85:313, 1974.

47. Edmonds, J., Morris, R. I., Metzger, A. L., et al.: *Follow-up of juvenile chronic polyarthritis with particular reference to histocompatibility antigen W27*. Ann. Rheum. Dis. 33:289, 1974.

48. Jordan, J. D.: *Cardiopulmonary manifestations of rheumatoid disease in childhood*. South. Med. J. 57:1273, 1964.

49. Friou, G. J., and Quismorio, F. P.: *The LE cell factor and antinuclear antibodies*, in Cohen, A. S.:

Laboratory Diagnostic Procedures in the Rheumatic Diseases, ed. 2. Little, Brown and Co., Boston, 1975.

50. BULKLEY, B. H., AND ROBERTS, W. C.: *The heart in systemic lupus erythematosus and the changes induced in it by corticosteroid therapy.* Am. J. Med. 58:243, 1975.

51. COHEN, A. S., REYNOLDS, W. E., FRANKLIN, E. C., ET AL.: *Preliminary criteria for the classification of systemic lupus erythematosus.* Bull. Rheum. Dis. 21:643, 1971.

52. SHARP, G. C., IRVIN, W. S., TAN, E. M., ET AL.: *Mixed connective tissue disease, an apparently distinct rheumatic disease syndrome with a specific antibody to an extractable nuclear antigen (ENA).* Am. J. Med. 52:148, 1972.

53. ESTES, D., AND CHRISTIAN, C. L.: *The natural history of systemic lupus erythematosus by prospective analysis.* Medicine (Baltimore) 50:85, 1971.

54. KEEFER, C. S., AND FELTY, A. R.: *Acute disseminated lupus erythematosus. Report of three fatal cases.* Bull. Johns. Hopkins Hosp. 35:294, 1924.

55. BRIDGEN, W., BYWATERS, E. G. L., LESSOFF, M. H., ET AL.: *The heart in systemic lupus erythematosus.* Br. Heart J. 22:1, 1960.

56. KONG, T. Q., KELLUM, R. E., AND HASERICK, J. R.: *Clinical diagnosis of cardiac involvement in systemic lupus erythematosus. A correlation of clinical and autopsy findings in thirty patients.* Circulation 26:7, 1962.

57. HEJTMANCIK, M. R., WRIGHT, J. C., QUINT, R., ET AL.: *The cardiovascular manifestations of systemic lupus erythematosus.* Am. Heart. J. 68:119, 1964.

58. CRUICKSHANK, B., in Dubois, E. L. (ed.): *Lupus Erythematosus.* University of Southern California Press, Los Angeles, 1974, p. 28.

59. WORTHINGTON, J. W., BAGGENSTOSS, A. H., AND HARGRAVES, M. M.: *Significance of hematoxylin bodies in the necropsy diagnosis of systemic lupus erythematosus.* Am. J. Pathol. 35:955, 1959.

60. STARKEY, R. H., AND HAHN, B H.: *Rapid development of constrictive pericarditis in a patient with systemic lupus erythematosus.* Chest 63:448, 1973.

61. JAMES, T. N., RUPE, C. E., AND MONTO, R. W.: *Pathology of the cardiac conduction system in systemic lupus erythematosus.* Ann. Intern. Med. 63:402, 1965.

62. KNODELL, R. G., AND MANDERS, S. C.: *Staphylococcal pericarditis in a patient with systemic lupus erythematosus.* Chest 65:103, 1974.

63. HARVEY, A. M., SHULMAN, L. E., TUMULTY, P. A., ET AL.: *Systemic lupus erythematosus: Review of the literature and clinical analysis of 138 cases.* Medicine (Baltimore) 33:291, 1954.

64. BONFIGLIO, T. A., BOTTI, R. E., AND HAGSTROM, J. W. C.: *Coronary arteritis, occlusion and myocardial infarction due to lupus erythematosus.* Am. Heart J. 83:153, 1972.

65. SHEARN, M. A.: *The heart in systemic lupus erythematosus.* Am. Heart J. 58:452, 1959.

66. DUBOIS, E. L., AND TUFFANELLI, D. L.: *Clinical manifestations of systemic lupus erythematosus. Computer analysis of 520 cases.* J.A.M.A. 190:104, 1964.

67. PURRIEL, P., MURAS, O., CANOSO, J. J., ET AL.: *Alteraciones pulmonares en las enfermedades llamadas del colágeno (mesenquinopatiás)* Torax (Montevideo) 13:139, 1964.

68. COOK, C. D., WEDGWOOD, R. J. P., CRAIG, J. M., ET AL: *Systemic lupus erythematosus. Description of 37 cases in children and a discussion of endocrine therapy in 32 of the cases.* Pediatrics. 26:570, 1960.

69. JACOBS, J. C.: *Systemic lupus erythematosus in childhood. Report of 35 cases with discussion of seven apparently induced by anticonvulsant medication, and of prognosis and treatment.* Pediatrics 32:257, 1963.

70. MEISLIN, A. G., AND ROTHFIELD, N.: *Systemic lupus erythematosus in childhood. Analysis of 42 cases, with comparative data on 200 adult cases followed concurrently.* Pediatrics 42:37, 1968.

71. DUBOIS, E. L.: *Lupus erythematosus.* University of Southern California Press, Los Angeles, 1974.

72. GREENBERG, J. H., AND LUTCHER, C. L.: *Drug-induced systemic lupus erythematosus. A case with life-threatening pericardial tamponade.* J.A.M.A. 222:191, 1972.

73. HUNDER, G. G., MULLEN, B. J., AND McDUFFIE, F. C.: *Complement in pericardial fluid of lupus erythematosus. Studies in two patients.* Ann. Intern. Med. 80:453, 1974.

74. GOLDENBERG, D., LEFF, G., AND GRAYZEL, A. I.: *Pericardial tamponade in systemic lupus erythematosus. With absent hemolytic complement activity in pericardial fluid.* N. Y. State J. Med. 75:910, 1975.

75. SEAMAN, A. J., AND CHRISTERSON, J. W.: *Demonstration of LE cells in pericardial fluid. Report of a case.* J.A.M.A. 149:145, 1952.

252

76. LERER, R. J.: *Cardiac tamponade as an initial finding in systemic lupus erythematosus.* Am. J. Dis. Child. 124:436, 1972.

77. WOLKOVE, N., AND FRANK, H.: *Lupus pericarditis.* Can. Med. Assoc. J. 111:1331, 1974.

78. CAREY, R. M., COLEMAN, M., AND FEDER, A.: *Pericardial tamponade: a major presenting manifestation of hydralazine-induced lupus syndrome.* Am. J. Med. 54:84, 1973.

79. CURTIS, A. C., AND HORNE, S. F.: *Disseminated lupus erythematosus with pericardial effusion.* Ann. Intern. Med. 30:209, 1949.

80. BERGEN, S. S., JR.: *Pericardial effusion, a manifestation of systemic lupus erythematosus.* Circulation 22:144, 1960.

81. SCHOENFELD, M. R., AND MESSELOFF, C. R.: *Cardiac tamponade in systemic lupus erythematosus.* Circulation 27:98, 1963.

82. ANDERSON, R. J., AND GENTON, E.: *Procainamide-induced pericardial effusion.* Am. Heart J. 83:798, 1972.

83. UTHMAN, S. M., AND TABBARA, R. A.: *Drug induced lupus syndrome presenting as pericardial effusion.* Lab. Med. J. 26:549, 1973.

84. GHOSE, M. K.: *Pericardial tamponade. A presenting manifestation of procainamide-induced lupus erythematosus.* Am. J. Med. 58:581, 1975.

85. YURCHAK, P. M., LEVINE, S. A., AND GORLIN, R.: *Constrictive pericarditis complicating disseminated lupus erythematosus.* Circulation 31:113, 1965.

86. MEDSGER, T. A., JR., MASI, A. T., RODNAN, G. P., ET AL.: *Survival with systemic sclerosis (scleroderma). A life-table analysis of clinical and demographic factors in 309 patients.* Ann. Intern. Med. 75:369, 1971.

87. CAMPBELL, P. M., AND LeRoy, E. C.: *Pathogenesis of systemic sclerosis: a vascular hypothesis.* Semin. Arth. Rheum. 4:351, 1975.

88. WEISS, S., STEAD, E. A., WARREN, J. V., ET AL.: *Scleroderma heart disease. With a consideration of certain other visceral manifestations of scleroderma.* Arch. Intern. Med. 71:749, 1943.

89. SACKNER, M. A., HEINZ, E. R., AND STEINBERG, A. J.: *The heart in scleroderma.* Am. J. Cardiol. 17:542, 1966.

90. D'ANGELO, W. A., FRIES, J. F., MASI, A. T., ET AL.: *Pathologic observations in systemic sclerosis (scleroderma). A study of fifty-eight autopsy cases and fifty-eight matched controls.* Am. J. Med. 46:428, 1969.

91. McWHORTER, IV, J. E., AND LeRoy E. C.: *Pericardial disease in scleroderma (systemic sclerosis).* Am. J. Med. 57:566, 1974.

92. BEDFORD, D. E.: *Chronic effusive pericarditis.* Br. Heart J. 26:499, 1964.

93. STEINBERG, I., AND ROTHBARD, S.: *Roentgen features of sclerodermal pericarditis with effusion.* Radiology 83:292, 1964.

94. NASSER, W. K., MISHKIN, M. E., ROSENBAUM, D., ET AL.: *Pericardial and myocardial disease in progressive systemic sclerosis.* Am. J. Cardiol. 22:538, 1968.

95. JAMES, T. N.: *De subitaneis mortibus. VIII. Coronary arteries and conduction system in scleroderma heart disease.* Circulation. 50:844, 1974.

96. MELTZER, J. I.: *Pericardial effusion in generalized scleroderma.* Am. J. Med. 20:638, 1956.

97. CANNON, P. J., HASSAR, M., CASE, D. B., ET AL.: *The relationship of hypertension and renal failure in scleroderma (progressive systemic sclerosis) to structural and functional abnormalities of renal cortical circulation.* Medicine (Baltimore) 53:1, 1974.

98. STEINBERG, I., AND ROTHBARD, S.: *Pericardial effusion and cor pulmonade in progressive systemic sclerosis (scleroderma).* Am. J. Cardiol. 9:953, 1962.

99. SHARP, G. C.: *Mixed connective tissue disease.* Bull. Rheum. Dis. 25:828, 1975.

100. BLOCH, K. J., BUCHANAN, W. W., WOHL, M. J., ET AL.: *Sjögren's syndrome. A clinical pathological and serological study of sixty-two cases.* Medicine (Baltimore) 44:187, 1965.

101. WHALEY, K., WILLIAMSON, J., CHISHOLM, D. M., ET AL.: *Sjögren's syndrome. I. Sicca components.* Q. J. Med. 42:279, 1973.

102. WHALEY, K., WILLIAMSON, J., CHISHOLM, D. M., ET AL.: *Sjögren's syndrome. 2. Clinical associations and immunological phenomena.* Q. J. Med. 42:513, 1973.

103. PASTOR, B. M., AND GEERKEN, R. G.: *Whipple's disease presenting as pleuropericarditis.* Am. J. Med. 55:827, 1973.

104. WHIPPLE, G. H.: *A hitherto undescribed disease characterized anatomically by deposits of fat and fatty*

acids in the intestinal and mesenteric lymphatic tissues. Johns Hopkins Hosp. Med. Bull. 18:382, 1907.

105. FARNAN, P.: *Whipple's disease. The clinical aspects.* Q. J. Med. 28:163, 1959.

106. COHEN, A. S.: *An electron microscopic study of the small intestine in Whipple's disease.* J. Ultrastruct. Res. 10:124, 1964.

107. SAIRANEN, E., PARONEN, I., AND MÄHÖNEN: *Reiter's syndrome: A follow-up study.* Acta Med. Scand. 185:57, 1969.

108. PAULUS, H. E., PEARSON, C. M., AND PITTS, W., JR.: *Aortic insufficiency in five patients with Reiter's syndrome. A detailed clinical and pathologic study.* Am. J. Med. 53:464, 1972.

109. GRAHAM, D. C., AND SMYTHE, H. A.: *The carditis and aortitis of ankylosing spondylitis.* Bull. Rheum. Dis. 9:171, 1958.

110. PARONEN, I.: *Reiter's disease: A study of 344 cases observed in Finland.* Acta Med. Scand. (suppl). 212, 1948.

111. CSONKA, G. W., AND OATES, J. K.: *Pericarditis and electrocardiographic changes in Reiter's syndrome.* Br. Med. J. 1:866, 1957.

112. BULKLEY, B. H., AND ROBERTS, W. C.: *Ankylosing spondylitis and aortic regurgitation. Description of the characteristic cardiovascular lesion from study of eight necropsy patients.* Circulation 48:1014, 1973.

113. CLARK, W. S., KULKA, J. P., AND BAUER, W.: *Rheumatoid aortitis with aortic regurgitation.* Am. J. Med. 22:580, 1957.

114. CRUICKSHANK, B.: *Pathology of ankylosing spondylitis.* Clin. Orthop. 74:43, 1971.

115. BREITENSTEIN, R. A., SALEL, A. F., AND WATSON, D. W.: *Chronic inflammatory bowel disease: acute pericarditis and pericardial tamponade.* Ann. Intern. Med. 81:406, 1974.

116. RHEINGOLD, O. J.: *Inflammatory bowel disease and pericarditis.* Ann. Intern. Med. 82:592, 1975.

117. MCKINLAY, C. A.: *Allergic carditis, pericarditis and pleurisy. Report of a case of serum sickness with predominant cardiac manifestations and symptomatic recovery.* Lancet 68:61, 1948.

118. GOLDMAN, M. J., AND LAU, F. Y. K.: *Acute pericarditis associated with serum sickness.* N. Engl. J. Med. 250:278, 1954.

119. GODMAN, G. C., AND CHURG, J.: *Wegener's granulomatosis. Pathology and review of the literature.* AMA Arch. Pathol. 58:533, 1954.

120. FAUCI, A. S., AND WOLFF, S. M.: *Wegener's granulomatosis: studies in eighteen patients and a review of the literature.* Medicine (Baltimore) 52:535, 1973.

121. ROSE, G. A., AND SPENCER, H.: *Polyarteritis nodosa.* Q. J. Med. 26:43, 1957.

122. CITRON, B. P., HALPERN, M., MCCARRON, M., ET AL.: *Necrotizing angiitis associated with drug abuse.* N. Engl. J. Med. 283:1003, 1970.

123. GOCKE, D. J., HSU, K., MORGAN, C., ET AL.: *Association between polyarteritis and Australia antigen.* Lancet 2:1149, 1970.

124. SERGENT, J. S., AND CHRISTIAN, C. L.: *Necrotizing vasculitis after acute serous otitis media.* Ann. Intern. Med. 81:195, 1974.

125. SINCLAIR, W., JR., AND NITSCH, E.: *Polyarteritis nodosa of the coronary arteries. Report of a case in an infant with rupture of an aneurysm and intrapericardial hemorrhage.* Am. Heart J. 38:898, 1949.

126. *Case records of Massachusetts General Hospital #23-1961.* N. Engl. J. Med. 264:664, 1961.

127. MILLER, J. P.: *Pericardial effusion and giant cell arteritis.* Proc. R. Soc. Med. 65:565, 1972.

128. LAMY, A., RIFLE, G., GUILLAUMIE, J., ET AL.: *Purpura rheumatoïde de l'adulte. Péricardite aiguë intercurrente.* Nouv. Press. Med. 2:2276, 1973.

129. PEARSON, C. M., AND CURRIE, S., IN WALTON, J. N. (ED.) *Disorders of Voluntary Muscle.* Churchill Livingstone, London, 1974.

130. BANKER, B. Q., AND VICTOR, M.: *Dermatomyositis (systemic angiopathy) of childhood.* Medicine (Baltimore) 45:261, 1966.

131. SIGEL, N., AND LARSON, R.: *Behçet's syndrome. A case with benign pericarditis and recurrent neurologic involvement treated with adrenal steroids.* Arch. Intern. Med. 115:203, 1965.

132. GODEAU, P., HERREMAN, G., BEN ISMAIL, M., ET AL: *Syndrome de Behçet. Atteintes pericardique et pulmonaire.* Nouv. Presse Med. 1:391, 1972.

133. HAMZA, M., ZRIBI, A., CHADLI, A., ET AL.: *La maladie de Behçet. Etude de 22 cas.* Nouv. Presse Med. 4:563, 1975.

134. O'DUFFY, J. D., CARNEY, J. A., AND DEODHAR, S.: *Behçet's disease. Report of 10 cases, 3 with new manifestations.* Ann. Intern. Med. 75:561, 1971.

135. CHAJEK, T., AND FAINARU, M.: *Behçet's disease. Report of 41 cases and a review of the literature.* Medicine (Baltimore) 54:179, 1975.

136. GALE, A., AND LEVIN, M. E.: *Pericarditis and auricular fibrillation. Occurrence in familial mediterranean fever.* Arch. Intern. Med. 112:234, 1963.

137. RAVIV, U., RUBINSTEIN, A., AND SCHONFELD, A. E.: *Pericarditis in familial mediterranean fever.* Am. J. Dis. Child. 116:442, 1968.

138. SOHAR, E., GAFNI, J., PRAS, M., ET AL.: *Familial mediterranean fever.* Am. J. Med. 43:227, 1967.

139. SOHAR, E., PRAS, M., AND GAFNI, J.: *Familial mediterranean fever and its articular manifestations.* Clin. Rheum. Dis. 1:195, 1975.

140. SCHWABE, A. D., AND PETERS, R. S.: *Familial mediterranean fever in Armenians. Analysis of 100 cases.* Medicine (Baltimore) 53:453, 1974.

141. COHEN, A. S.: *Amyloidosis.* N. Engl. J. Med. 277:522, 1967.

142. BRANDT, K., CATHCART, E. S., AND COHEN, A. S.: *A clinical analysis of the course and prognosis of forty-two patients with amyloidosis.* Am. J. Med. 44:955, 1968.

143. KYLE, R. A., AND BAYRD, E. D.: *Amyloidosis: review of 235 cases.* Medicine (Baltimore) 54:271, 1975.

144. LINDSAY, S.: *The heart in primary systemic amyloidosis.* Am. Heart J. 32:419, 1946.

145. BUJA, L. M., KHOI, N. B., AND ROBERTS, W. C.: *Clinically significant cardiac amyloidosis. Clinico-pathologic findings in 15 patients.* Am. J. Cardiol. 26:394, 1970.

146. CROCKETT, L. K., THOMPSON, M., AND DEKKER, A.: *Case report. A review of cardiac amyloidosis. Report of a case presenting as constrictive pericarditis.* Am. J. Med. Sci. 264:149, 1972.

147. PAULLEY, J. W., BARLOW, K. E., AND CUTTING, P. E. J.: *Acute gouty pericarditis.* Lancet 1:21, 1963.

Neoplastic Pericarditis

Joseph L. Cohen, M.D.

Tumor involvement of the heart and pericardium has been the source of numerous publications dealing with collected experiences and individual case reports in an attempt to describe the magnitude and dimensions of this uncommon clinical problem. DeLoach[1] cites a report of the first case of antemortem diagnosis of cardiac metastases published in 1924. Despite five decades of published experience of tumors involving the heart* and an evolving medical sophistication in the diagnosis of such diseases, only a small percentage of cases are diagnosed antemortem. The incidence of heart metastases among reported autopsy series ranges from 1.5 to 21 percent of patients dying with malignancy.[2, 3, 4, 5, 6, 7]

The reported incidence of heart involvement in patients dying with malignancy seems to have increased in frequency. Data prior to the early part of the 1940s record incidences generally well below 5 percent whereas data since 1945 report incidences between 10 and 20 percent.[2, 7] A report by Harrer,[5] reviewing the experiences at Thomas Jefferson Hospital, Philadelphia, between 1959 and 1969 in comparison with a prior report from the same institution in 1942, revealed an increased incidence of cardiac involvement. Their experience prior to 1942 established an incidence of 5.5 percent as compared with 14.1 percent for autopsies performed on patients with malignancies after 1959.

While it is quite possible that this difference in incidence reflects a longer life span for the cancer patient through various modes of palliative cancer therapy, the data most certainly reflect an improvement in our capacity to treat the complications of malignancy. The availability of antibiotics and other supportive measures during and after World War II has resulted in prolongation of the life of the patient with advanced cancer.

DISTRIBUTION OF PERICARDIAL METASTASES TO THE HEART

The pericardium is the most frequent site of metastatic involvement of the heart. In five reported series of cardiac metastases tabulated in Table 1, pericardial involvement was noted to occur in over 60 percent of the reported cases. The series of 36 cases of lymphoma metastatic to the heart reported by Madianos[10] represents the lowest incidence of pericardial involvement, 39 percent. Cham[9] and Onuigbo[11] both found pericardial involvement without myocardial metastases in approximately three-quarters of

---

*References to the heart will include pericardium since many authors fail to adequately differentiate myocardial from pericardial data. The distinction will be made only where such data exists and is pertinent.

Table 1. Distribution of cardiac metastases

	Pericardium	Myocardium	Both	No. of Cases	Tumor type
Kline[8]	15%	40%	46%	39	mixed
Cham*	74	3	24	38	mixed
Harrer[5]	34	35	31	147	mixed
Madianos[10]	11	62	28	36	lymphoma
Onuigbo[11]	74	0	26	27	lung

*Clinical diagnosis; other autopsy series.

their cases. Such findings have been reported by others,[8] to occur predominantly in association with breast and lung cancer. The detailed report of Onuigbo[11] of metastatic disease to the pericardium arising from primary lung cancer revealed a preponderance of parietal pericardial involvement (19/27 cases) as the only site of cardiac metastases, with an additional four cases involving both visceral and parietal pericardium but only 4 cases in which the visceral pericardium was the sole site of pericardial involvement.

ROUTE OF METASTATIC SPREAD TO THE HEART

There are three potential routes of dissemination of cancer: local extension, lymphatic invasion, and hematogenous spread. Most of the information regarding the route of metastatic involvement of the heart is inferred from the macroscopic and microscopic findings at autopsy. Kline[8] has performed detailed examination of 61 cases with cardiac involvement. Approximately one-half of the carcinoma patients had disease arising in the mediastinum or contiguous structures, primarily lung and breast cancer. The data presented suggests that the predominant route of metastatic spread is via retrograde lymphatic "permeation."[12] The latter term refers to a mode of lymphatic spread in which the tumor cells grow as solid intralymphatic columns in contrast to lymphatic "embolism."

The normal cardiac lymphatic flow arises in the endocardium and interstitial areas of the myocardium forming an initial or capillary lymphatic system. This fine network condenses in collecting lymphatics which lie subjacent to the myocardial fiber. The latter coalesce to form the tertiary level of lymphatic vessels, the lymphatic trunks which flow toward the epicardium through the septal lymphatic system. The subepicardial tissue has a diffuse lymphatic network. It appears that the flow of lymph from the endocardium and interstitium of the myocardium exists via the epicardial lymphatics to the mediastinal collecting system.[13]

Kline[8] found tumor replacement of the mediastinal nodes in all cases of gross cardiac metastases. Cases were observed of only epicardial involvement but there were no instances in this detailed study of myocardial lymphatic involvement without epicardial metastases. In addition, lymphatic dilatation was observed in the areas distal to the site of tumor involvement. These findings suggest that retrograde lymphatic permeation by cancer from involved mediastinal lymph nodes may account for the major pathway of cardiac involvement, certainly in lung and breast cancer, producing obstruction of the cardiac lymphatic system.[11]

Kline[8] was able to find only one case out of 61 malignant metastases to the heart where there was no evidence of mediastinal node involvement. He cites this as the only clear example of hematogenous spread. Six of his 61 cases could have been examples of direct extension as well as retrograde lymphatic permeation. Other authors have suggested that malignant melanoma, leukemia, and sarcomas metastasize to the heart via the blood stream.[14]

MALIGNANT PERICARDIAL EFFUSION

Cohen[6] reported that 22 percent of patients with cardiac involvement with metastatic disease had evidence of pericardial effusion. Thurber[4] found an incidence of 16 percent among the group of 55 cases of symptomatic malignancies of the heart. Experimental studies in the dog have demonstrated that substances placed in the pericardial sac are removed through the same lymphatic pathway described above for the endomyocardial lymphatic system.[15] It appears that the pericardial fluid exits via the subepicardial lymphatics. Additional studies in the dog demonstrated that obstruction of mediastinal lymphatics when coupled with epicardial (coronary sinus obstruction) obstruction produces a pericardial effusion. This laboratory evidence is consistent with the clinico-pathologic findings that: (1) mediastinal lymphatic obstruction does not initiate pericardial effusion despite evidence for resultant pleural effusions, and (2) involvement of the visceral, not the parietal, pericardium produces a pericardial effusion.[10, 16]

CLASSIFICATION OF CARDIAC TUMORS

Although the frequency of heart metastases found at autopsy varies from series to series depending mostly upon the nature of the institution and the patient referral, a range of 0.5 to 4 percent encompasses most large institutional experiences.[2] The same variability is to be expected and is observed when one attempts to establish an autopsy incidence for primary cardiac tumors. Table 2 lists the incidence of primary cardiac tumors in several series. It is apparent that the relative frequencies of primary and secondary cardiac tumors are at least two logs apart.

PRIMARY PERICARDIAL TUMORS (Table 3)

There appears to be an equal frequency of malignant and benign primary pericardial growths.[21] This is in contrast to the larger ratio of malignant tumors arising from myocardial and endocardial tissues.

Stromal tumors are most commonly primary mesotheliomas. This uncommon tumor in some series comprises as much as one half of the institutional experience with primary pericardial tumors.[22, 23] The subject of primary pericardial mesthoeliomas has been reviewed by Anderson,[22] who examined the world literature and was able to document 31 cases reported in the past 14 years. This review combined with the previous report by Mairot[24] of 61 cases published prior to 1960 provides a total of 92 reported primary pericardial mesotheliomas. The actual incidence is probably considerably greater since undoubtedly some cases remain unreported. In addition, the strict criteria established for case acceptability by Anderson[22] excludes an additional 64 alleged case reports since 1960. Major reasons for exclusion included incomplete autopsy information and evidence of penetration of the parietal pericardium or distant metastases. Both

Table 2. Primary cardiac tumors

	No. of autopsies	Incidence of primary cardiac tumors
Strauss[17]	60,000	0.0017%
Fine[18]	40,000	0.0028
Dahlgren[19]	1,000	0.1
Fine[20]	18,300	0.0012
Fine[20]	500,000	0.0022

Table 3. Classification of primary pericardial tumors

1. Stromal	3. Development rest
Fibroma	Intrapericardial bronchogenic cyst
Fibrosarcoma	Teratoma, benign or malignant
Mesothelioma, benign or malignant	Dermoid
Solitary	Thymoma
Diffuse	Thyroid
2. Vascular	Pericardial Cyst
Lymphangioma	4. Miscellaneous
Lymphangioepithelioma	Leiomyoma
Hemangioma	Lipoma
Malignant hemangioepithelioma	Neuroma
Hamartoma	Neurofibroma
	Rhabdomyosarcoma
	Granular cell myoblastoma

considerations were felt by the authors to confuse the issue of whether the described mesothelioma was primary or metastatic.

Patients with pericardial mesothelioma are divided nearly equally between males and females with an average age of 44 years. Reports of cases occurring as early as 1 year of age and as late as 79 years of age have been documented in the literature. The average duration of illness is approximately 5 months although surgical excision has on occasion been successful.

The tumor has been clinically associated with a hemorrhagic effusion in more than two-thirds of the reported cases but cytologic examination is negative in over three-fourths of the cases where specimens have been obtained. In an additional one-fourth of the cases the pericardial sac was obliterated. Reports of constrictive pericarditis secondary to pericardial mesothelioma have been described.[22]

The gross appearance of this tumor presents as either a localized mass or diffuse nodules. When diffuse it may appear as a confluent mass involving the visceral more frequently than the parietal pericardium, but generally both.

The relationship of pericardial mesothelioma to asbestos exposure and pulmonary asbestos is unknown. Obviously, too few cases are available for an epidemiologic study comparable to the pleural and peritoneal investigations.

Brunner[25] has reviewed the issues concerning the difficulty in histologic interpretation of pericardial mesotheliomas. Because of prior failure to recognize that mesotheliomas can assume various microscopic appearances and that elements of epithelioid and mesenchymal (especially fibroblastic) structures can exist in varying proportions, the literature frequently lists several synonyms for mesothelioma including endothelioma, coelothelioma, spindle sarcoma, round cell sarcoma, and giant cell sarcoma. The epithelioid structures can be divided into tubular, papilliform, trabecular, acinar, or solid elements. The World Health Organization (1965) classifies the histologic patterns into three categories: predominantly epithelioid, predominantly fibrous (spindle cell), and biphasic (mixed). About one-third of all cases are predominantly epithelioid and two-thirds mixed, whereas the pure fibrous (spindle) form is uncommon.

There is some doubt regarding the occurrence of a benign form of primary pericardial mesothelioma. Invasion of the myocardium and pericardial sac and frequent lymphatic extension are commonly observed.[22] Metastases have been reported in over one-third of the case reports.[20]

Vascular Tumors

This group of primary pericardial tumors are uncommon and only infrequently produce symptoms. The clinical and pathologic features of these tumors were reviewed in 1973 by Fine.[20]

Developmental Rest Tumors

This category of primary tumors is rare.[26] In a recent review of intrapericardial teratomas 31 reported cases were cited from the world literature, and only 21 cases of intrapericardial bronchogenic cysts were collected.[27] The teratomas are derived from all three germinal layers of the embryo and are equally distributed in males and females with two-thirds of the cases detected prior to one year of age and the rest described in adolescents and adults. This tumor like the other developmental rest tumors has a frequent association with other congenital anomalies. These tumors tend to be symptomatic when occurring in infants but appear generally as incidental asymptomatic findings in the older age groups. Pericardial effusion and tamponade are the most common clinical problems encountered in the infants. The most common pediatric pericardial tumors are mesotheliomas and hemangiomas.[28]

Pericardial cysts are most frequently encountered in adulthood, although pediatric presentation has been reported.[29] In most instances they are asymptomatic although various symptoms normally associated with pericardial disease have been described.[20] They are usually unilocular and located at the right cardiophrenic angle (90 percent), although they have been encountered adjacent to the left and right atrium in 10 percent of the cases. The smooth surface, ovoid shape, and stability of the mass over time are radiologic characteristics of this tumor.[21] The diameters of these cysts have ranged as large as 37 cm.

CANCER METASTATIC TO THE HEART AND PERICARDIUM

Numerically the most significant tumor involvement of the heart and pericardium is metastatic. While virtually every form of malignancy has the potential of metastasizing to the heart, breast and lung cancer primaries have been described as contributing to as much as half of the cases of malignant involvement of the heart.[4]

Table 4 lists the reports of several series of autopsies. The data illustrates the incidence of cardiac metastases for each of the primary sites listed. The series reported by Kline[8] had significant numbers (between 20 to 40 cases each) of cancer of the stomach, uterine cervix, ovary, urinary bladder, liver and bile duct, and endometrium. No metastatic involvement of the heart was noted in association with any of these sites. While cardiac metastases have been reported with these primaries, it is generally true that cancers arising below the diaphragm have a low order of frequency of metastasis to the heart.

Lung cancer is the most frequent cause of cancer in males. In the five autopsy series tabulated in Table 4, a total of 803 cases of lung cancer were examined. There was a total of 176 instances of cardiac metastases in these series for an overall frequency of 22 percent. In the series of 27 cases of lung cancer metastatic to the heart and pericardium reported by Onuigbo,[11] the parietal pericardium was the only area of involvement in 19 instances, the epicardium alone in 4, and both surfaces in 4. Other series generally report a more nearly equal involvement of both pericardial surfaces[7] but the myocardium is rarely the sole cardiac site of metastatic lung cancer. Thurber[4] found that 36 percent of lung cancer patients with pericardial metastases have functionally significant cardiac symptoms, an average slightly higher than his observed average of 29 percent for the series from all primary sites. Because of the proximity of the lung to the heart and the high incidence of mediastinal node involvement, direct extension and/or retrograde lymphatic permeation appear to account for most of the routes of cardiac spread. Mesotheliomas of the lung have also been associated with a high frequency of cardiac metastases.[5]

Carcinoma of the breast is the most frequent cancer in women and, like lung cancer, is associated with a high incidence of mediastinal lymph node involvement in the ad-

Table 4. Incidence of cardiac metastases for various cancer primary sites

	Lung	Breast	Melanoma	Colon/rectum	Head/neck	Sarcoma	Leukemia	Lymphoma	Renal	Pancreas	Esophagus
Kline[8]	20%	12%	(1/3)	2%	12%	7%	24%	8%	(0/8)	(0/34)	(0/19)
Harrer[5]	20	15	24%	2	17	9	20	9	21%	13%	15%
Nakayama[7]	18	25	(6/6)	8	44	–	12	21	(0/5)	–	4
Javier[2]	24	18	47	2	5	15	–	–	10	6	8
Misc. Refs.	27[11]		64[30]				37[31]	17[10]			

vanced cases. The series cited in Table 4 represent 555 autopsies on cases of breast malignancy in which 97 (18 percent) had evidence of heart metastases. Metastases are equally distributed between both the visceral and parietal pericardial tissues,[7] and similar to lung metastases, uncommonly involve the myocardium as a major site of metastatic deposit. The mechanism of spread appears to be identical to carcinoma of the lung. In both instances pericardial metastases have occurred in association with advanced metastatic disease state.[7]

Malignant melanoma tends to disseminate early in its course via the vascular pathways. Multiple nodules are frequently detected in lung, liver, and brain as well as unusual sites of metastatic spread such as bowel and spleen. It is therefore not surprising that this tumor should be associated with a high incidence of cardiac metastases. Unlike breast and lung cancer, however, it has been observed that this tumor frequently is associated with multiple nodules involving the more vascular epicardium and myocardium and less frequently involves the parietal pericardium, the less vascular of the two pericardial surfaces. In Nakayama's small series,[7] one-third of cardiac metastases from malignant melanoma predominantly involved the myocardium.

In contrast to the frequent cardiac metastases associated with lung and breast cancer and malignant melanoma, colorectal carcinomas have been consistently demonstrated to have a low occurrence of cardiac metastases despite the large number of advanced cases encountered. Table 4 presents the cumulative experience with 639 cases of colorectal carcinoma. Only 16 (2.5 percent) of these cases presented with cardiac metastases. This low association has been noted previously by others.[32]

Lymphoma involvement of the heart presents several interesting challenges.[33-39] The differential diagnosis and symptoms of pericarditis will frequently be complicated by a history of prior mediastinal irradiation raising the question of radiation pericarditis. In addition, the urgency of diagnosing lymphoma involvement is related to the radiosensitivity of these tumors and the potential for definitive local control with radiotherapy.[9, 34] Madianos[10] reported Roswell Park Memorial Institute's experience with cardiac metastases from lymphosarcoma and reticulum cell sarcoma and reviewed the reported frequencies of lymphoma metastases in other series. Of 274 cases of lymphosarcoma 51 (19 percent) had cardiac involvement. This compares with 53 (34 percent) of 105 cases of reticulum cell sarcoma and only 25 (10 percent) of 252 of Hodgkin's disease. These figures for incidence are comparable to the review of autopsy experience from the National Cancer Institute.[35] In that series 28 percent of 32 lymphosarcoma cases, 27 percent of 22 reticulum cell sarcoma cases, and 16 percent of 75 Hodgkin's disease autopsies were found to have cardiac metastases. Similar incidences were found for mycosis fungoides (33 percent). In the National Cancer Institute experience, approximately one half of the lymphoma cases had only microscopic metastases.

Both series, Madianos[10] and Roberts,[35] had an identical incidence (17 percent) of pericardial effusion. Myocardium and epicardium involvement was twice as frequent as parietal pericardial metastases. Roberts[35] was able to examine the epicardium and myocardium only and found 18 cases of only myocardial involvement and 23 cases where both tissues were involved. Of the 48 cases 20 had gross evidence of neoplastic pericarditis (6 fibrinous, 7 fibrinofibrous, 7 fibrous), and two others had focal areas of neoplastic pericarditis. It was observed that very few of the symptoms encountered could be attributed to the cardiac involvement. This was especially true for lymphosarcoma and reticulum sarcoma. A similar incidence of signs and symptoms including dyspnea, chest pain, effusions, murmurs, gallops, and ECG changes were noted in the lymphoma patients with or without cardiac involvement. The authors suggest that Hodgkin's disease is the lymphoma most likely to cause symptoms despite its low frequency of cardiac involvement in comparison with the other tumors. Pericardial constriction has been frequently encountered in Hodgkin's disease. In general, only 10 percent of cases of lymphoma involvement of the heart have signs or symptoms directly attributable to the neoplastic pericardial disease.

Signs and Symptoms

The antemortem diagnosis of cardiac metastases is made or suspected in less than 10 percent of autopsy-proven cases.[2, 4, 5, 6] In one series it was estimated that the diagnosis could have been suspected in 75 percent of the cases.[2] Thurber[4] considered that about one-third of 189 cases of cardiac metastases had significant clinical cardiac impairment. Whatever the figure is for symptomatic metastases, it remains considerably greater than the frequency of antemortem diagnosis.

The diagnosis of malignant pericardial involvement requires that the clinician maintain a heightened awareness and suspicion when a cancer patient develops cardiorespiratory signs or symptoms. The clinical setting in nearly all cases is that of a patient with active malignancy known to have metastasized to other organ sites. These other areas of metastic involvement are more frequently intrathoracic than extrathoracic sites.[4]

The most frequently encountered symptoms are those of dyspnea, cough, palpitations, and chest pains (Table 5). The lack of specificity of these symptoms is in part responsible for the infrequent antemortem diagnosis. Acute onset of these symptoms should, however, alert the physician. Other symptoms encountered are orthopnea, dizzy spells, syncope, weakness, and fatigue.

The most common signs noted are those of congestive heart failure, frequently acute in onset and usually minimally responsive to diuretic and cardiac management. Associated pleural effusion (usually bilateral), pulmonary rales, venous distension, hepatomegaly, and peripheral edema appear in approximately 10 to 15 percent of the cases (Table 5). In one retrospective analysis of 100 cases of metastatic cancer patients without cardiac involvement, the author was unable to document any instance of congestive heart failure while the records of 118 patients with cardiac metastases revealed findings of congestive heart failure in 6 percent of the cases.

Thurber[4] listed the causes of congestive heart failure, in order of decreasing frequency, as pericardial effusion, pericardial effusion in association with myocardial metastases, constrictive pericarditis, vascular obstruction, and myocardial metastases occurring alone. In 4 to 10 percent of cases of cardiac metastases, interference with cardiac function is the immediate cause of death.[4, 5]

Other signs less frequently encountered are a paradoxical pulse, new murmurs, dis-

Table 5. Signs and symptoms of cardiac metastases

Symptoms	Javier[2]	Cohen[6]	Harrer[5]	Thurber[4]
Dyspnea	~10%	–	11%	27%
Orthopnea	10	–	–	11
Cough	10	–	–	19
Chest pain	10	–	11	5

Signs				
Pleural effusion	12%	–	25%	15%
CHF	11	39%	33	11
Arrhythmia	13	23	–	7
Pericardial rub	1	2	3	<1
Paradoxical pulse	–	–	–	2
Murmur	4	–	–	3
Pericardial effusion	2	22	20	7
Distant heart sounds	3	–	–	<1

tant heart sounds, Ewart's sign, and arrhythmias frequently consisting of ectopic foci. A surprising observation is that a pericardial friction rub is documented quite infrequently.[4]

Cardiac tamponade occurred twice in 147 cases of cardiac metastases.[5] Conversely, however, Williams[40] reported that 7 out of 17 cases of tamponade were caused by metastatic cancer involving the pericardium. Other unusual complications of cardiac metastases include sudden death (c.f. incidence of arrhythmias, Cohen[6]) and myocardial infarction.[2, 5, 14,] Coronary artery erosion or obstruction has been described in association with epicardial metastases.

Diagnostic Tests

PERICARDIOCENTESIS. Information regarding the details of examination of pericardial fluid are scant. Examination of peritoneal and pleural effusions secondary to malignancy are generally characterized by their protein concentration, lactic acid dehydrogenase activity, glucose concentration, and white and red cell counts.[41] These characteristics help differentiate transudative from exudative effusions. Since causes of pericardial effusion almost invariably lead to an exudative process, such tests have limited value in pericardial disease. A scan of multiple reports of pericardial fluid associated with malignancy suggests that about one-third are serous and the remainder serosanguinous or grossly bloody.[2, 4, 6, 9, 14, 32, 42-49] In 24 of these cases where cytologic examination was reported, there were 11 positive specimens. This low yield of cytology for pericardial effusions contrasts with the report of Zipf,[50] reviewing the Duke experience with pericardial fluid cytology from 47 patients, in which specimens from 13 of 15 confirmed cases of metastatic pericardial effusion were positive. No false positive readings were reported. However, a reading of "suspicious" was made in 20 percent of the confirmed nonmalignant specimens. In most instances the characteristics of the cells obtained from the malignant effusions were sufficiently definitive to suggest a histologic type.

As carcinofetal tumor markers become more generally available, it will be possible to measure these proteins in the serous fluid. One case of metastatic lung carcinoma involving the pericardium was identified by measuring the cancer associated Regan isoenzyme of alkaline phosphatase in the pericardial fluid.[51]

ELECTROCARDIOGRAM. The electrocardiogram abnormalities associated with pericarditis have been extensively reviewed by Spodick.[52] Since in most series epicardial involvement is usually associated with myocardial implants, the spectrum of electrocardiographic abnormalities encompasses all possibilities. Conduction alterations,[9] electrical alternans,[53, 54] arrhythmias[2, 4, 6] (particularly atrial fibrillation), as well as low voltage T-wave abnormalities and ST-T changes have been extensively described in association with pericardial metastases.

RADIOLOGIC EXAMINATION. X-ray examination for neoplastic involvement of the heart has been extensively discussed by Abrams.[21] Pericardial metastases may produce changes in the heart contour and size and in the appearance of the pulmonary vascular bed. Fluoroscopy may indicate an altered cardiac pulsation. In particular, fluoroscopy may demonstrate adequate posterior pulsation, with dampened anteroposterior pulsation because of the tendency for pericardial effusions to accumulate anteriorly.[28] Special radiologic techniques which have been successfully employed to assess pericardial metastases include pneumopericardium[16, 28] and intracardiac CO_2.[16, 55] Angiocardiography is a more sophisticated approach to the diagnosis of pericardial effusion.[28] Shuford[55] compared intracardiac carbon dioxide with angiography in the diagnosis of pericardial effusion and described the pitfalls of both techniques. Pleural effusion which is common in association with malignant pericarditis can, by simulating a pericardial fluid band, interfere with the interpretation of the carbon dioxide study.[55]

Two more recent additions to the radiologist's diagnostic tools are cardiac scanning[32, 56] and echocardiography.[57] Both of these techniques have the advantage of simplicity, negligible morbidity, and a high yield of information regarding the presence of pericardial effusion. Neither of these techniques has the capacity to define detailed anatomic information.

MANAGEMENT OF MALIGNANT PERICARDIAL EFFUSIONS

The selection of the appropriate therapy for carcinomatous pericardial disease is complicated by the nature of the underlying disease state. Usually this complication occurs as a late event in a series of progressive physical deteriorations secondary to the metastatic cancer. As such, the goal of management has been short term palliation, in order to diminish symptoms, through the use of the least debilitating therapeutic procedure. However, with the increase in gains in systemic chemotherapy and hormonal therapy, the prognosis for remission even with advanced disease has become more favorable and more aggressive management can be considered. Smith[48] recently reviewed, retrospectively, the experience of 19 authors in the management of malignant pericardial effusions and concluded that control was more effective with nonsurgical measures than with pleuropericardial window. The mean survival of patients treated without surgery was approximately one year.

Surgical management has included radical pericardiectomy[58] and pleural pericardial window.[44] The window technique is technically simpler and would appear to offer adequate palliation in most conditions where a surgical procedure is indicated. These indications may be summarized as: (1) the presence of a severe constrictive component; (2) failure of control by radiotherapy, intrapericardial therapy, or repetitive pericardiocentesis; and (3) need for histologic documentation of etiology of the effusion.[59]

Pericardiocentesis provides the best form of management of the acute and subacute problem. In addition, the technique provides fluid for cytologic examination and culture and the potential for instillation of intracavitary compounds for more definitive treatment. Reaccumulation of fluid can be managed with repeated taps or with the use of an indwelling pericardial catheter for effective short term control of patients too ill for surgical management.[59] Long term control has been described by several authors following minimal intervention.[4, 59, 60]

Radiotherapy is probably the most frequently employed modality of therapy following the use of pericardiocentesis. Two-thirds of the cases reviewed by Smith[48] were treated with irradiation. Stewart[61] has reviewed the dose-time related tolerance of the heart through data culled from the experience of mediastinal irradiation in Hodgkin's disease and breast cancer. Radiation-induced pericarditis is negligible below 3500 rads generally administered over 28 days.[61, 62] Lymphoma involvement of the pericardium in particular, as well as carcinoma of the lung and breast cancer, is sufficiently radiosensitive to warrant consideration of this approach to the management of carcinomatous pericardial disease.[9, 34] Radiotherapy of lymphomas has produced long term control in some cases and provided control of effusion and reversal of arrhythmias in others.[34, 63] Terry[34] has recommended 1500 to 2000 rads in one and a half to two weeks for the treatment of the radiosensitive lymphomas. Cham[9] achieved improvement with radiotherapy in one-half of the carcinomas, lasting 1 to 36 months.

Intracavitary therapy includes instillation of radioactive colloidal gold (Au^{198})[42, 64, 65] or radioactive phosphorus as chromium phosphate $(CrP^{32}O_4)$.[65] Despite claims of 50 to 60 percent improvement with this therapy, the expense, radiation hazard to personnel handling the isotope, the short half-life $(Au^{198}T_{1/2} = 2.7$ days, $P^{32}T_{1/2} = 14.3$ days), and the availability of drugs capable of producing similar responses have resulted in infrequent use of these radioactive substances.[16, 66, 67]

Drugs which are effective when instilled intrapericardially include nitrogen mustard,[68] thiotepa,[69] 5-fluorouracil,[70] and quinacrine.[48] The use of these intracavitary drugs produces about 50 to 60 percent control of effusion, especially where the carcinomatous involvement of the pericardial surface is limited to small volume of cancer tissue.[16, 66, 67, 71] All, except for quinacrine, are associated with systemic toxicity, particularly marrow suppression, although the toxicity with intracavitary use is considerably less than a comparable dose administered systemically.

Finally, one should not ignore systemic management of the cancer through chemotherapy and hormonal therapy as an effective approach to long term management, particularly lymphomas and breast cancer. Combination chemotherapy has produced 50 to 80 percent complete remissions in advanced lymphomas and 40 to 60 percent remissions in breast cancer.

REFERENCES

1. DeLoach, J. F., and Haynes, J. W.: *Secondary tumors of the heart and pericardium.* Arch. Intern. Med. 91:224, 1953.

2. Javier, B. V., Youut, W. J., Hall, T. C., et al.: *The clinical implications of cardiac metastases from solid tumors. A clinical analysis of 292 cases proved at autopsy.* Neoplasma 14:561, 1967.

3. Scott, R. W., and Garvin, C. F.: *Tumors of the heart and pericardium.* Am. Heart J. 17:431, 1939.

4. Thurber, D. L., Edwards, J. E., and Achor, R. W. P.: *Secondary malignant tumors of the pericardium.* Circulation 26:228, 1962.

5. Harrer, W. V., and Lewis, P. L.: *Metastatic tumors involving the heart and pericardium.* Pa. Med. 74: 57, 1971.

6. Cohen, G. U., Peery, T. M., and Evans, J. M.: *Neoplastic invasion of the heart and pericardium.* Ann. Intern. Med. 42:1238, 1955.

7. Nakayama, R., Yoneyama, T., Takatani, O., et al.: *A study of metastatic tumors to the heart, pericardium and great vessels. Incidences of metastases to the heart, pericardium and great vessels.* Jap. Heart J. 7:227, 1966.

8. Kline, I. K.: *Cardiac lymphatic involvement by metastatic tumor.* Cancer 29:799, 1972.

9. Cham, W. C., Freiman, A. H., Carstens, P. H. B., et al.: *Radiation therapy of cardiac and pericardial metastases.* Radiology 114:701, 1975.

10. Madianos, M., and Sokal, J. E.: *Cardiac involvement in lymphosarcoma and reticulum cell sarcoma.* Am. Heart J. 65:322, 1963.

11. Onuigbo, W. I. B.: *The spread of lung cancer to the heart, pericardium and great vessels.* Jap. Heart J. 15:234, 1974.

12. Onuigbo, W. I. B.: *Cancer permeation: process, problems, and prospects-A review.* Cancer Res. 33: 633, 1973.

13. Kline, I. W.: *Lymphatic pathways in the heart.* Arch. Pathol. 88:638, 1969.

14. Bartecchi, C. E., and Howe, J. J.: *Cardiogenic shock.* Rocky Mt. Med. J. 68:51, 1971.

15. Miller, A. J.: *Some observations concerning pericardial effusions and their relationship to the venous and lymphatic circulation of the heart.* Lymphology 3:76, 1970.

16. Lokich, J. J.: *The management of malignant pericardial effusions.* J.A.M.A. 224:1401, 1973.

17. Strauss, R., and Merliss, R.: *Primary tumors of the heart.* Arch. Path. 39:74, 1945.

18. Fine, G.: *Neoplasms of the pericarcium and heart,* in Gould, S. E.: (ED): *Pathology of the Heart.* Charles C Thomas, Springfield, Ill., 1960.

19. Dahlgren, S., and Nordenstrom, B.: *Primary fibrous hamartoma of the heart.* Acta Pathol. Microbiol. Scand. 63:355, 1965.

20. Fine, G.: *Primary tumors of the pericardium and heart.* Cardiovasc. Clin. 5(1):208, 1973.

21. Abrams, H. L., Adams, D. F., and Grant, H. A.: *The radiology of tumors of the heart.* Radiol. Clin. No. Am. 9(2):299, 1971.

22. Anderson, J. A., and Hansen, B. F.: *Primary pericardial mesothelioma.* Danish Med. Bull. 21:195, 1974.

23. Argianas, E., Mellisinos, K., Drivas, G., et al.: *Mesothelioma of the pericardium with cholesterol pericarditis.* Angiology 25:297, 1974.

24. MAIROT, A.: *Contribution a l'etude des tumeurs primitives due pericarde.* Combier Macon. 1960.

25. BRUNNER, P.: *Papillary-polypous mesothelioma of the pericardium of a dog (at the same time a contribution to the question as to primary tumors arising from serous cover cells).* Virchows Arch. Abt. A. Pathol. Anat. 357:275, 1972.

26. HEATH, D.: *Pathology of cardiac tumors.* Am. J. Cardiol. 21:315, 1968.

27. DEENADAYALU, R. P., TUURI, D., DEWALL, R. A., ET AL.: *Intrapericardial teratoma and bronchogenic cyst.* J. Thorac. Cardiovasc. Surg. 67:945, 1974.

28. STOLZ, J. L., BORNS, P., AND SCHWADE, J.: *The pediatric pericardium.* Radiology 112:159, 1974.

29. LILLIE, W. I., McDONALD, J. R., AND CLAGETT, O. I.: *Pericardial coelomic cysts and pericardial diverticulae: concept of etiology and report of case.* J. Thorac. Surg. 20:494, 1950.

30. GLANCY, D. L., AND ROBERTS, W. C.: *The heart in malignant melanoma.* Am. J. Cardiol. 21:555, 1968.

31. ROBERTS, W. C., BODEY, G. P., AND WERTLAKE, P. T.: *The heart in acute leukemia. A study of 420 autopsy cases.* Am. J. Cardiol. 21:388, 1968.

32. STEINER, R. M., BULL, M. I., KUMPEF, F., ET AL.: *The diagnosis of intracardiac metastases of colon carcinoma by radioisotopic and roentgenographic studies.* Am. J. Cardiol. 26:300, 1970.

33. HAGANS, J. A.: *Hodgkin's granuloma with pericardial effusion.* Am. Heart J. 40:624, 1950.

34. TERRY, L. N., AND KLIGERMAN, M. M.: *Pericardial and myocardial involvement by lymphomas and leukemias. The role of radiotherapy.* Cancer 25:1003, 1970.

35. ROBERTS, W. C., GLANCY, D. L., AND DeVITA, V. T.: *Heart in malignant lymphoma (Hodgkin's disease, lymphosarcoma, reticulum cell sarcoma and mycosis fungoides).* Am. J. Cardiol. 22:85, 1968.

36. JAKOB, H. G., AND ZIRKIN, R. M.: *Hodgkin's disease with involvement of the heart and pericardium.* J.A.M.A. 73:82, 1960.

37. *Case 49-1974. Case Records of the Massachusetts General Hospital. Weekly Clinicopathological Exercises.* New Engl. J. Med. 291:1297, 1974.

38. BYHARDT, R., BRACE, K., RUCKDESCHEL, J., ET AL.: *Dose and treatment factors in radiation-related pericardial effusion associated with the mantle technique for Hodgkin's disease.* Cancer 35:795, 1975.

39. GLICKMAN, A. S., AND NICKSON, J. J.: *Acute and late reactions to irradiation in the treatment of Hodgkin's disease.* Arch. Intern. Med. 131:369, 1973.

40. WILLIAMS, C., AND SOUTTER, L.: *Pericardial tamponade: diagnosis and treatment.* AMA Arch. Intern. Med. 94:571, 1954.

41. LIGHT, R. W., MacGREGOR, M. I., LUCHSINGER, P. C., ET AL.: *Pleural effusions: the diagnostic separation of transudates and exudates.* Ann. Intern. Med. 77:507, 1972.

42. BACHMAN, K. P., FOSTER, C. G., JACKSON, M. A., ET AL.: *Radioactive gold instilled intrapericardially: report of a case.* Arch. Intern. Med. 40:811, 1954.

43. CHIA, B. L., DaCOSTA, J. L., AND RANSOME, G. A.: *Cardiac tamponade due to leukaemic pericardial effusion.* Thorax 28:657, 1973.

44. HILL, G. J., AND COHEN, B. I.: *Pleural pericardial window for palliation of cardiac tamponade due to cancer.* Cancer 26:81, 1970.

45. KUSNOOR, V. S., D'SOUZA, R. S., BHANDARKAR, S. D., ET AL.: *Case Reports: Malignant pericardial effusion.* J. Assoc. Physicians India 21:101, 1973.

46. McFADDEN, R. R., AND DAWSON, P. J.: *Adenocarcinoma arising in a Ghon complex presenting with massive pericardial effusion.* Chest 62:520, 1972.

47. MISCIA, V. F., HOLSINGER, J. W., MATHERS, D. H., ET AL.: *Primary pericardial tumor masquerading as constrictive pericarditis.* J.A.M.A. 230:722, 1974.

48. SMITH, F. E., LANE, M., AND HUDGINS, P. T.: *Conservative management of malignant pericardial effusion.* Cancer 33:47, 1974.

49. THIJS, L. G., KROON, T. A. J., AND VAN LEEUWEN, TH. M.: *Leiomyosarcoma of the pulmonary trunk associated with pericardial effusion.* Thorax 29:490, 1974.

50. ZIPF, R. E., AND JOHNSTON, W. W.: *The role of cytology in the evaluation of pericardial effusions.* Chest 62:593, 1972.

51. STOLBACH, L. L.: *Clinical application of alkaline phosphatase isoenzyme analysis.* Ann. N.Y. Acad. Sci. 166:760, 1969.

52. SPODICK, D. H.: *Differential diagnosis of acute pericarditis.* Prog. Cardiovasc. Dis. 14:192, 1971.

53. McGREGOR, M., AND BASKIND, E.: *Electric alternans in pericardial effusion.* Circulation 11:837, 1955.

54. WHEELER, R. C., AND ABELMANN, W. H.: *Cardiomyopathy associated with systemic disease.* Cardiovasc. Clin. 4(1):284, 1972.

55. SHUFORD, W. H., SYBERS, R. G., ACKER, J. J., ET AL.: *A comparison of carbon dioxide and radiopaque angiocardiographic methods in the diagnosis of pericardial effusion.* Radiology 86:1064, 1966.

56. CHARKES, N. D., AND SKLAROFF, D. M.: *Radioisotope photoscanning as a diagnostic aid in cardiovascular disease.* J.A.M.A. 186:134, 1963.

57. SOULEN, R. L., LAPAYOWKER, M. S., AND GIMENEZ, J. L.: *Echocardiography in the diagnosis of pericardial effusion.* Radiology 86:1047, 1966.

58. ITURRINO, J. L., AND HOLLAND, R. H.: *The emergency surgical management of acute pericarditis.* J. Thorac. Cardiovasc. Surg. 45:324, 1963.

59. FLANNERY, E. P., GREGORATOS, G., AND CORDER, M. P.: *Pericardial effusions in patients with malignant disease.* Arch. Intern. Med. 135:976, 1975.

60. HIRSH, D. M., NYDICK, I., AND FARROW, I. H.: *Malignant pericardial effusion secondary to metastatic breast carcinoma. A case of long term remission.* Cancer 19:1296, 1966.

61. STEWART, J. R., AND FAJARDO, L. F.: *Dose reponse in human and experimental radiation-induced heart disease.* Radiology 99:403, 1971.

62. STEWART, J. R., COHN, K. E., FAJARDO, L. F., ET AL.: *Radiation-induced heart disease.* Radiology 89: 302, 1967.

63. STEINBERG, I.: *Angiography in diagnosis of pericardial effusion and pulmonary stenosis in Hodgkin's disease.* Am. J. Roentgenol. 102:619, 1968.

64. ROSE, R. G.: *Intracavitary radioactive colloidal gold: results in 257 cancer patients.* J. Nucl. Med. 3: 323, 1962.

65. O'BRYAN, R. M., TALLEY, R. W., BRENNAN, M. J., ET AL.: *Critical analysis of the control of malignant effusions with radioisotopes.* Henry Ford Hosp. Med. J. 16:3, 1968.

66. DOLLINGER, M. R.: *Management of recurrent malignant effusions.* Cancer 22:138, 1972.

67. ROSATO, F. E., WALLACH, M. W., AND ROSATO, E. F.: *The management of malignant effusions from breast cancer.* J. Surg. Oncol. 6(5):441, 1974.

68. WEISBERGER, A. S.: *Direct instillation of nitrogen mustard in the management of malignant effusions.* N.Y. Acad. Sci. 68:1091, 1958.

69. ULTMANN, J. E., HYMAN, G. A., CRANDALL, C., ET AL.: *Triethylenethiophosphoramide (thio-TEPA) in the treatment of neoplastic disease.* Cancer 10:902, 1957.

70. SUHRLAND, L. G., AND WEISBERGER, A. S.: *Intracavity 5-Fluorouracil in malignant effusions.* Arch. Intern. Med. 116:431, 1965.

71. FARBER, L. R.: *Correctable complications of neoplastic disease: III. Neoplastic effusions.* Conn. Med. 35:411, 1971.

Congenital Diseases of the Pericardium

William K. Nasser, M.D.

Congenital malformations of the pericardium, according to Edwards,[1] can be classified as follows: (1) defect or absence of the pericardium or (2) cysts, diverticulum, and benign teratoma of the pericardium.

DEFECTS OR ABSENCE OF THE PERICARDIUM

Congenital pericardial defects are uncommon and can be classified embryologically into those due to deficiency in the development of the pleuropericardium which includes partial defects (foramen type) and complete absence of the pericardium, and those due to deficiency in the development of the pericardioperitoneal communication.

Defects in the Pleuropericardium

Until recent years, the diagnosis of absence of the pericardium, partial or complete, had rarely been made prior to postmortem examination or thoracotomy. There are presently approximately 153 cases reported in the literature.[2]

History

M. Realdus Columbus[3] is credited with the first reported case in 1559. However, the first unquestionable example of this condition was reported by Baille in 1793.[4] In 1936, Ladd[5] was the first to diagnose an antemortem case when he accidentally discovered absence of the left pericardium during repair of a diaphragmatic hernia.

In 1937, Dahl[6] inferred the presence of a communication between the pericardial space and left pleural space after artificial pneumothorax which resulted in pneumopericardium in a young man being treated for bilateral exudative pulmonary tuberculosis. In 1938, Southworth and Stevenson[7] were first to describe adequate clinical findings in their excellent postmortem description. However, it was not until 1959 that Ellis and coworkers[8] described the characteristic roentgenologic findings on plain chest radiographs and diagnostic pneumothorax. In 1960, Dimond and associates[9] described the first case of partial defect diagnosed by cineangiography which demonstrated herniation of the left atrial appendage through a foramen in the pericardium. Since that time, an increasing number of cases have been reported in the literature.

Incidence

The rarity of this anomaly is indicated by the fact that only 2 instances were encountered by Versé in 13,000 autopsies[10] and only one by Southworth and Stevenson in 14,000 autopsies at the Johns Hopkins Hospital.[7] According to Saint Pierre and Froement,[2] who collected 153 cases of pericardial defect, the percentage of each variety was as follows: total absence of the pericardium, 9 percent; left-sided defects, partial 35 percent, total 35 percent; right-sided defects, partial 4 percent, total 0 percent; diaphragmatic pericardial aplasia, 17 percent.

Etiology

The etiology of this congenital defect is unknown. Embryologic evidence suggests that pleuropericardial defects of the pericardium may result from premature atrophy of the left duct of Cuvier, resulting in a compromised vascular circulation to the pleuropericardial membrane which would eventually become the left pericardium.[11] Support for this theory is based on postmortem studies[7] showing that congenital pleuropericardial defects almost invariably involved the entire left side of the heart. Right-sided lesions and total defects of the pericardium are extremely rare (vida supra).

Associated Cardiac Defects

Associated congenital anomalies of the heart and lungs such as patent ductus arteriosus,[12-18] atrial septal defects,[19, 20] mitral stenosis,[16, 21, 22] tetralogy of Fallot,[23] bronchogenic cysts,[24-28] pulmonary sequestration,[29, 30] and tricuspid insufficiency[31] occur in approximately one third of the reported cases. Deficiency of the pericardium has a male to female ratio of approximately 3 to 1.

Symptoms and Physical Findings

Most of the reported cases of patients with pleuropericardial defects but without associated cardiac anomalies have been asymptomatic.[8, 32] However, symptoms may occur. The most common symptom is a vague nonspecific chest pain; dyspnea, dizziness, and syncope have occasionally been present. It has been suggested that chest pain may be attributed to the following:[19] (1) undue torsion or strain on the great vessels which serve as the only anchor for the heart, (2) lack of cushioning effect of the pericardium, (3) tension on the pleuropericardial adhesions, and (4) pressure of the rim of remaining pericardium on cardiac vessels.

This latter factor is well demonstrated in a case report by Lajos and coworkers[33] in which the left anterior descending coronary artery had a localized area of narrowing precisely beneath the anterior rim of the pericardial defect. This was demonstrated angiographically and was confirmed by operative intervention.

Figure 1 demonstrates localized narrowing of the left anterior descending coronary artery in a 50-year-old white woman who presented to our hospital with fairly typical angina pectoris. The circumflex and right coronary arteries were angiographically free of atheromatous disease. Despite the lack of response to optimum medical management, she refused surgical intervention. This case is also felt to represent an example of localized narrowing in the anterior descending coronary artery secondary to compression by the fibrous rim of the anterior pericardial defect, especially since the remaining coronary vessels did not reveal evidence for atheromatous changes.

Physical findings are not usually helpful. Systolic ejection murmurs, noted in most patients, are generally heard at the second interspace along the left sternal border. These

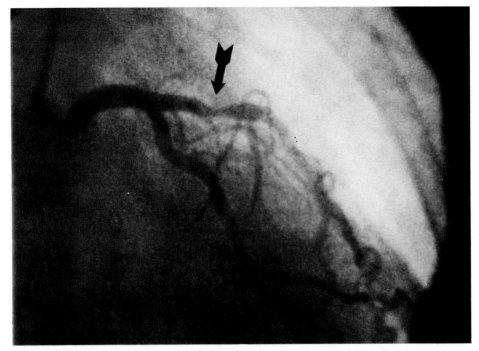

Figure 1. Arteriography demonstrates localized narrowing of the left anterior descending coronary artery in a 50-year-old white woman with fairly typical angina pectoris. The area of localized narrowing is felt to be secondary to compression by the fibrous rim of the anterior pericardial defect, especially since the circumflex and right coronary arteries are angiographically free of atheromatous disease.

murmurs may be the result of turbulence set up by various mechanical deformities at the base of an unusually mobile heart.[8] Precordial activity may be conspicuous and the apical impulse may be shifted to the left, especially in pericardial deficiency of the entire left side. Unusual mobility of the heart was demonstrated in one patient with marked posterior rotation of the heart in which the apical impulse was palpable medial to the left scapula.[34] Pectus excavatum deformities may be present. Aside from these few observations, the physical findings are dependent upon the underlying cardiac disorder.

Electrocardiographic Changes

ECG alterations usually reflect the unusual intrathoracic position of the heart which is permitted by absence of the restraining pericardium.[35] Electrocardiographic abnormalities are more commonly seen in cases of complete left pericardial defects and usually consist of right axis deviation, incomplete right bundle branch block pattern, and leftward displacement of the transition zone in the precordial leads.[12, 14, 35] Sinus bradycardia is not an uncommon finding. Complete heart block, presumably congenital, was reported in a single patient.[36]

Differential Diagnosis

The differential diagnosis of a left-sided pericardial defect is usually based on lesions causing prominence of the left hilum, pulmonary artery, or both. Mimicking lesions in-

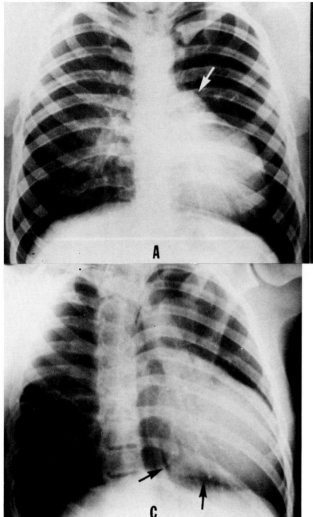

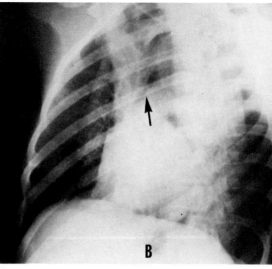

Figure 2. Roentgenograms in posteroanterior (A), left anterior oblique (B), and right anterior oblique (C) views of a patient with complete absence of the left pericardium. A, The heart is shifted to the left (levo position), the right heart border is hidden by the spine, the trachea is in the midline, the pulmonary artery segment is prominent (arrow), and there is interposition of the lung between the left hemidiaphragm and inferior border of the heart. B, The arrow points to a "tongue" of lung separating the aorta and main pulmonary artery. The arrows point to interposition of the lung between the left hemidiaphragm and inferior border of the heart. (From Nassar, et al.[44] with permission.)

clude aneurysm, tumor of the lung or heart, mitral valve disease, atrial septal defect, pulmonary stenosis, idiopathic dilatation of the pulmonary artery, and hilar lymphadenopathy. It is essential to correctly diagnose complete left-sided pericardial defects since these conditions are usually benign in the absence of associated disease of the heart or lungs, and the patient is spared a needless thoracotomy.

X-Ray Findings

Roentgenologic findings are usually characteristic when the left side of the pericardium is completely absent. These findings include the following: levoposition of the heart associated with midline trachea, prominence of the pulmonary artery segment, an indistinct right heart border that is usually hidden by the spine, a "tongue" of lung projecting between the aorta and pulmonary artery, and interposition of lung between the left hemidiaphragm and inferior border of the heart (Fig. 2).

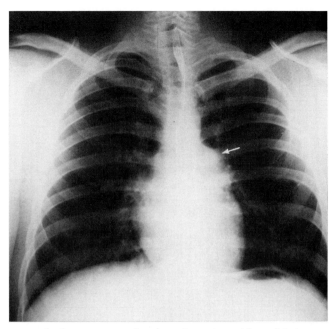

Figure 3. Roentgenograms in the posteroanterior view of a patient with partial absence of the left pericardium. The arrow indicates prominence of the upper left heart border representing the pulmonary artery and left atrial appendage in the absence of levo position of the cardiac silhouette. (From Nasser, et al.[47] with permission.)

In partial pericardial defects, the heart is usually in its normal position and the abnormality consists of prominence of the pulmonary artery, left atrial appendage, or both (Fig. 3). Cineangiography, demonstrating herniation of the left atrial appendage beyond the left heart border (Fig. 4) is considered diagnostic of partial absence of the left side of the pericardium by several authors.[32, 37-41] This procedure is usually not diagnostic for complete left-sided pericardial defects.

Pneumopericardium, after the induction of artificial pneumothorax, has been considered the procedure of choice for the diagnosis of complete absence of the left side of the pericardium (Fig. 5). However, since the x-ray findings are so strikingly similar, some authors[19, 20, 39] feel that diagnostic pneumothorax, with its possible hazards, may no longer be necessary to establish the diagnosis. Also, the absence of pneumopericardium after artificial pneumothorax does not rule out absence of the pericardium since, in some cases, adhesions could conceivably prevent the accumulation of air in the pericardial space.[8, 14, 18, 20, 39]

Prognosis

Disturbance of normal cardiac function does not appear to occur in patients with complete pleuropericardial defects. This observation is suggested by normal heart catheterization studies in many of these patients[8, 19, 20, 32, 42-44] without intrinsic disease of the heart or lungs. However, three reports have been published of sudden death due to herniation and strangulation of the heart through a partial pericardial defect.[37, 45, 46] In a hemodynamic study involving 6 patients (two with partial and four with complete left-sided defects), it was noted that all 6 patients had normal resting intracardiac pressures.[47] However, the 2 patients with partial pericardial defects had elevation of the

275

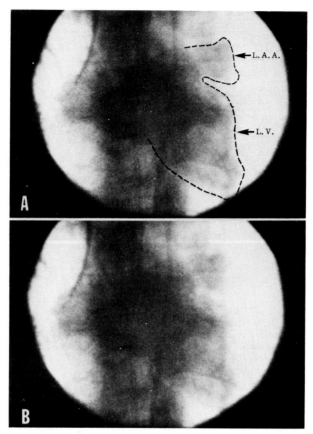

Figure 4. Radiopaque contrast medium is injected into the right atrium. Cineangiogram with follow through of dye to the left side demonstrates herniation of the left atrial appendage (LAA) through a pericardial foramen (A). B represents the same frame (not outlined). LV = left ventricle. (From Nasser, et al.[47] with permission.)

pulmonary artery and left ventricular end-diastolic pressures during mild exercise in the recumbent position, which suggests that this type of defect is not totally innocuous. These authors concluded "in view of the unusual and extreme cardiac mobility of this condition, it is conceivable that a portion of the heart could herniate and transiently incarcerate through the partial pericardial defect during exercise."

Treatment

Surgical intervention for partial pericardial defects has been undertaken in recent years in an attempt to relieve symptoms and prevent herniation and strangulation of the left atrium and ventricle through the defect. The presence of symptoms and the possibility of sudden death in partial defects, accompanied by angiographic evidence of herniation of the left atrial appendage through a pericardial foramen, argues strongly for surgical correction of this lesion.[14, 18, 32, 47-50]

A 45-year-old white woman with a partial pericardial defect was admitted to our hospital with complaints of vague chest discomfort and dyspnea. Cardiac catheterization revealed normal resting intracardiac pressures. During mild exercise in the recumbent position, there was elevation of the pulmonary artery, pulmonary capillary wedge, left

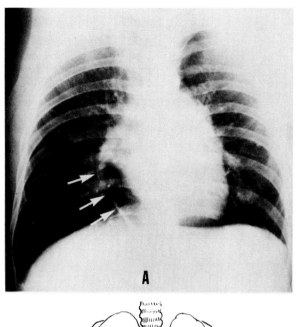

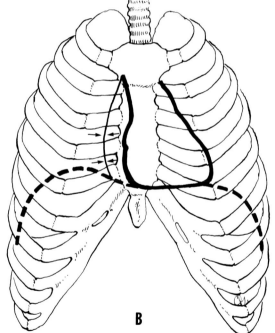

Figure 5. Diagnostic pneumothorax after the injection of 500 ml. of air into the left pleural space. In the left lateral decubitus view of the chest (A), pneumopericardium is produced and the right pleural pericardium (arrows) is outlined against air in the right lung. B is a line drawing of A. (From Nasser, et al.[44] with permission.)

atrial and left ventricular end-diastolic pressures. Her coronary arteriograms were normal. Because of our previous experience,[47] surgical intervention was recommended. Her partial pericardial defect was extended (Fig. 6). Although the patient has not had repeat cardiac catheterization, she is symptomatically improved.

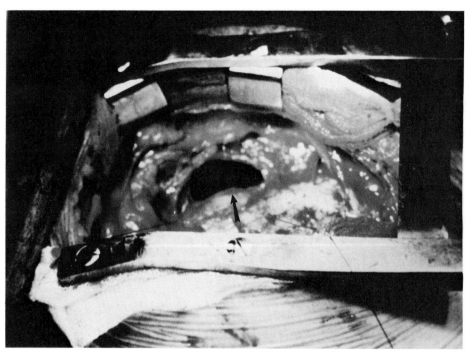

Figure 6. An example of partial pericardial defect (arrow) as viewed at surgery in a 45-year-old white woman. The partial pericardial defect was extended.

Conclusion

Absence of the pleuropericardium is not as rare as once believed. This entity can and should be diagnosed during life.[51] The clinician, surgeon, and radiologist should be aware of the possibility of this condition.

Defects in the Diaphragmatic Pericardium

Congenital defects in the diaphragmatic portion of the pericardium are extremely rare. These defects are the result of a deficiency in the development of the pericardio-peritoneal communication.

In 1958, Cantrell and associates[52] established the following criteria for this syndrome of five associated anomalies: (1) mid-line supraumbilical abdominal defect; (2) defect of the lower sternum; (3) deficiency of the diaphragmatic pericardium; (4) deficiency of the anterior diaphragm; (5) congenital intracardiac abnormality.

Crittenden and coworkers[53] in 1959 expanded upon the syndrome by including the feature of malrotation of the heart with dextroposition. One year later, the same authors[54] described left ventricular diverticulum in three additional cases and concluded that a left ventricular diverticulum was a definite component of this syndrome rather than an incidental anomaly as previously suspected.

The most critical abnormality of this entity appears to be a defect in the anterior diaphragm which is contributed embryologically by the septum transversum. Because of the close contact of the diaphragmatic pericardium to the septum transversum, a defect in this portion of the pericardium occurs in nearly all cases. Therefore, the majority of

278

patients with this striking syndrome will have defects of the ventral diaphragm and basilar pericardium. The occurrence of this syndrome has been confirmed by a number of authors.[55-66]

The prognosis is usually dependent upon the extent of the omphalocele and the severity of the underlying cardiac abnormality. Because the lesion is potentially curable and often fatal, surgical correction when possible would appear to be the treatment of choice.[59, 60, 63, 64, 67, 68]

CONGENITAL PERICARDIAL CYSTS AND DIVERTICULA

An extensive review of the literature reveals considerable confusion concerning the topic of congenital pericardial cysts and diverticula. The first and major aspect of controversy involves a difference in description of the two entities. By definition, a diverticulum of the pericardium should contain all of the layers of the pericardium and communicate freely with the pericardial cavity. A "true" cyst is usually encapsulated and should not communicate directly with the pericardial cavity. Lillie, in an excellent monograph,[69] believes that persistence of the ventral parietal recess results in a pericardial celomic cyst when it is "pinched off" from the pericardium, and a pericardial diverticulum when it remains connected with pericardial cavity (Table 1).

Another major source of confusion occurs when authors use the term pericardial cyst and pericardial diverticulum interchangeably within the same manuscript in a discussion of the same patient. In recent literature, authors refer to pericardial cysts when they are discussing this topic. For this reason, and since pericardial diverticulum is clinically indistinguishable from a pericardial cyst, discussion in this chapter will consider the two as a single entity.

A host of terms have been used to describe pericardial cysts. Most are descriptive of the site, contents, or histology. Other terms imply a conception of pathogenesis. Some of the terms used are hydrocele of the mediastinum, serosal cyst, spring-water cyst,[70] pleuropericardial cysts,[71] pericardial celomic cysts,[72] mesothelial mediastinal cysts,[73] and pericardial diverticulum.[74, 75] Since nomenclature appears to be another source of confusion, this discussion will be concerned with congenital pericardial cysts in an effort to avoid more confusion.

History

In 1934, Pickhardt[76] was the first to describe the successful removal of a congenital pericardial cyst. Prior to this report, cysts were occasionally recorded as chance findings at necropsy.[77-81] Kienböck and Weiss, in 1934, described the radiographic appearances of a pericardial cyst.[82] An occasional report of pericardial cysts appeared in the literature.[83-90]

Table 1. Lesions which may result when the ventral parietal process persists

Embryonic condition	Resultant lesion
1. The ventral parietal process persists intact	1. Diverticulum of pericardium with wide base
2. Proximal portion constricted	2. Diverticulum of pericardium with narrow base
3. Proximal portion completely constricted	3. Cysts with pedicle which extends to pericardium
4. Completely pinched off	4. Cysts in the cardiophrenic angle
5. Completely pinched off and left cephalad as the septum transversum moves caudally	5. Mesothelial-lined cysts found higher in the mediastinum than the cardiophrenic angle

In 1940, Lambert[72] reviewed the literature, added three more cases, and suggested a theory for pathogenesis. Following this report, several authors became interested in the subject and described their findings in detail.[91-117]

Incidence

Despite the rarity of this entity, there are approximately 130 cases reported.[1] One in 3400 admissions to Johns Hopkins Hospital over an 8 year period of time was for a primary tumor or cyst of the mediastinum.[118] During this period, 101 tumors were recognized and 2 of these were pericardial cysts (2 percent). Of all congenital thoracic cysts, it has been found that the proportion of congenital pericardial cysts comprises between 4 and 7 percent. Rubush and coworkers[119] reported 186 cases of mediastinal tumors. Of these patients, 34 (18.3 percent) had tumors of the middle mediastinum. They concluded that the most frequently encountered tumor of the middle mediastinum was a congenital pericardial cyst (8 patients). In 1952, Loehr[120] classified pericardial cysts into true, acquired, and pseudocysts, but no figures are available on the incidence of congenital pericardial cysts as compared with other types, that is, inflammatory and so forth.

An incidence of three pericardial cysts among 300,000 people was found in a mass x-ray program in Edinburg in 1958.[121] From these figures, it has been estimated that approximately 1 in every 100,000 people in the population at large may have a pericardial cyst.[121]

Etiology

The etiology of pericardial cysts is unknown. Several theories have been proposed. Three major theories appear repeatedly in the literature.

LACUNAR THEORY.[72] The pericardium is derived from a number of lacunae or spaces which form in the cephalad region of the embryo. These lacunae later join to form the primitive pericardial celom. Failure of union of one or more of the lacunae would be manifested in later life as a diverticulum.

VENTRAL PARIETAL RECESS THEORY.[69] This theory presupposes that persistence of a ventral recess results in a pericardial celomic cyst when it is "pinched off" from the pericardium, and a pericardial diverticulum when it remains connected to the pericardial cavity.

CONGENITAL WEAKNESS THEORY.[84] This theory suggests that a potential weakness in the pericardium exists where vessels and nerves enter the pericardium. An increase in such weakness would lead to a pericardial diverticulum or cyst.

There are statements for and against each theory. LeRoux[121] favored the ventral parietal recess theory. He states, "If this theory is correct, it is felt that a relationship is established between the pericardial celomic cysts and diverticulum of the pericardium which are of developmental and not of inflammatory origin. This theory has the advantages that it is based upon the existence of a definite embryologic structure at a fairly advanced stage of development; and it explains the existence of cysts in the costophrenic angle, where they are most common." Therefore, it seems justifiable, according to this author, to refer to these as "pericardial celomic cysts".

Edwards and Ahmad[122] concluded that a satisfactory explanation of the development of a pericardial cyst from the visceral pericardium is best afforded by Lambert's lacunar theory of failed coalescence of pericardial lacunae. They felt that this theory is acceptable for the etiology of pericardial cysts, both inside and outside the pericardial cavity.

Pathology

Congenital true pericardial cysts may be celomic (mesodermal), lymphangiomatous, bronchial, or teratomatous.

The cyst is usually unilocular, round, or ellipsoid, but may on occasions be multilocular. They may or may not be pedunculated and may vary in size. The weight ranges between 100 and 300 gm. One unusual case[108] revealed a cyst which contained 1 liter of fluid and measured 25×37 cm. The fluid is usually clear and has been compared to rock-water, hence the name spring-water cyst. Biochemically, the fluid is a transudate rather than lymph or exudate.

The cysts are composed of fibrous connective tissue, lined by a single layer of flat cells similar to serosal and endothelial cells.

Clinical Manifestations

Most cases are asymptomatic. When symptoms are present, chest discomfort is the most common presenting complaint. This is usually described as a tightness, aching, or pain in the chest. Dyspnea and cough have also been reported. Occasional patients have presented with hemoptysis, atelectasis, palpitations, and venous obstruction.

Pericardial cysts occur with a male to female ratio of approximately 3 to 2. Cysts have been reported at all ages from early adolescence to an advanced age. The majority of these cysts have been detected in the fourth decade of life.

Diagnosis

Pericardial cysts are usually found during the course of a routine chest x-ray in an asymptomatic patient. The cyst usually presents as a mass on either side of the cardiac silhouette. These are usually located in the costophrenic angles. Most cysts occur on the right side but they are not infrequently left-sided. When a chest x-ray reveals tumor to be present in the right or left supradiaphragmatic area in communication with the cardiac silhouette, a pericardial cyst should always be suspected. Malignant tumors are usually located higher in the mediastinum, frequently in the posterior mediastinum. Thyroid or thymic cysts are found in the anterosuperior mediastinum.

Sometimes the cysts (or diverticula) alter their shape or size by variations in respiration or posture of the patient, that is, positions favoring drainage of the diverticula into the pericardial cavity.[121] The cardiac flouroscopist will note a sharply-outlined or lobulated, semi-circular, oval, or polygonal area protruding from the cardiac silhouette. This may or may not pulsate with changes in the cardiac cycle. Calcification in these cysts may develop after many years.

Some authors have suggested needle aspiration of the contents and/or injection of air directly into the cyst.[123] In the past, authors have advocated the creation of a pneumothorax or pneumoperitoneum by injecting air and placing the patient in the Trendelenburg position. An x-ray at that time should theoretically enable the physician to determine whether the tumor has an intra- pulmonary or extrapulmonary location. These tests are of little diagnostic value and may be hazardous. Most recent authorities have advocated exploratory thoracotomy when a pericardial cyst is suspected.

Differential Diagnosis

The differential diagnosis includes a mass lesion in the thorax that closely approximates the cardiac silhouette. Congenital thoracic cysts involve the thyroid, thymus,

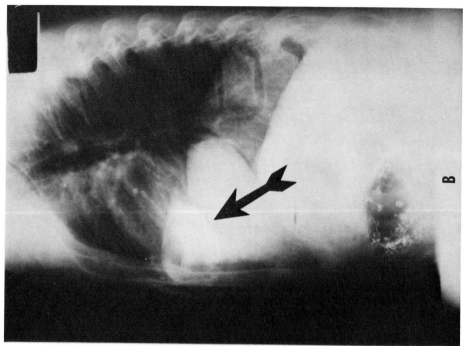

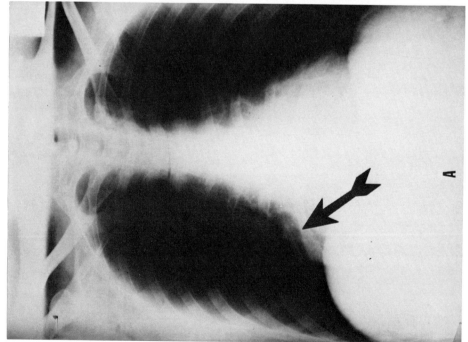

Figure 7. Posteroanterior (A) and lateral (B) views of a right pericardial cyst. The arrows point to the pericardial cyst. (With the kind permission of Dr. Eugene Klatte, Chairman, Department of Radiology, Indiana University School of Medicine.)

esophagus, gastric, pulmonary, bronchus, or lymph tissue. Cystic hygromas are usually multilocular. A Morgagni hernia, in its usual location, may closely simulate a pericardial cyst. Thoracic tumors, malignant or benign, must also be differentiated. Cardioangiography may be of value in ruling out a ventricular aneurysm.

Treatment

The major significance of a pericardial cyst or diverticulum is that it mimics a mediastinal tumor. Thus, surgical exploration is likely to be necessary to provide a definitive diagnosis.[75, 120] The operation is simple, and the morbidity and mortality are extremely low.[121] Patients with symptoms may experience marked improvement postoperatively.

From a prognostic standpoint, a complete review of the literature fails to disclose a single episode of recurrence following surgical extirpation of a pericardial cyst or diverticulum.

REFERENCES

1. EDWARDS, J., in GOULD, S. E. (ED.): *Pathology of the Heart and Blood Vessels*, ed. 3. Charles C Thomas, Springfield, Ill., 1968.

2. SAINT PIERRE, A., AND FROEMENT, R.: *Absenes totales et partielles du péricarde*. Arch. Mal. Coeur. 63:638, 1970.

3. COLUMBUS (MATTHEAUES REALDUS) (1494–1559): *De re anatomica Libre XV. 3 p. 1, 269 pp 1 1.4°*. Venetiis, ex typog N. Beuilacquae 1559.

4. BAILLE, M.: *On the want of a pericardium in the human body*. Trans. Soc. Improve. Med. Chir. Knowl. 1:91, 1793.

5. LADD, W. E.: *Congenital absence of pericardium, with report of case*. N. Engl. J. Med. 214:183, 1936.

6. DAHL, E.: *Case of congenital defect of pericardium revealed after application of sinistrolateral pneumothorax*. Med. Rev. (Bergen) 54:312, 1937.

7. SOUTHWORTH, H., AND STEVENSON, C. S.: *Congenital defects of pericardium*. Arch. Intern. Med. (Chicago) 61:223, 1938.

8. ELLIS, K., LEEDS, N. E., AND HIMMELSTEIN, A.: *Congenital deficiencies in partial pericardium: review with two new cases including successful diagnosis by plain roentgenography*. Am. J. Roentgenol. 82: 125, 1960.

9. DIMOND, E. G., KITTLE, C. F., AND VOTH, D. W.: *Extreme hypertrophy of left atrial appendage; a case of giant dog ear*. Am. J. Cardiol. 5:122, 1960.

10. VERSÉ, M.: *Fall van kongenitalem defekt des Herzbeutels*. Munch. Med. Wochenschr. 56:2665, 1909.

11. PERNA, G.: *Sopra un arresta di Sviluppo della sierosa pericardica nell'uomo*. Anat. Anz. 35:389, 1961.

12. BROADBENT, J. D., CALLAHAN, J. A., KINCAID, O. W., ET AL.: *Congenital deficiency of pericardium*. Chest 50:237, 1966.

13. BOR, I., AND KAFKA, V.: *Aplasia of pericardium*. J. Cardiovasc. Surg. (Torino) 2:389, 1961.

14. CHANG, C. H., AND LEIGHT, T. F.: *Congenital defect of pericardium associated with herniation of left atrial appendage*. Am. J. Roentgenol. 86:512, 1961.

15. KJELLBERG, S. R., MANNHEIMER, E., RUDHE, U., ET AL.: *Diagnosis of Congenital Heart Disease*. Year Book Publishers, Inc., Chicago, 1955, p. 571.

16. INADA, K., NAKANISHI, S., AND YOKOYAMA, T.: *Congenital defect of pericardium with special reference to radiodiagnosis*. Jap. J. Thorac. Surg. 16:619, 1963.

17. LINDSKOG, G. J., AND LIEBOW, A. A.: *Thoracic and Cardiovascular Surgery with Related Pathology*. Appleton-Century-Crofts, New York, 1962, p. 959.

18. SCHUSTER, B., ALEXJANDRINO, S., YAVUZ, F., ET AL.: *Congenital pericardial defect: report of patient with associated patent ductus arteriosus*. Am. J. Dis. Child. 110:199, 1965.

19. FISHER, J. D., AND EHRENHAFT, J. L.: *Congenital pericardial defect*. J.A.M.A. 188:78, 1964.

20. TABAKIN, B. S., HANSON, J. S., TAMPAS, J. P., ET AL.: *Congenital absence of left pericardium*. Am. J. Roentgenol. 94:122, 1965.

21. SATO, T., ITO, T., KOMATSU, S., ET AL.: *A case of congenital absence of left pericardium.* Sapporo Med. J. 21:78, 1962.

22. WOLFE, W., PORSTMANN, W., AND ALBERT, M.: *Perikardaplasie.* Thoraxchirurgie 11:338, 1964.

23. HIPONA, F. A., AND CRUMMY, A. B., JR.: *Congenital pericardial defect associated with tetralogy of Fallot: herniation of normal lung into pericardial cavity.* Circulation 29:132, 1964.

24. RUSBY, N. L., AND SELLORS, T. H.: *Congenital deficiency of pericardium associated with bronchogenic cyst.* Br. J. Surg. 32:357, 1945.

25. HORIIDE, R., ISHIKAWA, N., AND OGATA, K.: *Case of mediastinal bronchogenic cyst associated with partial pericardial defect and cured by excision.* Jap. J. Thorac. Surg. 16:46, 1963.

26. JONES, P. H.: *Developmental defects in lungs.* Thorax 10:205, 1955.

27. MUKERJEE, S.: *Congenital partial left pericardial defect with bronchogenic cyst.* Thorax 19:176, 1964.

28. VORNOV, A. A., AND GAVRILOV, S. G.: *Congenital absence of pericardium in combination with bronchogenic cyst of left lung.* Grudn. Khir. 4:78, 1962.

29. HAMILTON, I. C.: *Congenital deficiency of pericardium: case report of complete absence of left pericardium.* Radiology 77:984, 1961.

30. WARNER, C. L., BRITT, R. L., AND RILEY, H. D., JR.: *Bronchopulmonary sequestration in infancy and childhood.* J. Pediatr. 53:521, 1958.

31. MOORE, T. C., AND SHUMACKER, H. B., JR.: *Congenital and experimentally produced pericardial defects.* Angiology 4:1, 1953.

32. HERING, A. C., WILSON, J. S., AND BALL, R. E., JR.: *Congenital deficiency of pericardium.* J. Thorac. Cardiovasc. Surg. 40:49, 1960.

33. LAJOS, T. Z., BUNNELL, I. L., COLKATHIS, B. P., ET AL.: *Coronary artery insufficiency secondary to congenital pericardial defect.* Chest 58:73, 1970.

34. GLANCY, D. L., SANDERS, C. V., AND PORTA, A.: *Posterior chest wall pulsation in congenital complete absence of the left pericardium.* Chest 65:564, 1974.

35. CALLAHAN, J. A., BROADBENT, J. C., KINCAID, O. W., ET AL.: *Electrocardiogram in congenital defect of the pericardium.* Circulation 22 (Suppl. 21):63, 1965.

36. VARRIALE, P., ROSSI, P., AND GRACE, W. J.: *Congenital absence of the left pericardium and complete heart block.* Chest 52:405, 1967.

37. BRUNIG, E. G. H.: *Congenital defect of pericardium.* J. Clin. Pathol. 15:133, 1962.

38. CUCCURULLO, L.: *Agenesis of pericardium—etiopathogenic considerations of case found by chance in autopsy.* Riv. Anat. Patol. Oncol. 23:537, 1963.

39. ROGGE, J. D., MISHKIN, M. E., AND GENOVESE, P. D.: *Congenital partial pericardial defect with herniation of left atrial appendage.* Ann. Intern. Med. 64:137, 1966.

40. SWANSON, G. E., AND STEINBERG, I.: *Roentgen features of atrial appendages.* Am. J. Roentgenol. 91: 311, 1964.

41. GLOVER, L. B., BARCIA, A., AND REEVES, T. J.: *Congenital absence of the pericardium.* Am. J. Roentgenol. 106:542, 1969.

42. KAVANAGH-GRAY, D., MUSGROVE, E., AND STANWOOD, D.: *Congenital pericardial defects: report of case.* N. Engl. J. Med. 26:692, 1961.

43. DUFFIE, E. R., JR., MOSS, A. J., AND MALONEY, J. W., JR.: *Congenital pericardial defects with herniation of heart into pleural space.* Pediatrics 30:746, 1962.

44. NASSER, W. K., FEIGENBAUM, H., AND HELMEN, C.: *Congenital absence of left pericardium.* Circulation 34:100, 1966.

45. SUNDERLAND, S., AND WRIGHT-SMITH, R. J.: *Congenital pericardial defects.* Br. Heart J. 6:167, 1944.

46. BOXALL, R.: *Incomplete pericardial sac: Escape of heart into pleural cavity.* Trans. Obstet. Soc. (London) 28:209, 1887.

47. NASSER, W. K., HELMEN, C., TAVEL, M. E., ET AL.: *Congenital absence of the left pericardium: clinical, electrocardiographic, radiographic, hemodynamic, and angiographic findings in six cases.* Circulation 41:469, 1970.

48. FOSBURG, R. A., JAKUBIAK, J. V., AND DELANEY, T. B.: *Congenital absence of the pericardium.* Ann. Thorac. Surg. 5:171, 1968.

49. PERNOT, D., HOEFFEL, J. C., HENRY, M., ET AL.: *Partial left pericardial defect with herniation of the left atrial appendage.* Thorax 27:246, 1972.

50. NASSER, W. K.: *Congenital absence of the left pericardium.* Am. J. Cardiol. 26:466, 1970.

51. LIND, T. A., PITT, M. J., GROVES, B. M., ET AL.: *The abnormal left hilum.* Circulation 51:183, 1975.

52. CANTRELL, G. R., HALLER, J. A., AND RAVITCH, M. N.: *Syndrome of congenital defects involving abdominal wall, sternum, diaphragm, pericardium and heart.* Surg. Gynecol. Obstet. 107:602, 1958.

53. CRITTENDEN, I. H., ADAMS, F. H., AND MULDER, D. G.: *Syndrome featuring defects of heart, sternum, diaphragm and anterior abdominal wall.* Circulation 20:396, 1959.

54. MULDER, D. G., CRITTENDEN, I. H., AND ADAMS, F. H.: *Complete repair of syndrome of congenital defects involving the abdominal wall, sternum, diaphragm, pericardium and heart; excision of left ventricular diverticulum.* Ann. Surg. 151:113, 1960.

55. EDGETT, J. W., JR., NELSON, W. P., HALL, R. J., ET AL.: *Diverticulum of heart: part of syndrome of congenital cardiac and midline thoracic and abdominal defects.* Am. J. Cardiol. 24:580, 1969.

56. GALIOTO, J. M., JR., REITMAN, M. J., VARGO, T. A., ET AL.: *Congenital diverticulum of left ventricle.* Am. Heart J. 87:109, 1974.

57. LOWE, J. D., WILLIAMS, J. C. P., ROBB, D., ET AL.: *Congenital diverticulum of left ventricle.* Br. Heart J. 21:101, 1959.

58. MURPHY, D. A., ABERDEEN, E., DOBBS, R. H., ET AL.: *Surgical treatment of syndrome consisting of thoraco-abdominal wall, diaphragmatic, pericardial and ventricular septal defects; and left ventricular diverticulum.* Ann. Thorac. Surg. 6:528, 1968.

59. PEREZ-ALVAREZ, J. J., PEREZ-TREVINO, C., AND DOMENE-FLOR, R.: *Successful total correction of ventricular septal defect, diverticula of left ventricle, and anomaly of thoraco-abdominal wall in 11 year old boy with cardiac dextroversion.* J. Thorac. Cardiovasc. Surg. 52:386, 1966.

60. SYMBAS, P. N., AND WARE, R. E.: *Syndrome of defects of thoracoabdominal wall, diaphragm, pericardium and heart: one-stage surgical repair and analysis of syndrome.* J. Thorac. Cardiovasc. Surg. 65:914, 1973.

61. TOYAMA, W. M.: *Combined congenital defects of anterior abdominal wall, sternum, diaphragm, pericardium and heart: case report and review of syndrome.* Pediatrics 50:778, 1972.

62. VAZQUEZ-PEREZ, J., GAUTIER, M., MERTIER, J. N., ET AL.: *Diverticulum of left ventricle: á propos of three cases.* Arch. Mal. Coeur 62:922, 1969.

63. VERGER, P., BRICAND, H., FONTAN, F., ET AL.: *Congenital diverticulum of left ventricle: report of case treated successfully by surgery.* Ann. Pediatr. 17:24, 1970.

64. WAGNER, M. L., SINGLETON, E. B., AND LEACHMAN, R. D.: *Congenital left ventricular diverticulum.* Am. J. Roentgenol. Rad. Ther. Nucl. Med. 122:137, 1974.

65. HAIDER, R., THOMAS, D. G. T., ZIADY, G., ET AL.: *Congenital pericardio-peritoneal communication with herniation of omentum into the pericardium.* Br. Heart J. 35:981, 1973.

66. CASEY, B. M., NEIMAN, H., GALLAGHER, T., ET AL.: *Syndrome of mesodermal defects involving the abdominal wall, diaphragm, sternum, heart and pericardium.* Br. J. Radiol. 48:52, 1975.

67. POTTS, W. J., DEBOER, A., AND JOHNSON, F. R.: *Congenital diverticulum of left ventricle: case report.* Surgery 33:301, 1953.

68. SKAPINKER, S.: *Diverticulum of left ventricle of heart: review of literature and report of successful removal of diverticulum.* Arch. Surg. 63:629, 1951.

69. LILLIE, W. I., McDONALD, J. R., AND CLAGETT, O. T.: *Pericardial celomic cysts and pericardial diverticula — a concept of etiology and reports of cases.* J. Thorac. Surg. 20:494, 1950.

70. GREENFIELD, I., STEINBERG, I., AND TOUROFF, A. S. W.: *Pericardial celomic cysts.* J. Thorac. Surg. 12:495, 1943.

71. DeROOVER, P. H., MIASEN, J., AND LACQUET, A.: *Congenital pleuropericardial cysts.* Thorax 18:346, 1963.

72. LAMBERT, A. V.: *Etiology of thin-walled thoracic cysts.* J. Thorac. Surg. 10:1, 1940.

73. CHURCHILL, E. D., AND MALLORY, T. B.: *Pericardial coelomic cysts, Cabot case 23492.* N. Engl. J. Med. 217:958, 1937.

74. WARE, G. W. AND CONRAD, H. A.: *Diverticula of the pericardium.* Am. J. Surg. 88:918, 1954.

75. MAIER, H. C.: *Diverticulum of the pericardium — with observations on mode of development.* Circulation 16:1040, 1957.

76. PICKHARDT, O. C.: *Pleuro-diaphragmatic cyst.* Ann. Surg. 99:814, 1934.

77. BRISTOWE, J. S.: *Diverticulum from the pericardium.* Trans. Pathol. Soc. London 20:101, 1869.

78. BRISTOWE, J. S.: *Diverticulum from heart.* Trans. Pathol. Soc. London 19:42, 1887.

79. DUFOUR, H., AND MOURRUT: *Pericardial coelomic cysts.* Bull. Soc. Med. Hop. Paris 2:1482, 1929.

80. EDWARDS, A. T.: *Pericardial coelomic cysts.* Br. J. Surg. 14:607, 1927.

81. ELLIOTT, R.: *Pericardial coelomic cysts.* Am. J. Anat. 48:355, 1931.

82. KIENBÖCK, R., AND WEISS, K.: *Fortschr, a.d. Geb. d.* Roentgenstr. 40:389; 50:422, 1934.

83. CUSHING, E. H., AND MORITZ, A.: *Diverticulum of the pericardium.* Arch. Intern. Med. 60:482, 1937.

84. HAAS, L.: *Diverticulum pericardii.* Acta Radiol. 20:228, 1939.

85. HART, T.: *An account of hernia pericardii.* Dublin J. M. Sc. 2:365, 1937.

86. YATER, W. M.: *Cyst of the pericardium.* Am. Heart J. 6:710, 1931.

87. D'ABREU, A. L.: *Pericardial coelomic cysts.* Br. J. Surg. 25:317, 1937.

88. FREEDMAN, E., AND SIMON, M. A.: *Pericardial coelomic cysts.* Am. J. Roentgenol. 35:53, 1936.

89. GOETSCH, E.: *Pericardial coelomic cysts.* Arch. Surg. 36:394, 1938.

90. SKINNER, G. G., AND HOBBS, M. E.: *Pericardial celomic cysts.* J. Thorac. Surg. 6:98, 1936.

91. ADDEY, W.: *Pericardial coelomic cysts.* Br. J. Radiol. 13:180, 1940.

92. ALEXANDER, J.: *Pericardial coelomic cysts.* J.A.M.A. 119:395, 1942.

93. BARRETT, N. R., AND BARNARD, W. G.: *Pericardial coelomic cysts.* Br. J. Surg. 32:447, 1945.

94. BATES, J. C., AND LEAVER, F. Y.: *Pericardial coelomic cysts.* Radiology 57:330, 1951.

95. BLADES, B.: *Pericardial coelomic cysts.* Ann. Surg. 123:749, 1946.

96. BRADFORD, M. L., MAHON, H. W., AND GROW, J. B.: *Pericardial coelomic cysts.* Surg. Gynecol. Obstet. 85:467, 1947.

97. BROWN, R. K., AND ROBBINS, L. L.: *Pericardial celomic cysts.* J. Thorac. Surg. 13:84, 1944.

98. BUYERS, R. A., AND EMERY, J. B.: *Pericardial coelomic cysts.* Arch. Surg. 60:1002, 1950.

99. CRADDOCK, W. L.: *Pericardial coelomic cysts.* Am. Heart J. 40:619, 1950.

100. CURRERI, A. R., AND GALE, J. W.: *Pericardial coelomic cysts.* Ann. Surg. 113:1086, 1941.

101. DAVIS, D., DORSEY, J., AND SCANLON, E.: *Pericardial coelomic cysts..*A.M.A. Arch. Surg. 67:110, 1953.

102. DRASH, E. C., AND HYER, H. J.: *Pericardial celomic cysts.* J. Thorac. Surg. 19:755, 1950.

103. FORSEE, J. H., AND BLAKE, H. A.: *Pericardial coelomic cysts.* Surgery 31:753, 1952.

104. GROSS, R. E., AND HURWITT, E. S.: *Pericardial coelomic cysts.* Surg. Gynecol. Obstet. 87:599, 1948.

105. HARLEY, H. R. S., AND DREW, C. E.: *Pericardial coelomic cysts.* Thorax 5:105, 1950.

106. HIS, W.: *Pericardial coelomic cysts.* Arch. Anat. 1950, p. 303.

107. KISNER, W. H., AND REGANIS, J. C.: *Pericardial celomic cysts.* J. Thorac. Surg. 19:799, 1950.

108. LAM, C. R.: *Pericardial coelomic cysts.* Radiology 48:239, 1947.

109. LEAHY, L. J., AND CULVER, G. J.: *Pericardial celomic cysts.* J. Thorac. Surg. 16:695, 1947.

110. SCHEIN, G. J.: *Pericardial coelomic cysts.* Am. J. Surg. 78:411, 1949.

111. WEIG, C. G., AND FUGO, W. W.: *Pericardial coelomic cysts.* Dis. Chest 26:110, 1954.

112. YELIN, G., AND ABRAHAM, A.: *Pericardial coelomic cysts.* Dis. Chest 23:285, 1953.

113. BISHOP, L. F., JR., KIRSCHNER, P. A., AND PESSAR, T.: *Diverticulum of the pericardium.* Circulation 1: 813, 1950.

114. NICHOL, W. W., AND DEAN, G. O.: *Pericardial coelomic cysts.* U.S.A. Armed Forces Med. J. 2:473, 1951.

115. RIENHOFF, W. J., JR., JACKSON, R. L., AND MOORE, M. W.: *Pericardial coelomic cysts: Review of the literature and report of a case.* Bull. School Med. Univ. Maryland 36:1, 1951.

116. DAVIS, C., JR., DORSEY, J., AND SCANLON, E.: *Cysts about the pericardium.* A.M.A. Arch. Surg. 28: 110, 1954.

117. MAZER, M. L.: *True pericardial diverticulum.* Am. J. Roentgenol. 55:27, 1946.

118. SABISTON, D. C., AND SCOTT, H. W.: *Pericardial coelomic cysts.* Am. J. Roentgenol. 136:777, 1952.

119. RUBUSH, J. L., GARDNER, I. R., BOYD, W. C., ET AL.: *Mediastinal tumors; review of 186 cases.* J. Thorac. Cardiovasc. Surg. 65:216, 1973.

120. LOEHR, W. M.: *Pericardial cysts.* Am. J. Roentgenol. 68:584, 1952.

121. LEROUX, B. T.: *Pericardial coelomic cysts.* Thorax 14:27, 1959.

122. EDWARDS, M. H., AND AHMAD, A.: *Epicardial cyst—a case report.* Thorax 27:503, 1972.

123. FUNCH, R. B., AND WENGER, D. S.: *Preoperative diagnosis of pericardial celomic cysts.* Am. J. Roentgenol. 73:584, 1955.

Surgery of the Pericardium

Dwight Emary Harken, M.D.

"A most disconcerting thing about constrictive *pericarditis is that whenever we make the diagnosis and ask the surgeon to correct it . . . he always finds it. I must conclude therefore, that the diagnosis is frequently missed."*

C. Sidney Burwell, M.D.

HISTORICAL NOTE

Pericardial disease has been a subject of interest, conjecture, awe, and challenge since Galen. He knew pericarditis occurred in animals and suspected it in man. Its protean forms are abundantly reviewed elsewhere in this monograph. By 1756 Morgagni recognized the dangers of tamponade but Laennec as of 1819 despaired of its correction. About that time Romero is alleged to have performed pericardiocentesis but, characteristic of the doubters, the nihilists, and the timid who have always constituted the controlling majority, his Faculty of Medicine suppressed reporting the triumph lest it be interpreted as sanction. So, characteristically, the surgeon, this time Napoleon's surgeon, Baron Larrey, inserted a catheter and drained "three beakers of wine colored fluid" from a soldier's pericardial sac.

Weil recognized the effects of constrictive pericarditis in 1895 and forecast surgical therapy. Pick's name is associated with a type of cirrhosis, mediastinopericarditis and *constrictive pericarditis.* The late Kalkstein reported in 1937 to me that one of his German docents knew Pick as a clinician. He alleged that Pick considered the *small* quiet heart as essential to the diagnosis and clinical syndrome of Pick's disease or constrictive pericarditis. Furthermore, Pick had a large heart of undiagnosed nature and at autopsy after Pick's death in 1896, it was found that his death had been from Pick's disease, that is, constrictive pericarditis.

The wide variety of causes, effects, and diagnostic methods involved in pericarditis are discussed elsewhere in this monograph. This presentation is confined to mechanical procedures and clinical references only to clarify some mechanical effects of pericardial disease. Perhaps nowhere else is kinetic pathology more directly observed by the surgeon and the correction of that pathologic state more clearly visible.

In reviewing these procedures it is hoped that the physician will gain a better insight into the truly remarkable diagnostic and therapeutic surgical armamentarium available to his patient and the thoracic surgeon entering the field, a skeleton blueprint on which to organize his thoughts.

PERICARDIOCENTESIS

This procedure of immense diagnostic and therapeutic value is at once too little used and too often badly performed. Rapid accumulation of blood in stab wounds, contusion, or accumulation of effusion can be promptly fatal. Large amounts of fluid can accumulate with minimal hemodynamic alteration and then, suddenly, small additional volume can cause tamponade with rising venous pressure, paradoxical and narrowed pulse, lowered blood pressure, quiet heart and an anxious, sweating, "shocky," patient. What is essential for successful use of pericardiocentesis is to suspect need, which is the case in most therapeutic triumphs. The prompt skillful intervention with pericardiocentesis is often rewarded with marked hemodynamic improvement, even when only a small volume has been aspirated. Masquerading hypovolemia or acute heart failure may be difficult to distinguish from acute tamponade.

TECHNIQUE. Simplicity is the keynote. The patient is elevated to 45 degrees (semi-Fowler's position) and the skin preparation and drapes are standard for exposure of the left costoxiphoid area. Blood pressure and electrocardiographic monitoring are used. The operator, if right handed, stands at the patient's right side and, after administration of suitable local anesthesia, directs a 3 inch #17 gauge needle with sheathed catheter upward, inward, and to the right, slowly exerting aspirating force through the 10 cc. syringe. The law of "45s" is applied; that is, the patient's chest is elevated 45 degrees, the aspirating needle is inserted through the left costoxiphoid angle at 45 degrees from the abdominal wall, with syringe 45 degrees from the midline with needle pointing toward the right shoulder. As the needle traverses the pericardiophrenic structures, resistance is overcome gently while guarding against sudden advance, by the restraining left thumb and forefinger on the needle. As fluid is encountered and the operator becomes convinced that the needle is in the pericardial sac rather than the right ventricle, the catheter sheathing the needle is advanced as the needle is withdrawn. The fluid, blood, effusion, or pus is withdrawn for culture and appropriate examination. The hemodynamic effect is assessed as fluid is withdrawn and as the fluid is exhausted a small amount of air (10 to 15 cc.) is allowed to enter the pericardial sac. Appropriate antibiotics are instilled and the catheter is withdrawn.

The hazards involve damage to the right ventricle or atrium. The often mentioned but rarely encountered damage to coronary vessels is mentioned here to keep this discussion conventional rather than to raise serious concern.

In the case of stab wounds, preparation must be made for thoractomy and definitive treatment of a heart wound. Often the aspiration of even a small amount of blood is sufficient therapy; the judgment for or against exploratory thoractomy is delicate and beyond this discussion. However, the late breakdown of hemoglobin three or four days later, increasing the hydroscopic oncotic effect with recurrence of tamponade, must be borne in mind.

The advent of antibiotics has dramatically reduced the incidence of suppurative pericarditis. Whereas 30 years ago bacterial pericarditis including tuberculous pericarditis was commonly encountered, these disorders have diminished to be replaced by viral and uremic forms. Indeed chronic dialysis programs have made the occurrence of uremic pericarditis familiar to many physicians. However, these forms of chronic and recurring effusion lend themselves to thoractomy and *pericardiectomy*. Pericardiectomy is used advisedly because a timid little fenestration is often insufficient. Wide pericardial resection anterior and posterior to the left phrenic nerve is only slightly more traumatic and vastly more effective.

From the foregoing it is apparent that elective, nonemergency pericardiocentesis must be carefully planned and monitored, with antibiotics ready for instillation.

PERICARDIAL BIOPSY, EXPLORATION, AND DRAINAGE

Techniques for biopsy of the pericardium range from needle biopsy (for the most part to be condemned), through direct xiphoid exposure, to transpleural approaches. The selection of method is contingent upon the further purpose to which the operation might need to be extended. For example, if it is possible that the biopsy might need to be extended to drain suppurative pericarditis, the choice might be the left subcostal, xiphoid approach via Larrey's angle. Conversely, if the biopsy is to clarify the cause of a recurring effusion, the transthoracic approach makes possible resection of sufficient pericardium to drain the pericardial sac into the pleural space. Here the word and concept *fenestration* has crept into use. Again the physician and inexperienced surgeon are reminded that a window may close or incompletely drain; therefore, wide resection of pericardium in front of and behind the phrenic nerve is scarely more traumatic and is more likely to be definitive.

The *subcostal, xiphoid approach for biopsy* or drainage via Larrey's angle is described for completeness. A 10 cm. incision is made over the xiphoid cartilage and just below the left costal symphysis. The rectus sheath is divided obliquely and the medial rectus fibers divided and retracted laterally. The xiphoid process is excised. The transversalis fascia is followed by blunt dissection to the anterior diaphragmatic surface. The pericardium is then identified and exposed. Needle aspirations may clarify the depth and direction of exploration. Generous biopsy is then taken. If suppurative process is encountered, the pericardial biopsy and pericardial exploration site must be extended to admit exploring fingers and catheter for irrigation. If adequate drainage is to be effected through this surgical site, it is mandatory to sweep an exploring finger around the heart daily to break up loculations and to irrigate thoroughly via catheters with fibrinolytic and bacteriocidal solutions.

The *transthoracic biopsy* can be rendered flexible when the nature of a recurrent effusion is to be clarified and when that recurring effusion needs pleural drainage. In that situation it is again emphasized that wide pericardial resection of the pericardium anterior and posterior to the left phrenic nerve may be indicated if there is a recurring effusion. This approach is generally carried through the left fourth or fifth interspace in the anterior axillary area. The patient is in the full lateral decubitus position so that the incision can be extended anteriorly or posteriorly, as needed.

This very *atraumatic* exploration is conducted under the usual formal thoracotomy conditions. It has largely replaced the subcostal xiphoid approach as it affords opportunity to biopsy and to explore when differentiations between constrictive pericarditis and myocardial disease must be made or when drainage with or without decompression is desired. It must be borne in mind that the pericardium can be drained almost ideally into the pleural space, that the pleura like the peritoneum can withstand even a massive septic insult if not repetitive, and, finally, that the pleura can and must be thoroughly drained with two intercostal tubes through the same interspace.

PERICARDIECTOMY FOR CONSTRICTIVE PERICARDITIS
(DECORTICATION OF THE HEART)

Adequate correction of the various forms of constrictive pericarditis demands complete familiarity with the several forms of constriction. It also requires that the surgeon and hemodynamacist appreciate the fact that even though sophisticated pressure and echo studies have increased diagnostic accuracy, there remains a wide zone of error, especially in some forms of *myocardial, endocardial,* and *epicardial* diseases. Unfortunately, these may masquerade as constrictive pericarditis. *Constrictive epicarditis* has been observed without significant pericardial constriction. It is diagnostically indistinguishable from some patterns of constrictive pericarditis. It is occasionally combined with constricive pericarditis and generally lends itself to surgical excision. When a constricting epicardium is removed, there is much more surface blood loss than in ideal pericardiectomy, and special care must be exercised to avoid coronary vessel damage.

While I have considered various methods of relieving tamponade by endocardial fibroelastosis I have never attempted it. To our knowledge the only person who has accomplished this is DuBost of Paris.

The several forms or patterns of constrictive pericarditis must be understood in order to correct them adequately. Once such spectrum of disease is in surgeon's ken, and the actual technical correction is reasonable procedure and generally extraordinarily rewarding.

The most common form of constrictive pericarditis is the diffuse concentric form. Next most frequent in our experience has been the atrioventricular groove constriction extending around the pulmonary artery and aortic bases (observed 6 times in 67 patients). The rare forms have been pure left ventricular constriction, pulmonary vein constrictions, and caval obstruction (twice in each category). In Burwell's vast experience with this disease, he saw only three instances of the caval form and my two patients were also two of Burwell's. The pulmonary vein obstruction occurs at the point the veins pass through the pericardium into the left atrium. The A-V groove constriction can masquerade as mitral or pulmonic stenosis; I have had one of each and both responded dramatically to excision.

Much has been written about the approaches for decortication of the heart in constrictive pericarditis. Some of these approaches are quite incomprehensible to this surgeon. Some approaches are simply unnecessary; others are clearly inadequate. If a surgeon knows what he is trying to accomplish and has a clear understanding of what he must look for additionally in that endeavor, he can select an appropriate surgical exposure.

The anterior third, fourth, or fifth interspace exposures are mentioned only to condemn them. The anterolateral fifth interspace incision has proved inadequate. The median sternotomy seems to have the most widespread acceptance but to me is unacceptable because of the poor exposure of the very important portion of left ventricle back of the left phrenic nerve. The transverse bilateral sternal dividing incision has never been used (and never will be used) by me as it seems to combine all of the previously described limitations and compounds them into a much more traumatic procedure.

My choice is the full lateral thoracotomy with extensive decortication in front of and behind the left phrenic nerve. Freeing the layers of onion skin fibrocalcific peel until the emancipated myocardium bulges through the constricting scar is essential to determining the proper plane. This plane is patiently pursued with minimal epicardial laceration. It is extended past the atrioventricular groove by clearing the pulmonary artery level and extending that down to the groove. The left pulmonary veins are identified and freed if compromised. The intrapericardial lysis and dissection can be carried to both cavae without difficulty, anteriorly for the superior cava and on the diaphragmatic surface posteriorly and inferiorly for the inferior cava.

Unless the atria are readily stripped, no great effort at decortication is made. I find some reason in Sir Thomas Holmes Sellors' answer when asked if he also removed the pericardium from the auricles. He replied, "Any fool could but only a bloody fool would."

In conclusion, no better message can be left with the internist and surgeon than that implied by Burwell: a low threshold of suspicion will extend discovery in the spectrum of acute and chronic tamponade. The simple and sophisticated diagnostic methods will sort out the protean forms of that tamponade. Finally, the surgeon's mastery of straightforward techniques offers many patients definitive and gratifying relief.

Index